Occupational and Environmental Medicine: Assessment and Management

Occupational and Environmental Medicine: Assessment and Management

Editor: Kirk Anderson

AMERICAN
MEDICAL PUBLISHERS
www.americanmedicalpublishers.com

AMERICAN
MEDICAL PUBLISHERS
www.americanmedicalpublishers.com

Cataloging-in-Publication Data

Occupational and environmental medicine : assessment and management / edited by Kirk Anderson.
p. cm.
Includes bibliographical references and index.
ISBN 978-1-63927-450-5
1. Medicine, Industrial. 2. Environmental health. 3. Occupational diseases. 4. Occupational therapists.
5. Pharmaceutical services. I. Anderson, Kirk.
RC963.3 .O23 2021
616.980 3--dc23

American Medical Publishers,
41 Flatbush Avenue,
1st Floor, New York,
NY 11217, USA

ISBN 978-1-63927-450-5 (Hardback)

Contents

Preface

Occupational health is a multidisciplinary field that deals with the safety, health and welfare of people at work. Fostering a safe and healthy work environment is the primary goal of this domain. It also aims to protect co-workers, family members, employers, etc., who have chances of getting affected by the workplace environment. Occupational health has a strong focus on primary prevention of physical, biological and psychosocial hazards. Environmental health is the domain of public health that deals with all types of the natural and built environment that affect the human health. Environmental epidemiology, toxicology, exposure science, environmental engineering and environmental law are the five basic subsets that contribute to the branch of environmental health. The objective of this book is to give a general view of the different areas of these fields and its applications. It explores all the important aspects of occupational and environmental health in the present day scenario. This book with its extensive content provides the readers with a thorough understanding of the subject.

The information contained in this book is the result of intensive hard work done by researchers in this field. All due efforts have been made to make this book serve as a complete guiding source for students and researchers. The topics in this book have been comprehensively explained to help readers understand the growing trends in the field.

I would like to thank the entire group of writers who made sincere efforts in this book and my family who supported me in my efforts of working on this book. I take this opportunity to thank all those who have been a guiding force throughout my life.

Editor

1

Comet assay based DNA evaluation of fuel filling stations and automobile workshops workers from Khyber Pakhtunkhwa province, Pakistan

Muhammad Khisroon[1*†], Aisha Gul[1†], Ajmal Khan[1†], Naheed Ali[1], Farah Zaidi[1], Syed Basit Rasheed[1], Ahmadullah[1] and Huma Akbar[2]

Abstract

Background: Fuel filling stations workers and automobile workshops mechanics are consistently exposed to gasoline hydrocarbons during their occupation, this may cause DNA damage. Objective of this study was to evaluate the level of DNA damage in subjects occupationally exposed to these hydrocarbons.

Methods: Comet assay was performed on blood lymphocytes of exposed subjects to assess the probable DNA damage. 100 cells per individual were scored and graded by comet tail length. Exposed group consisted of 98 subjects (age 25.4 ± 7.2 years), of which 68 were CNG/Petrol filling men and 30 were automobile workshop workers, selected randomly from different service stations and automobile workshops of populated and adjacent cities of Peshawar, Mardan and Nowshera of Khyber Pakhtunkhwa province, while control group included 92 subjects (age 26.7 ± 11.8 years) were also from the same areas.

Results: Significantly high level of DNA damage was found in the subjects exposed to gasoline hydrocarbons as compared to control subjects (173.2 ± 50.1 and 61.0 ± 25.0, $P = 0.001$, respectively). Period of exposure and use of tobacco also showed considerable effects ($P < 0.05$) on DNA damage, while effect of age and daily working hours on total comet score (TCS) were non-significant ($P > 0.05$).

Conclusions: The results of our study concluded that petroleum hydrocarbons have the potential to cause DNA damage in the exposed subjects. The study also suggested that protective strategies should be implemented by the concerned authorities to minimize exposure to fuel hydrocarbons.

Keywords: Gasoline hydrocarbons, DNA damage, Comet assay, Blood lymphocytes

Background

Gasoline (Petrol) is a complex man-made compound that does not exist naturally in the environment. Most of its chemicals are present around the human settlement in a number of physical states i.e. liquid, gaseous or in some other form. Gasoline is extracted in the refining process of crude petroleum [1]. Liquid gasoline in petroleum chemicals is one of the known complex mixtures to which human is exposed. It contains more than 150 hydrocarbons with a boiling range of 40 °C to 180 °C. Hydrocarbons of gasoline are alkanes (paraffins), isoparaffins, alkenes (olefins) and naphthenics in a ratio of about 50 % to 70 %, while its aromatic compounds are benzene, toluene, ethylbenzene and xylene, present in a ratio of 30 % to 40 %, all of which are significantly hazardous carcinogenic chemicals. More than 1,000 possible chemical substances are found in gasoline [2].

The significant release of vapours from gasoline resulted in direct human exposure to these vapours at various contact points and most importantly in the large number of retail service stations and adjoining settled areas [3]. The vapour form of gasoline, when present in

* Correspondence: m_khisroon@upesh.edu.pk
†Equal contributors
[1]Department of Zoology, University of Peshawar, Peshawar, Pakistan
Full list of author information is available at the end of the article

the atmosphere can dispensed at any time, especially at fuel filling service stations, so the people who are working in fueling and refueling of vehicles are more exposed and are at higher risk to its adverse health effects [4].

A number of epidemiological and experimental studies have shown that fumes of petrol and diesel engines are carcinogenic and mutagenic to both humans and animals [5]. All places where refinery products are manufactured, processed or soled are potentially carcinogenic to humans [6].

Benzene a widely spread environmental pollutant, constitutes about 1–5 % of petrol [7]. It is classified as a known carcinogen to human [6]. Persons working at filling stations, motor mechanic, tanker crew and traffic personnel are more susceptible to benzene exposure due to their occupation [8]. Benzene also affects hematopoiesis in the bone marrow [9]. It lowers the number of peripheral white blood cells and platelet, specifically decreases T-cells, B-cells and granulocytes [10]. Due to metabolism of benzene in human liver, its metabolites repress the production of DNA, RNA and various other cellular proteins [11, 12]. Due to its clastogenic property benzene can produce disorders like micronuclei, chromosomal aberrations and sister chromatid exchange [13]. Thus for the improvement of health and occupational safety, monitoring of occupational exposure to chemicals is important both for the evaluation of risks and for the implementation of strategies [14].

A number of techniques such as sister chromatid exchange, chromosomal aberration and micronucleus assay are normally used for investigating genetic damages. However, these methods are economically costly, time consumable and require proliferating cells. Therefore, the use of single cell gel electrophoresis (SCGE) or comet assay for genotoxicity studies have greatly increased during the past few decades [15–17].

Considering the hazardous effects of gasoline hydrocarbons and lack of awareness among our study group, the aim of present study was to assess the level of DNA damage in retail service stations attendants and automobile workshops mechanics and of corresponding unexposed control subjects.

Methods

Study population

The study population was consisted of 190 people, of which 98 were exposed subjects and 92 control group. Among the exposed subjects, 68 were CNG/Petrol filling men while 30 were automobile workshops workers, selected from different retail service stations and automobile workshops located in Peshawar, Nowshera and Mardan cities of Khyber Pakhtunkhwa province. All exposed subjects were males with mean age of 25.4 ± 7.2 years. All the subjects were healthy, with no history of diseases, and were not taking any kind of medications which could cause the DNA damage. Control group was also selected from the same area with mean age of 26.7 ± 11.8 years and no exposure to petroleum fumes or other potentially genotoxic substances. The study was approved from Ethical Committee of the Department of Pharmacy, University of Peshawar (42/Pharm, Dated: 12.05.2014).

Questionnaire

Information were collected from all the subjects on a questionnaire according to their own consent, which included demographic data of the subjects, medical history, addiction of tobacco or alcohol and complete details of their occupation i.e. daily duty hours, years of exposure, use of protective devices etc. Samples were collected from all the subjects at their workplaces on the working days.

Blood sample collection and lymphocyte separation

3 ml of venous blood sample was collected from each subject using sterilized syringes and then transferred to K-EDTA containing tubes. The samples were labeled, transported to the laboratory and processed within 3 to 4 h. Lymphocytes were isolated from the blood by Ficoll-1077 density gradient centrifugation and washed in phosphate buffered saline (PBS). The viability of the cells was tested by Trypan blue and was kept greater than 90 %.

Alkaline comet assay

We used the standard procedure of alkaline comet assay described by Singh et al. [15] with slight modifications. Duplicate slides per sample were prepared. For the preparation of pre-coated slides, the conventional glass slides were dipped into hot normal melting agarose (NMA) (0.7 %), laid in a tray to air dry and then wiped from the underside to remove the extra agarose. Slides were generally prepared one day before use, labeled and then stored at room temperature. 15 μl of cell suspension was mixed with 70 μl of low melting point agarose (LMPA) (0.7 %), spread on top of pre-coated slides and kept at 0 °C for 5 min with cover slip on it. After that the cover slip was removed and a second layer of 85 μl LMPA was added to fill any residual holes and again kept at 0 °C for 5 min to solidify, with cover slip on it.

Lysing of slides

After solidification, the cover slips were removed and slides were gently immersed in freshly prepared cold-lysing solution [(2.5 M NaCl, 100 mM Na_2EDTA, 10 mM Tris, pH 10) with 1 % Triton X-100 and 10 % DMSO added just before use] for at least 2 h at 4 °C.

Electrophoresis and neutralization

After lysing, the slides were immersed in electrophoresis buffer (300 mM NaOH and 1 mM EDTA, pH 13) and left for 20 min to allow the unwinding of DNA and expression of alkali-labile sites. The slides were then subjected to electrophoresis for 25 min at 300 mA and 25 V. To prevent any kind of unintentional DNA damage, the slides were protected from direct exposure to light. The steps were conducted at 4 °C. After electrophoresis, the slides were neutralized by washing three times with neutralization buffer (400 mM Tris, pH 7.5) for 5 min each.

Staining, scoring and visualization of slides

The slides were stained with 70 µl Acridine orange dye (20 µg/ml) and kept for 5 min. Cover slips were placed on it, and viewed at 200x of fluorescent microscope (Nikon Eclipse 80 i) equipped with 450-490 nm excitation filter. In order to calculate DNA damage, 100 cells per sample were chosen randomly and analyzed visually according to comet appearance. 5 classes, i.e. from class 0 (no DNA damage) to class 4 (maximum DNA damage) give sufficient declaration (Fig. 1). Visual scoring is a reliable, simple and rapid method for scoring the comets [18]. Total comet score (TCS) was then calculated according to the formula, TCS = 0(n) +1(n) +2(n) +3(n) +4(n), where "n" indicates number of cells in each class [18].

Statistical analysis

Statistical analysis was performed, using SPSS V.20.0. Mean and standard deviation values of the data were determined. Student's *t*–test (two-tailed) was used to calculate mean differences, where P value was kept at 0.05 for statistical significance. The comet assay data, which was non-normally distributed, were analyzed using non-parametric Mann-Whitney *U*-test (two-tail). Correlation was calculated for the duration of occupational exposure and TCS using online software [19].

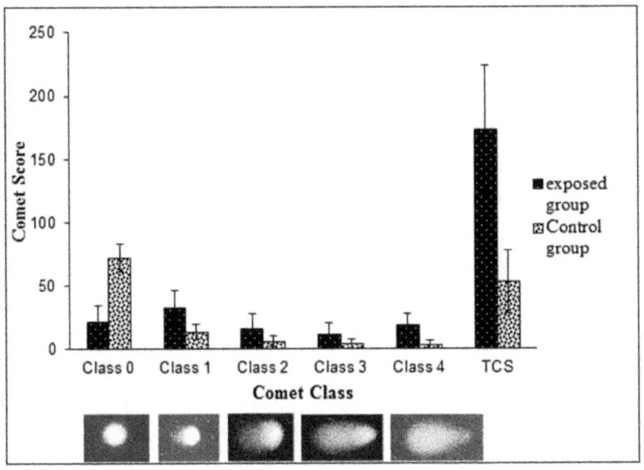

Fig. 1 DNA damage assessed using the comet assay. Mean comet score and comet classes in control and exposed groups. The cells were assessed visually and received class 0 (undamaged) to 4 (maximally damaged), according to the size and shape of the tail. Score were obtained using the mean score of three independent, blind evaluators

Results

The effect of occupational exposure due to petroleum hydrocarbons on the DNA in fuel filling station/automobile workers and control subjects was assessed by the comet assay. The main characteristics including age, tobacco consumption, duration and nature of occupation of the studied population are given in Table 1. The age of exposed and control groups had no significant difference (i.e. $P > 0.05$). The exposed and control subjects were healthy having no such disease which could cause DNA damage.

The mean total comet score (TCS) in 100 lymphocytes of study group is shown in Table 2. The cells with DNA damaged had the appearance of a comet, while undamaged cells had an intact nucleus without a tail (Fig. 1). DNA damage observed in persons working in CNG/ Petrol pumps, and automobile workshops (TCS = 173.2 ± 50.1) were significantly higher than that observed in the control group (TCS = 61.0 ± 25.0, $P \leq 0.001$) (Table 2). Comet class 3 (11.3 ± 9.9 cells) and class 4 (18.7 ± 9.4 cells) were observed more frequently in exposed group than in the control group (5.3 ± 4.1 and 3.7 ± 2.3 cells, respectively). The opposite results were observed with undamaged cells; comet class 0 was observed more frequently in the control group (67.7 ± 13.0) as compared to the persons working in CNG/ Petrol Pumps, and automobile workshops (21.6 ± 13.4 cells) (Table 2). Figure 1 shows the graphical representation of the mean TCS and Comet classes in both persons working in CNG/Petrol pumps, and automobile workshops and control groups.

A positive correlation ($r = 0.96$, $P \leq 0.02$) was observed between the duration of occupational exposure and TCS. Among the study group, the lowest TCS value (160.7 ± 42.0) was observed in the subject working for

Table 1 Distribution of the main characteristics of persons working in CNG/petrol pumps and automobile workshops and control group

Main characteristics	Exposed group	Control group
N	98	92
Mean Age (Years)	25.4 ± 7.2	26.7 ± 11.8
Mean Duration of Job (Years)	4.4 ± 4.8	
Nature of Job		
Fuel filling station workers	68 (69.4 %)	
Automobile Workshop workers	30 (30.6 %)	
Smoking		
No	71 (72.4 %)	70
Yes	27 (27.6 %)	22

N, Number of subjects

Table 2 Mean frequency of each comet class per 100 cells (± standard deviation) and overall mean comet score (± standard deviation) of persons working in CNG/petrol pumps, automobile workshops (exposed group) and control group

Comet class	0	1	2	3	4	TCS
Exposed group	21.6 ± 13.4	32.5 ± 14.2	15.8 ± 11.9	11.3 ± 9.9	18.7 ± 9.4	173.2 ± 50.1*
Control group	67.7 ± 13.0	16.2 ± 8.0	7.1 ± 4.4	5.3 ± 4.1	3.7 ± 2.3	61.0 ± 25.0

*Difference significant relative to control group at $P \leq 0.001$ (student's t-test); TCS, total comet score

less than a year, while the exposed individuals who worked for 1 to 5 years had the TCS of 173.5 ± 52.4. The highest TCS value (183.7 ± 45.9) was observed in those working for more than 6 to 10 years (Table 3). The results indicate that the TCS increased with increasing exposure duration of job.

No significant effect of age and per day exposure hours on TCS was observed. The effect of smoking on TCS value was evaluated.

Smoking habits had significant effect on TCS value among the exposed and the control subjects (Table 4). A significant increase ($P \leq 0.001$) in TCS values was observed in smokers when compared with non-smokers in both control and exposed groups (Table 4).

The automobile workshop mechanics had significantly higher TCS (204.0 ± 59.3, P = 0.001) than CNG/Petrol pumps filler men (169.7 ± 48.1) (Table 5).

Discussion

According to petroleum industry the highest occupational exposure to gasoline vapours typically occurs amongst marine loading operators, truck drivers, service station attendants and bulk terminal operators [20]. Retail service stations attendants are workers who experience chronic exposure to petroleum products mainly through inhalation due to their occupational exposure [21]. As these workers are exposed to gases such as CO_2, CO, NO_2, Hydrocarbons, Nitro aromatics, Benzopyrene, Benzene, 1, 3 Butadiene etc, all these gases are chemical mutagens [22]. Similarly in engine repair workshops engine exhaust and used engine oils are also major sources of polycyclic aromatic hydrocarbons (PAH) [23].

The Current research work showed a significant DNA damage in the exposed subjects as compared to control group. This study correlates with the study done in Thailand, which showed greater DNA damage in fifty workers of gasoline stations than that in control group [24]. Santos-Mello et al. [25] have demonstrated hematopoietic malignancy and chromosomal deletions in lymphocytes of workers exposed to petrol. In a study from North India, genotoxicity in retail service stations attendants showed significantly higher level of DNA damage in exposed subjects as compared to control subjects [26]. Another study from India showed higher level of genotoxicity in filling station attendants exposed to petroleum hydrocarbons as compared to control group [27].

We observed an increase in TCS with an increase in exposure duration. Similarly Schnatter et al. [28] found a close relationship between duration of occupation and genotoxicity. Keretetse et al. [29] in their pilot study on petrol attendants showed that subjects exposed for 5-10 years or >10 years have the highest ratio of DNA damage. Subjects exposed for 1-3 years also had increased DNA damage as compared to those exposed for less than a year. A research work done by Shastri and Pant [30] claimed that occupational exposure to the chemicals such as heavy metals, contained in brake fluids, degreasers, detergents, lubricants, metal cleaners, paints, fuel, solvents, found in the garage environment, can cause DNA damage and the genotoxic effects increases with increase in duration of exposure. On the other hand the study conducted by Rekhadevi et al. [27] showed no significant association with the duration of exposure.

Smoking is one of the first exposure parameters to which researchers give their attention, as this is an agent that has been supposed to produce harmful effects [31]. Tobacco consumption affected the results for DNA damage used in this study, a significant increase in TCS values was observed in smokers when compared with non-smokers in both control and exposed groups (Table 4). Similarly, from Italy a research on 200 individuals showed

Table 3 Comet score distributed according to duration of occupational exposure

Duration	N	TCS
<1 year	20	160.7 ± 42.0
1 to 5 years	52	173.5 ± 52.4
6 to 10 years	26	183.7 ± 45.9

$r = 0.96$, $P \leq 0.02$

Table 4 Effect of tobacco use on TCS (mean ± SD)

Subject	N	TCS
Control		
Smokers	22	71.6 ± 23.2
Nonsmokers	70	53.0 ± 25.0
Exposed		
Smokers	27*	177.0 ± 51.3
Nonsmokers	71*	143.0 ± 46.5

*Difference significant relative to control group at $P \leq 0.001$ (Mann–Whitney *U*-test, two-tail)

Table 5 TCS (mean ± SD) according to nature of job in CNG/ petrol pumps and automobile workshops

Nature of Job	N	TCS
Automobile workshop workers	30	204.0 ± 59.3
CNG/Petrol filling men	68	169.7 ± 48.1

P ≤ 0.001; SD, standard deviation

that the extent of DNA migration increased up to 10 % in lymphocytes of smokers, but they detected no effect or no relationship to the amount of cigarettes being smoked per day [32]. Many other occupational studies from France [33], Poland [34] and Turkey [35, 36] have also reported damaging effects of smoking. A study from China revealed that in a cigarette factory both employees and smokers had more DNA damage as compared to control non-smokers that were not occupationally exposed to any kind of tobacco dust [37].

Several earlier epidemiological studies have reported that gasoline stations attendants and garage mechanics have an increased risk of haematological malignancy. In Washington State, Milham [38] analyzed death certificates (from 1950-79) of four occupational groups with petrol or fuel exposures, and have found higher risks for numerous haematopoietic cancers. Car mechanics were found to have significantly higher level of lymphatic leukemia, and other lymphomas, and non-significantly higher level of Hodgkin's disease, unspecified leukemia and acute leukemia. The workshop mechanics continuously wash their hands with petrol during car or engine repair; therefore these workers inhale petrol gases which contain genotoxic substances, like benzene and the products derived from engine ignition. Hadnagy and Seemayer [39] showed that, when these products enter the blood circulation cause genotoxic and cytotoxic properties. Karahalil et al. [40] used sister chromatid exchange test and micronucleus assay on peripheral blood lymphocytes of oil and petrol engine repair garages workers. The exposed group showed a significant high ($P < 0.05$) value of Micronuclei as compared to control group i.e. 1.87 ± 0.04 and 1.56 ± 0.06, respectively. These investigations are in line with our results, in which the automobile workshop mechanics showed higher level of DNA damage as compared to fuel filling station attendants.

Conclusions

Pakistan is a developing country and there are no provisions for the safe use of petroleum at work places in Pakistan. As a result the workers' health is negatively affected. The study results concluded that gasoline and its various chemicals impose genotoxic effects and cause increase DNA damage in exposed workers during their occupational exposure, as compared to control. This DNA damage may be attributed to the extensive exposure to petrol without any protective strategy.

Abbreviations

CA: Comet assay; CNG: Compressed natural gas; DMSO: Dimethyl sulfoxide; EDTA: Ethylenediaminetetraacetic acid; IARC: International Agency for Research on Cancer; LMPA: Low melting point agarose; MN: Micronuclei; NMA: Normal melting agarose; PBS: Phosphate buffered saline; SCGE: Single cell gel electrophoresis; TCS: Total comet score.

Competing interests

The authors declare that they have no competing interests.

Authors' contributions

AK and AG prepared samples for analysis and performed lymphocyte isolation and the comet assay. MK designed and prepared the initial draft of the study. A and HA collected the samples and interviewed the subjects. FZ and SBR arranged, statistically analyzed and interpreted the results of lab work. NA was involved in extensive writing/editing of the paper and correcting draft versions of the manuscript. All the authors read and approved the final manuscript.

Acknowledgments

We are thankful to the University of Peshawar for providing funds and research facilities to complete this research work.

Author details

[1]Department of Zoology, University of Peshawar, Peshawar, Pakistan.
[2]Institute of Chemical Sciences, University of Peshawar, Peshawar, Pakistan.

References

1. Harper C, Liccione JJ. Toxicological profile for automotive gasoline. U.S. Department of Health and Human Services, Agency for Toxic Substances and Disease Registry. Washington, DC: GPO; 1995.
2. Page NP, Mehlman MA. Health effects of gasoline refueling vapours and measured exposures at service stations. Toxicol Lnd Health. 1989;5:369–890.
3. Mehlman MA. Dangerous properties of petroleum refining products: Carcinogenicity of motor fuels (Gasoline). Teratogenesis Carcinog Mutagenesis. 1990;10:399–408.
4. Lewne M, Nise G, Lind ML, Gustavsson P. Exosure to particles and nitrogen dioxide among taxi, bus lorry drivers. Int Arch Occup Environ Health. 2006;79:6–220.
5. Crebelli R, Conti L, Crochi B, Carera A. The effect of fuel composition on the mutagenicity of diesel engine exhaust. Mutat Res. 1995;346:167–72.
6. IARC (International Agency for Research on Cancer). Monographs on the evaluation of the carcinogenic risks to humans. Occupational exposures in petroleum refining; crude oil and major petroleum fuels. Lyon. 1989;45:41–57.
7. Gupta S, Dogra TD. Air pollution and human health hazards. Indian. J Occup Environ Med. 2002;6:89–93.
8. Carrieri M, Bonfiglio E, Scapellato ML, Macca I, Tranfo G, Faranda P, et al. Comparison of exposure assessment methods in occupational exposure to benzene in gasoline filling-station attendants. Toxicol Lett. 2005;162:146–52.
9. Wallace LA. Major sources of benzene exposure. Environ Health Perspect. 1989;82:165–9.
10. Lan Q, Zhang L, Hakim F, Shen M, Memon S, Li G, et al. Lymphocytes toxicity and T cell receptor excision circles in workers exposed to benzene. Chem Biol Interact. 2005;153–154:111–5.
11. Fishbein L. Benzene: uses, occurrence and exposure. World Health Organ Int Agency Res Cancer. 1988;85:67–96.
12. Irons RD, Stillman WS, Colagiovanni DB, Henry VA. Synergistic action of the benzene metabolite hydroquinone on myelopoietic stimulating activity of granulocyte/macrophage colony-stimulating factor in vitro. Proc Natl Acad Sci USA. 1992;89:3691–95.
13. Snyder R, Witz G, Goldstein BD. The toxicology of benzene. Environ Health Perspect. 1993;100:293–306.
14. Moller P. The alkaline comet assay: towards validation in biomonitoring of DNA damaging exposures. Basic Clin Pharmacol Toxicol. 2006;98:336–45.
15. Singh NP, McCoy MT, Tice RR, Schneider LL. A simple technique for quantitation of low levels of DNA damage in individual cells. Exp Cell Res. 1988;175:184–91.

16. Tice RR, Andrews PW, Hirai O, Singh NP. The single cell gel (SCG) assay: an electrophoretic technique for the detection of DNA damage in individual cells. In: Witmer CM, Snyder RR, Hollow DJ, Kalf GF, Kocsis JJ, Sipes JG, editors. Biological Reactive Intermediates. IV. Molecular and Cellular Effects and their impact on Human Health. New York: Plenum Press; 1991. p. 157–64.
17. Olive PL. DNA damage and repair in individual cells: applications of the comet assay in radiobiology. Int J Radiat Biol. 1999;75:395–405.
18. Collins AR. The comet assay for DNA damage and repair: principles, applications, and limitations. Mol Biotechnol. 2004;26:249–61.
19. Wessa P. Free statistical software. Office for Research Developmental Education. 2011. Version 1.1.23-r7. http://www.wessa.net/rankcorr.wasp [Accessed 22 March 2014].
20. Verma DK, Julian JA, Beebee G, Cheng WK, Holborn K, Shaw L. Hydrocarbon exposures at petroleum bulk terminals and agencies. Am Ind Assoc J. 1992;10:645–56.
21. Celik A, Akbas E. Evaluation of sister chromatid exchange and chromosomal aberration frequencies in peripheral blood lymphocytes of gasoline station attendants. Ecotoxicol Environ Saf. 2005;60:106–12.
22. Bukvic N, Bavaro P, Elia G, Cassano F, Fanelli M, Guanti G. Sister chromatid exchange (SCE) and micronucleus (MN) frequencies in lymphocytes of gasoline station attendants. Mutat Res. 1998;415:25–33.
23. International Agency for Research on Cancer. Polynuclear aromatic compounds, part 1, chemical, environmental and experimental data. IARC Monogr Eval Carcinog Risk Chem Hum. 1983; 32:1–453.
24. Navasumrit P, Chanvaivit S, Intarasunanont P, Arayasiri M, Lauhareungpanya N, Parnlob V, et al. Enviromental and occupational exposure to benzene in Thailand. Chem Biol Interact. 2005;153:75–83.
25. Santos-Mello R, Cavalcante B. Cytogenetic studies on gas station attendants. Mutat Res. 1992;280:285–90.
26. Pandey AK, Bajpayee M, Parmar D, Kumar R, Rastogi SK, Mathur N, et al. Multipronged evaluation of genotoxicity in Indian petrol pump workers. Environ Mol Mutagen. 2008;49:695–707.
27. Rekhadevi PV, Rahman MF, Mahboob M, Grover P. Genotoxicity in filling station attendants exposed to petroleum hydrocarbons. Ann Occup Hyg. 2010;54:944–54.
28. Schnattear AR, Katz AM, Nicolich MJ, Theriault G. A retrospective mortality study among Canadian petroleum marketing and distribution workers. Environ Health Perspect. 1993;6:85–99.
29. Keretetse GS, Laubscher PJ, Du Plessis JL, Pretorius PJ, Vander Westhuizen FH, Van Deventer E, et al. DNA Damage and Repair detected by the Comet Assay in lynphocytes of African petrol attendants: A pilot study. Ann Occup Hyg. 2008;52:653–62.
30. Shastri NM, Pant H. Genotoxic Profile of Motor Garage Workers. Am J Infect Dis. 2011;7:55–60.
31. Moller P, Knudsen LE, Loft S, Wallin H. The comet assay as a rapid test in biomonitoring occupational exposure to DNA-damaging agents and effect of confounding factors. Cancer Epidemiol Biomarkers Prev. 2000;9:1005–15.
32. Betti C, Davini T, Giannessi L, Loprieno N, Barale R. Comparative studies by comet test and SCE analysis in human lymphocytes from 200 healthy subjects. Mutat Res. 1995;343:201–7.
33. Lebailly P, Vigreux C, Lechevrel C, Ledemeney D, Godard T, Sichel F, et al. DNA damage in mononuclear leukocytes of farmers measured using the alkaline comet assay: discussion of critical parameters and evaluation of seasonal variations in relation to pesticide exposure. Cancer Epidemiol Biomark Prev. 1998;7:917–27.
34. Palus J, Dziubaltowska E, Rydzynski K. DNA damage detected by the comet assay in white blood cells of workers in a wooden furniture plant. Mutat Res. 1999;444:61–74.
35. Sardas S, Aygun N, U nal Y, U nal N, Berk N, Karakaya AE. Use of alkaline Comet assay (single cell gel electrophoresis technique) to detect DNA damage in lymphocytes of operating room personnel occupationally exposed to anaesthetic gases. Mutat Res. 1998;418:93–100.
36. Sardas S, Aygun N, Karakaya AE. Genotoxicity studies on professional hair colorists exposed to oxidation hair dyes. Mutat Res. 1997;394:153–61.
37. Zhu CQ, Lam TH, Jiang CQ, Wei BX, Lou X, Liu WW, et al. Lymphocyte DNA damage in cigarette factory workers measured by the Comet assay. Mutat Res. 1999;444:1–6.
38. Milham SJr. Occupational mortality in Washington State 1950-1979. Washington, DC: DHHS publication no. (NIOSH) 83–116,1983.
39. Hadnagy W, Seemayer HN. Cytotoxic and genotoxic effects of extract of particulate emission from a gasoline-powered engine. Environ Mol Mutagen. 1988;12:385–396.
40. Karahalil B, Burgaz S, Fisek G, Karakaya AE. Biological monitoring of young workers exposed to polycyclic aromatic hydrocarbons in engine repair workshops. Mutat Res. 1998;412:261–9.

2

Two cases of hard metal lung disease showing gradual improvement in pulmonary function after avoiding dust exposure

Hiroya Terui[1], Satoshi Konno[1*], Kichizo Kaga[2], Yoshihiro Matsuno[3], Kanako C. Hatanaka[3], Hiromi Kanno[3], Hiroshi Moriyama[4], Motohiro Uo[5] and Masaharu Nishimura[1]

Abstract

We present herein two cases of hard metal lung disease (HMLD) with distinct pathological findings. Both cases showed gradual improvements in pulmonary function over a period of a few years (Case 1: 30 months; Case 2: 12 months) after the avoidance of dust exposure, while improvements on high-resolution computed tomography were modest. The increased lymphocytes and decreased CD4/CD8 ratio in BALF observed at initial diagnosis normalized after the avoidance of dust exposure in one case. To the best of our knowledge, this is the first report demonstrating continual follow-up of pulmonary function and radiographic findings, and a comparison of BALF findings before and after avoidance of hard metal dust exposure.

Keywords: Hard metal lung disease, Pulmonary function, Dust exposure, Avoidance, BALF

Background

Hard metal lung disease (HMLD) is a rare occupational lung disease that can occur in workers engaged in the manufacture, utilization, or maintenance of tools composed of hard metal, a synthetic compound composed of tungsten carbide and cobalt [1, 2]. Although giant cell interstitial pneumonitis (GIP) is known as a typical pathological finding for this disease [3–5], some cases without GIP have also been reported [6, 7]. The clinical course of this disease varies, with some cases requiring corticosteroid treatment and others showing spontaneous improvement simply by avoiding exposure to hard metal [5, 8–12]. We report two cases of HMLD with distinct pathological findings: one as typical GIP; and the other characterized by peribronchial fibrosis without typical features of GIP. Continual follow-up of pulmonary function and radiological findings as well as comparisons of bronchoalveolar lavage fluid (BALF) findings before and after dust exposure were obtained.

* Correspondence: satkonno@med.hokudai.ac.jp
[1]First Department of Medicine, Hokkaido University School of Medicine, Kita-15 Nishi-7 Kita-Ku, Sapporo, Hokkaido 060-8638, Japan
Full list of author information is available at the end of the article

Case presentation

Case 1

A 50-year-old non-smoking woman presented with a 6-month history of nonproductive cough, which had started 8 years after she began working with a hard metal grinder without using a dust protective mask. High-resolution computed tomography (HRCT) of the chest showed diffuse centrilobular micronodular opacities and curved linear shadows in the dorsum (Fig. 1a). Pulmonary function test results were almost within normal levels for vital capacity (VC) (2.20 L; percentage predicted VC (%VC), 86.6 %), forced expiratory volume in 1 s (FEV_1) (2.07 L; percentage predicted FEV_1 (%FEV_1), 95.4 %), total lung capacity (TLC) (3.33 L; percent predicted TLC (%TLC), 87.2 %), and diffusing capacity of the lung for carbon monoxide (%DL_{CO}; 77.8 %). BALF obtained from the right middle lobe (S^5) showed an increased percentage of lymphocytes (55.0 %) and a decreased CD4/CD8 ratio (0.40) (Table 1). Multinucleated giant cells were not observed in BALF. Thoracoscopic lung biopsy (video-assisted thoracoscopic surgery (VATS)) of the right upper and lower lobes was performed, and microscopic examination revealed peribronchiolar fibrosis with lymphocytic infiltration. Although a

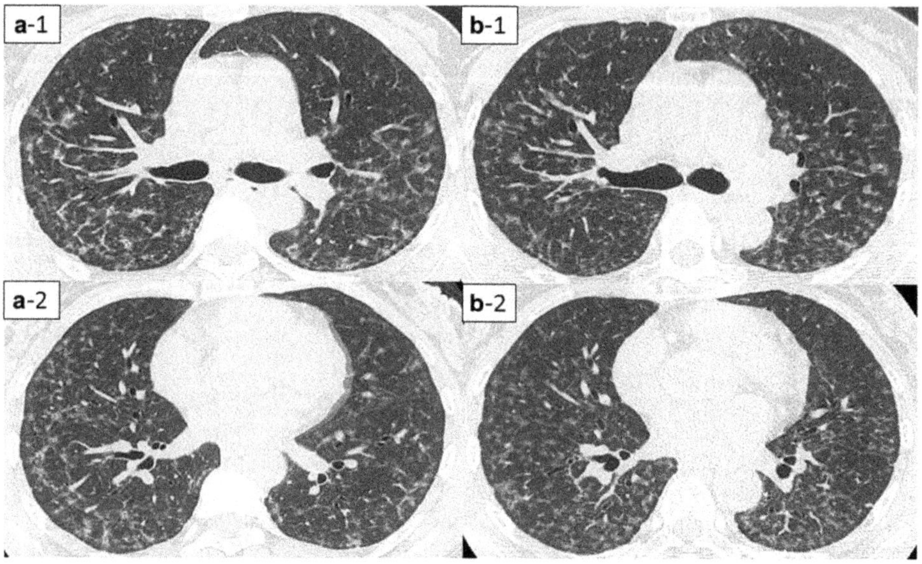

Fig. 1 High-resolution computed tomography (HRCT) findings before and after the avoidance of dust exposure in Case1. Bilateral diffuse centrilobular micronodular opacities and curved linear shadows in the dorsum. **a**: before the avoidance (a-1: upper lobe; a-2: lower lobe); **b**: after the avoidance (b-1: upper lobe; b-2: lower lobe)

few multinucleated giant cells were observed, no features diagnostic of GIP were evident (Fig. 2). Elemental analysis of the lung tissue using an electron probe microanalyzer with a wavelength-dispersive spectrometer (EPMA-1610; Shimadzu Ltd, Kyoto, Japan) revealed the presence of tungsten and cobalt in the peribronchial fibrotic region (Fig. 3). Furthermore, X-ray absorption fine structure (XAFS) analysis confirmed that the tungsten present in the samples was in the form of tungsten carbide (data not shown). These results clearly indicated that the subject had inhaled hard metal, leading to the diagnosis of HMLD.

Table 1 Results from bronchoalveolar lavage fluid (BALF) in Case 1

	Before avoidance of dust exposure	After avoidance of dust exposure
Lavaged area	rt. S^5	rt. S^5
Total cell count (/ml)	3.36×10^5	4.04×10^5
Macrophages (%)	43.8	72.6
Lymphocytes (%)	55.0	26.3
Neutrophils (%)	0.6	1.0
Eosinophils (%)	0.0	0.2
CD4/CD8 ratio	0.40	1.72
Multinucleated giant cells	(-)	(-)

After reaching this diagnosis, we recommended the patient quit her job or transfer to a different workplace to completely avoid exposure to hard metal dust. However, she continued working at the same place without using a dust protective mask for financial reasons, and nonproductive cough continued. In addition, pulmonary function continued to worsen. Finally, 18 months after diagnosis, she obtained a transfer to a different department where she was completely isolated from exposure to hard metal dust. Her cough improved and had completely disappeared by 2 months after ending exposure to hard metal dust. A series of pulmonary function tests revealed continuous improvements over the course of 30 months without exposure to hard metal dust (Fig. 4), although improvements in HRCT findings were modest (Fig. 1b). BALF findings obtained at 21 months after ceasing hard metal dust exposure showed a decreased percentage of lymphocytes (26.3 %) and an increase in the CD4/CD8 ratio (1.72) compared to the initial findings (Table 1). She did not take any corticosteroids or other immunosuppressive drugs during this follow-up period.

Case 2

A 45-year-old non-smoking man presented with a 2-year history of dyspnea, which had started 11 years after he began a job mixing raw materials for manufacturing hard metal tools without using a dust protective mask. Chest HRCT showed diffuse centrilobular micronodular

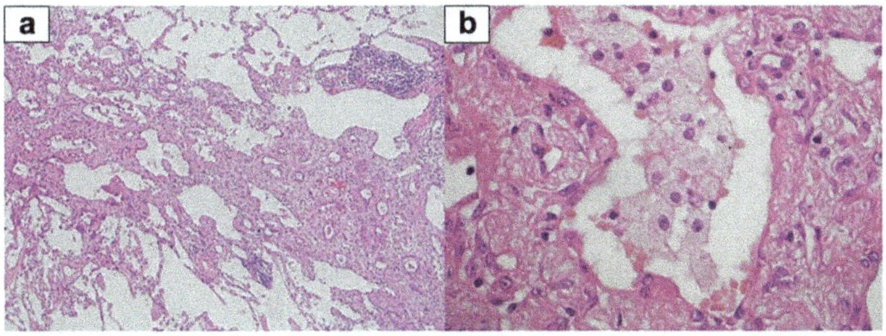

Fig. 2 Histological findings from biopsy specimens in Case 1. Peribronchiolar fibrosis and lymphocytic infiltration are marked, but multinucleated giant cells are barely apparent (**a**: hematoxylin and eosin [HE] stain × 100; **b**: HE × 400)

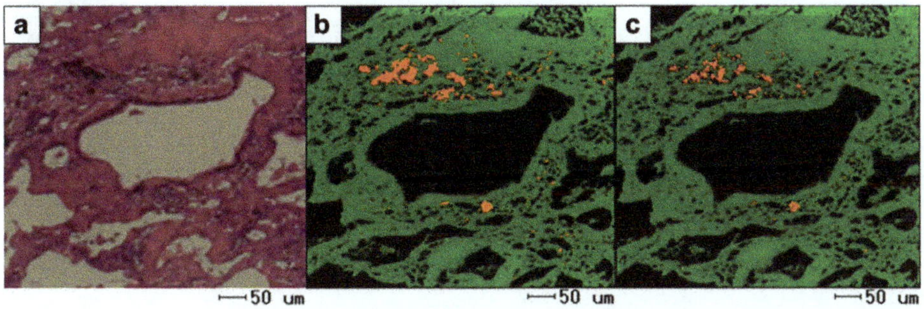

Fig. 3 Images of EPMA in Case 1. The presence of tungsten and cobalt in the peribronchial fibrotic region was observed (**a**: HE stain; **b**: tungsten; **c**: cobalt)

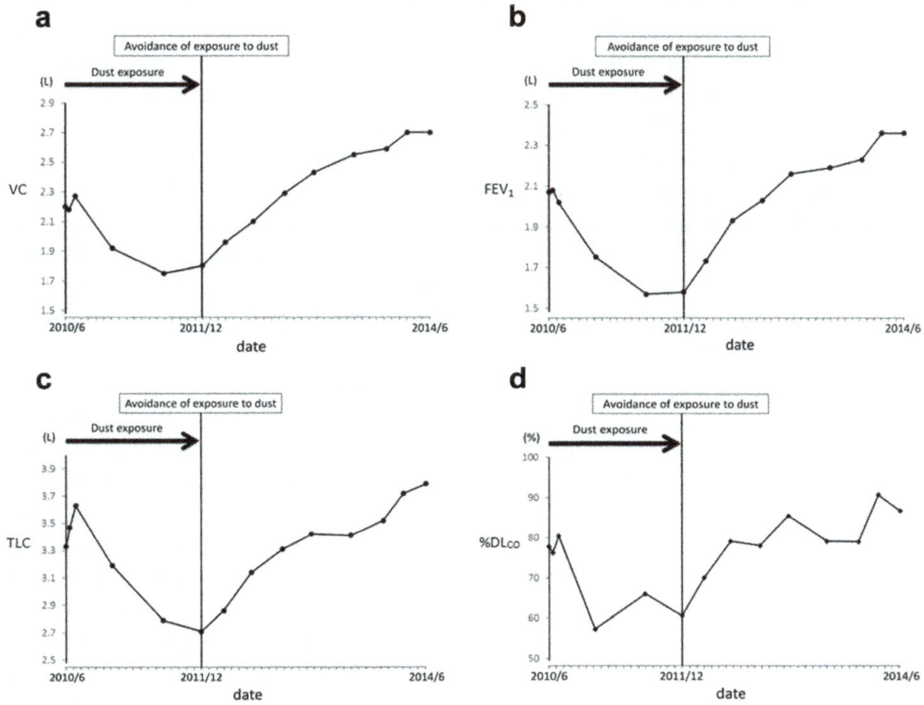

Fig. 4 Serial changes in pulmonary function in Case 1. **a**: vital capacity (VC), **b**: forced expiratory volume in 1 s (FEV1), **c**: total lung capacity (TLC), **d**: diffusing capacity of the lung for carbon monoxide (%DL_{CO})

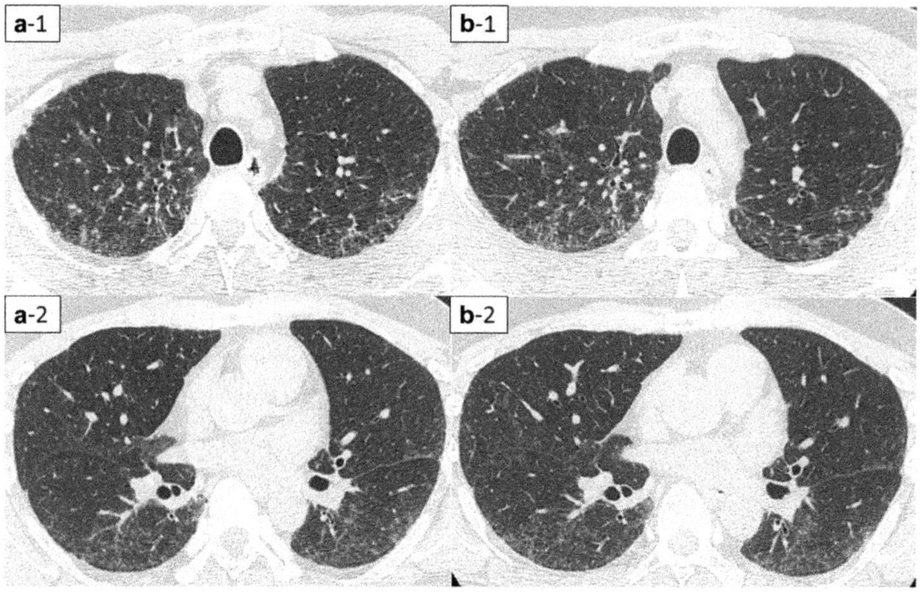

Fig. 5 HRCT findings before and after the avoidance of exposure in Case 2. Bilateral diffuse centrilobular micronodular opacities and reticular shadows. **a**: before the avoidance (a-1: upper lobe; a-2: lower lobe); **b**: after the avoidance (b-1: upper lobe; b-2: lower lobe)

and reticular shadows (Fig. 5a). Pulmonary function testing showed a low VC (2.10 L; %VC, 46.0 %), FEV_1 (1.61 L; $\%FEV_1$, 41.9 %), TLC (3.32 L; %TLC, 55.9 %), and DL_{CO} ($\%DL_{CO}$, 65.0 %). Although BALF obtained from the right middle lobe (S^5) demonstrated normal cell counts, multinucleated giant cells were observed (Table 2). VATS of the left upper and lower lobes were performed, and histopathological examination revealed interstitial fibrosis accompanied by multinucleated giant cell infiltration into peribronchiolar and alveolar tissues, leading to a diagnosis of GIP (Fig. 6). Elemental analysis of the lung tissue revealed the presence of tungsten in the bronchioles and alveoli (Fig. 7), and XAFS analysis confirmed the presence of tungsten carbide (data not shown), thus leading to the clinical diagnosis of HMLD.

Three weeks after his first visit, the patient obtained a transfer to a different department with reduced (but not eliminated) exposure to dust. Dyspnea gradually improved after reducing the dust exposure. Although a series of pulmonary function tests revealed improvements over the course of a year (Fig. 8), improvements in HRCT findings were modest (Fig. 5b). Multinucleated giant cells remained observable in BALF a year after reducing dust exposure, and cell differentiation was similar to that before the avoidance of dust exposure (Table 2). The patient did not take any corticosteroids or other immunosuppressive drugs during this follow-up period.

Table 2 Results from bronchoalveolar lavage fluid (BALF) in Case 2

	Before avoidance of dust exposure	After avoidance of dust exposure
Lavaged area	rt. S^5	rt. S^5
Total cell count (/ml)	1.66×10^5	6.40×10^4
Macrophages (%)	86.9	84.4
Lymphocytes (%)	10.7	13.8
Neutrophils (%)	2.1	0.6
Eosinophils (%)	0.3	1.2
CD4/CD8 ratio	1.85	1.22
Multinucleated giant cells	(+)	(+)

Discussion

The clinical features of HMLD are known to be heterogeneous in several respects, such as pathological findings, BALF findings, and clinical course. In the two cases we encountered, thoracoscopic lung biopsy revealed distinct pathological findings, with one case characterized by typical GIP, and the other by diffuse centrilobular fibrosis around the respiratory bronchioles without GIP. In a study of 100 cases of HMLD, Asghar et al. [6] described 41 cases not showing GIP findings, and some cases only showed infiltration of lymphocytes and fibrosis in peribronchial lesions similar to that noted in our

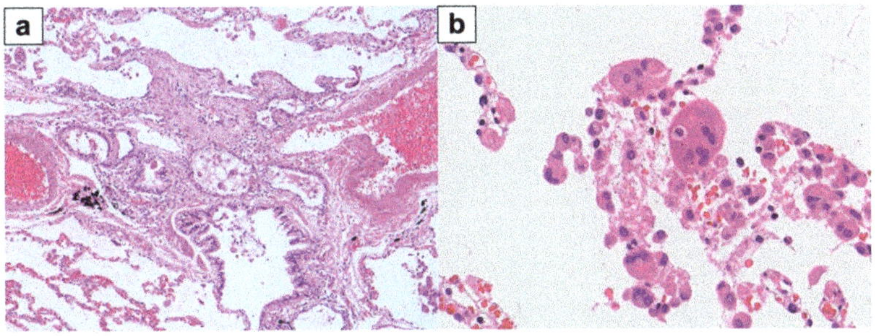

Fig. 6 Histological findings from biopsy specimens in Case 2. Marked peribronchiolar fibrosis accompanies multinucleated giant cells in the bronchioles and alveoli (**a**: HE stain × 100; **b**: HE stain × 400)

Case 1. Tanaka et al. [7] recently examined 19 cases of HMLD diagnosed in Japan and described various pathological findings, including typical GIP, centrilobular fibrosis, and usual interstitial pneumonia (UIP) pattern. In the present cases, differences in the type of job (Case 1: grinder of hard metal; Case 2: mixer of raw materials) and/or genetic backgrounds of the two patients may have been involved in the different pathological findings observed.

Avoidance of exposure to hard metal dust is central to preventing deterioration of this disease in any case, and improvements of the symptoms and/or radiological findings after avoiding exposure have been reported in several previous studies [5, 8–10]. However, to the best of our knowledge, no previous reports have provided continuous follow-up information on pulmonary function and radiological findings after reducing exposure to hard metal dust exposure. Of note, pulmonary function displayed gradual improvement after reducing dust exposure in both cases, while improvements in HRCT findings were more modest. As shown in Case 1, the improvement in pulmonary function was continuing even 2 years after starting avoidance of hard metal dust. Clinicians should thus keep in mind that gradual improvement of pulmonary function can be expected over the course of years, despite the lowered pulmonary function before the avoidance of dust exposure. Immunological responses to hard metal ingredients trapped in the bronchioles and/or to cobalt dissolved in the lungs might gradually diminish after marked reductions in exposure. We therefore speculate that the persistence of hard metal in the lung may determine the clinical course of the disease after the avoidance of dust exposure.

In some previously reported cases, respiratory failure progressed to death despite suspending exposure to the dust [11, 12], while in others, the symptoms and/or radiological findings improved with the avoidance of exposure [8–10]. The pathogenesis of HMLD is thus considered to encompass a wide spectrum of cases, from mimicking hypersensitivity pneumonitis to those similar to typical pneumoconiosis generally caused by silica and asbestos, progressing even after the avoidance of dust exposure.

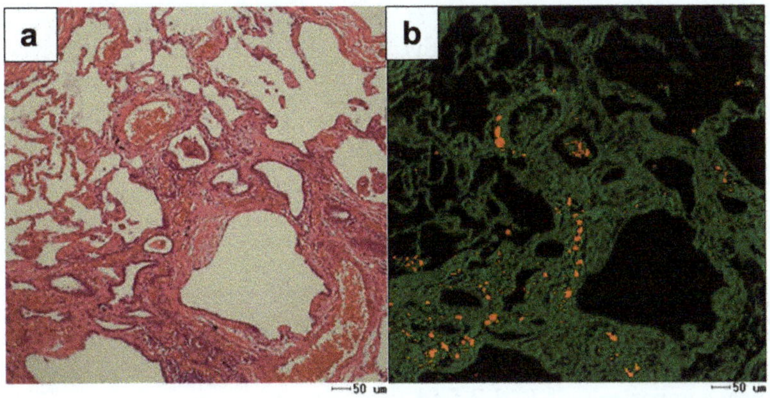

Fig. 7 Images of EPMA in Case 2. The presence of tungsten in the bronchioles and alveoli was observed (**a**: HE stain; **b**: tungsten)

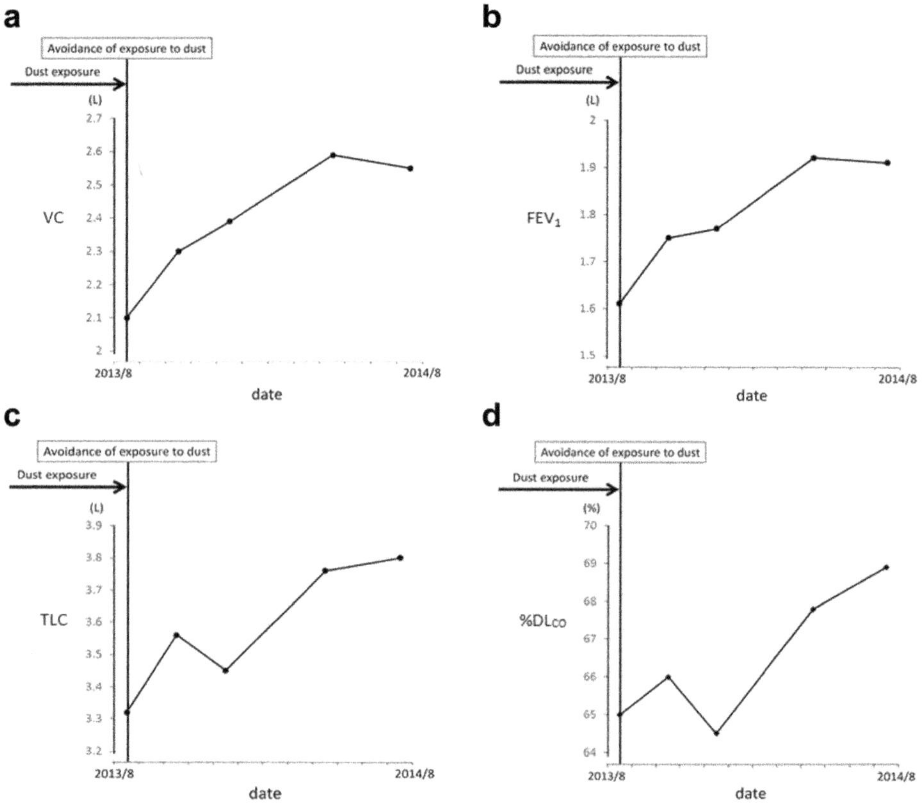

Fig. 8 Serial changes in pulmonary function in Case 2. **a**: VC; **b**: FEV_1; **c**: TLC; **d**: $\%DL_{CO}$

Although previous studies have suggested that increased lymphocytes and decreased CD4/CD8 ratio are characteristic BALF findings in subjects with HMLD [7, 9, 12, 13], this does not always seem to be the case. In fact, in the present study, BALF findings from Case 2 showed normal cell differentiation and CD4/CD8 ratio. To date, no reports have compared BALF findings of subjects with HMLD before and after the avoidance of dust exposure similar to that encountered in the present study. The increased lymphocytes and decreased CD4/CD8 ratio observed at initial diagnosis in our Case 1 normalized by 9 months after reducing dust exposure, indicating altered immune cellular responses to hard metal in the pathogenesis of this case.

Conclusion

We have presented two cases of HMLD with continuous follow-up of pulmonary function and radiological findings before and after avoidance of hard metal dust exposure. The clinical courses of the two cases were presented, together with a comparison of BALF findings before and after avoidance of dust exposures.

Consent

Written informed consent was obtained from both patients for the publication of this case report and the accompanying images.

Competing interests

The authors declare that they have no competing interests.

Authors' contributions

HT, SK, and MN wrote the manuscript. HT and SK contributed to the treatment of both patients. KK was involved in performing the thoracoscopic lung biopsy. YM, KH, and HK performed pathological diagnosis. HM and MU were involved in performing the elemental analysis. All authors have read and approved the final manuscript.

Acknowledgement

We would like to express our sincere gratitude to Dr. Takeshi Hosokawa, former Assistant Professor of the First Department of Medicine, Hokkaido University School of Medicine, who passed away on January 17th, 2013. We are also thankful to Dr. Yasuhiro Hida (Cardiovascular and Thoracic Surgery, Hokkaido University Hospital) for performing thoracoscopic lung biopsy, and to Drs. Akira Isada, Takashi Inomata (First Department of Medicine, Hokkaido University School of Medicine), Kenzo Okamoto, and Kiyonobu Kimura (Hokkaido Chuo Rosai Hospital) for their valuable discussions.

Author details

[1]First Department of Medicine, Hokkaido University School of Medicine, Kita-15 Nishi-7 Kita-Ku, Sapporo, Hokkaido 060-8638, Japan. [2]Cardiovascular and Thoracic Surgery, Hokkaido University School of Medicine, Sapporo, Hokkaido 060-8638, Japan. [3]Department of Surgical Pathology, Hokkaido

University Hospital, Sapporo, Hokkaido 060-8638, Japan. [4]Niigata University Medical & Dental Hospital Bioscience Medical Research Center, Niigata, Niigata 951-8520, Japan. [5]Advanced Biomaterials, Department of Restorative Sciences, Division of Oral Health Sciences, Graduate School of Medical and Dental Sciences, Tokyo Medical and Dental University, Bunkyo-ku, Tokyo 113-8549, Japan.

References

1. Coates EO, Watson JHL. Diffuse interstitial lung disease in tungsten carbide workers. Ann Intern Med. 1971;75:709–16.
2. Nemery B. Metal toxicity and the respiratory tract. Eur Respir J. 1990;3:202–19.
3. Cugell DW. The hard metal disease. Clin Chest Med. 1992;13:269–79.
4. Ohori NP, Sciurba FC, Owens GR, et al. Giant-cell interstitial pneumonia and hard-metal pneumoconiosis. Am J Surg Pathol. 1989;13:581–7.
5. Nemery B, Verbeken EK, Demedts M. Giant cell interstitial pneumonia (hard metal lung disease, cobalt lung). Semin Respir Crit Care Med. 2001;22:435–48.
6. Asghar H, Hunt A, Bryan R, Abraham JL. Pathologic spectrum and lung dust burden in giant cell interstitial pneumonia (Hard metal disease/cobalt pneumonitis): Review of 100 cases. Arch Environ Occup Health. 2008;63:51–70.
7. Tanaka J, Moriyama H, Terada M, et al. An observational study of giant cell interstitial pneumonia and fibrosis in hard metal lung disease. BMJ Open. 2014;4:e004407.
8. Okuno K, Kobayashi K, Kotani Y, Ohnishi H, Ohbayashi C, Nishimura Y. A case of hard metal lung disease resembling a hypersensitive pneumonia in radiological images. Intern Med. 2010;49:1185–9.
9. Kinoshita M, Sueyasu Y, Watanabe H, Tanoue S, Okubo Y, Koga T, et al. Giant cell interstitial pneumonia in two hard metal workers: the role of bronchoalveolar lavage in diagnosis. Respirology. 1999;4:263–6.
10. Demedts M, Gheysens B, Nagels J, Verbeken E, Lauweryns J, van den Eeckhout A, et al. Cobalt lung in diamond polishers. Am Rev Respir Dis. 1984;130:130–5.
11. Seike M, Usuki J, Uematsu K, Enomoto T, Shinoda K, Yoshimori K, et al. Giant cell interstitial pneumonia in a metal grinder with an abnormally high level of serum CA19-9. Nihon Kyobu Shikkan Gakkai Zasshi (Article in Japanese). 1995;33:894–9.
12. Nemery B, Nagels J, Verbeken E, Dinsdale D, Demedts M. Rapidly fatal progression of cobalt lung in a diamond polisher. Am Rev Respir Dis. 1990;141:1373–8.
13. Forni A. Bronchoalveolar lavage in the diagnosis of hard metal disease. Sci Total Environ. 1994;150:69–76.

3

Diesel engine exhaust and lung cancer risks – evaluation of the meta-analysis

Peter Morfeld[1,2*] and Michael Spallek[3,4]

Abstract

Background: Vermeulen et al. 2014 published a meta-regression analysis of three relevant epidemiological US studies (Steenland et al. 1998, Garshick et al. 2012, Silverman et al. 2012) that estimated the association between occupational diesel engine exhaust (DEE) exposure and lung cancer mortality. The DEE exposure was measured as cumulative exposure to estimated respirable elemental carbon in μg/m^3-years. Vermeulen et al. 2014 found a statistically significant dose–response association and described elevated lung cancer risks even at very low exposures.

Methods: We performed an extended re-analysis using different modelling approaches (fixed and random effects regression analyses, Greenland/Longnecker method) and explored the impact of varying input data (modified coefficients of Garshick et al. 2012, results from Crump et al. 2015 replacing Silverman et al. 2012, modified analysis of Moehner et al. 2013).

Results: We reproduced the individual and main meta-analytical results of Vermeulen et al. 2014. However, our analysis demonstrated a heterogeneity of the baseline relative risk levels between the three studies. This heterogeneity was reduced after the coefficients of Garshick et al. 2012 were modified while the dose coefficient dropped by an order of magnitude for this study and was far from being significant ($P = 0.6$). A (non-significant) threshold estimate for the cumulative DEE exposure was found at 150 μg/m^3-years when extending the meta-analyses of the three studies by hockey-stick regression modelling (including the modified coefficients for Garshick et al. 2012). The data used by Vermeulen and colleagues led to the highest relative risk estimate across all sensitivity analyses performed. The lowest relative risk estimate was found after exclusion of the explorative study by Steenland et al. 1998 in a meta-regression analysis of Garshick et al. 2012 (modified), Silverman et al. 2012 (modified according to Crump et al. 2015) and Möhner et al. 2013. The meta-coefficient was estimated to be about 10–20 % of the main effect estimate in Vermeulen et al. 2014 in this analysis.

Conclusions: The findings of Vermeulen et al. 2014 should not be used without reservations in any risk assessments. This is particularly true for the low end of the exposure scale.

Keywords: Diesel, DEE, Lung cancer, Epidemiology, Meta-analysis

* Correspondence: peter.morfeld@evonik.com
[1]Institute and Policlinic for Occupational Medicine, Environmental Medicine and Prevention Research of Cologne University, Kerpener Str. 62, 50937 Köln, Germany
[2]Institute for Occupational Epidemiology and Risk Assessment (IERA) of Evonik Industries AG, Rellinghauser Str. 1-11, D-45128 Essen, Germany
Full list of author information is available at the end of the article

Background

Vermeulen et al. [1] published a meta-regression analysis of three major epidemiological US studies [2–4] which investigated the association between diesel engine exhaust (DEE) exposure – based on the cumulative exposure to respirable elemental carbon (REC) in μg/m^3-years – and lung cancer mortality. The authors reported that some of them worked as members of the IARC Working Group (see [5]), which produced a review of the carcinogenic effect of DEE (hazard assessment) and classified DEE as a human carcinogen (IARC Group 1) in 2012. With this follow-up analysis, Vermeulen et al. [1] aimed to continue these considerations and contribute to the quantitative risk assessment based on the major studies. From the data of the three studies, the authors' main result was a common exposure-risk curve without a threshold and concluded: "We estimated a lnRR of 0.00098 (95 % CI: 0.00055, 0.0014) for lung cancer mortality with each 1-μg/m^3-year increase in cumulative EC based on a linear meta-regression model. Corresponding lnRRs for the individual studies ranged from 0.00061 to 0.0012. Estimated numbers of excess lung cancer deaths through 80 years of age for lifetime occupational exposures of 1, 10, and 25 μg/m^3 EC were 17, 200, and 689 per 10,000, respectively. For lifetime environmental exposure to 0.8 μg/m^3 EC, we estimated 21 excess lung cancer deaths per 10,000. Our estimates suggest that stringent occupational and environmental standards for DEE should be set." So the paper describes elevated risks of cancer even at very low DEE exposures. As a result, the Vermeulen et al. [1] paper will play an important role in the ongoing DEE limit value discussions. The US National Institute for Occupational Health (NIOSH) has already attempted to derive estimates from this using its standard procedure (excess case calculation) [6]: Based on Vermeulen et al. [1], Dr. Park calculated an estimate for the 8 h DEE threshold at the workplace of 0.59 μg/m^3.

In contrast, the EU's ACSH [7] recommended a limit value of 100 μg/m^3 for DEEE (diesel engine exhaust emissions), measured as elemental carbon. This recommendation is not health-based but reflects mainly socioeconomic considerations. Cherrie et al. [8] concluded that only 2 % of workers exposed to DEEE are estimated to be exposed above this level in the EU. In addition, the authors wrote: "There is a case for introducing an OEL [occupational exposure limit] for DEE particulate, but the OEL would need to be much lower than the typical European OEL that we tested (0.1 mg/m^3)". The proposal derived by Park [6] using Vermeulen et al. [1] is such a proposal that is much lower than the recommendation of the EU's ACSH [7]. A critical analysis of the meta-regression approach by Vermeulen et al. [1] is indicated to understand whether the Vermeulen et al. analysis presents evidence to support such a low limit value, far-off the 100 μg/m^3 limit value recommendation of ACSH [7].

Throughout this paper, we use "dose" as an abbreviation for "cumulative exposure to respirable elemental carbon (REC) in μg/m^3-years".

Material

Vermeulen et al. 2014: input data for primary analysis

The meta-regression analysis of Vermeulen et al. [1] included three epidemiological US studies (Steenland et al. 1998 [2], Garshick et al. 2012 [3], Silverman et al. 2012 [4]) that estimated the association between occupational DEE exposure, measured as cumulative REC exposure in μg/m^3-years (dose), and lung cancer mortality.

Steenland et al. [2] is a nested case–control study on workers in the US trucking industry (994 lung cancer deaths and 1085 controls). The dose values were lagged 5 years when calculating the odds ratios (OR). Lagging is an evaluation technique which discards the exposure data of the last years (in this case the last 5 years) to take cancer latency phenomena into account [9]. This is the oldest study in the analysis, as it is based on the data from the case–control study by Steenland et al. [10]: "all cases and controls had died in 1982–1983." The measurements for elemental carbon by Zaebst et al. [11], which were not collected until 1990, were used as the basis for exposure estimation for the period from 1949 to 1983. Accordingly, the measurements were taken approx. 8 years after the death of the persons in the study, and therefore even later after the end of their exposure phase. Steenland et al. [2] attempted to extrapolate these data back "dependent on very broad assumptions". The authors evaluated this key limitation of their research as follows: "Our results should be regarded with appropriate caution because our exposure estimates are based on broad assumptions rather than actual measurements" and they noted the following in the abstract: "Our results depend on estimates about unknown past exposures, and should be viewed as exploratory."

Garshick et al. [3] is a cohort study independent of this on the US trucking industry (31,135 male employees, 779 lung cancer deaths). Date of death and cause-specific mortality was obtained from 1985 through 2000. Historical trends in ambient terminal REC were estimated based on historical trends in the coefficient of haze available for 1971 through 2000, a measurement of particulate matter based on optical density, assumed to be predictive of ambient REC. Vermeulen et al. [1] used this cohort data after excluding mechanics, and also used dose values lagged by 5 years. Those risk estimates (hazard ratios) from the Garshick study were used which were adjusted for duration of exposure.

Silverman et al. [4] is the case–control study of the US DEMS (DEMS = Diesel Exhaust in Miners Study). The underlying cohort [12] totalled 12,315 miners from 8 non-metal mining operations and included both surface and underground workers (no ore or coal mining). The case–control study included 198 lung cancer deaths and 562 controls based on mortality follow-up through December 31, 1997. Unlike the other two studies, the authors used a lag of 15 years to calculate the odds ratios. The exposures to REC were estimated in a complicated manner based on measurements of carbon monoxide (CO) and REC made in 1998–2000 and estimates of diesel equipment horsepower used through 1997 and mine ventilation.

The supplement to Vermeulen et al. [1] contains most of the input data to the Vermeulen meta-analyses (mean dose estimate for each dose category of the studies incorporated and the corresponding relative risk RR with a 95 % confidence interval). The data were extracted and transferred to a Stata file. Gaps were filled, where the original individual study publications contained the missing information.

Table 1 shows the input data as incorporated in the primary analysis by Vermeulen et al. [1]. The three studies included [2–4] reported cumulative exposure to DEE as respirable elemental carbon (dose) with relative risks and the corresponding 95 % confidence intervals. While the dose is reported using different categorizations, all three papers use μg/m^3-years as the dose unit. Table 1 lists ORs and HRs uniformly as relative risks.

For a more detailed description of the studies incorporated, we refer to Vermeulen et al. [1] and the original publications.

Corrected estimates: Garshick et al. 2012 (modified)

All analyses in Vermeulen et al. [1] applied the risk estimates (hazard ratios) from the Garshick study that were additionally adjusted for duration of exposure. An important aspect in this context is evident from the Letter to the Editor by Morfeld [13] (including the authors' answer) on adjustment errors in the coefficients used by Vermeulen et al. [1]. Morfeld criticised that the cumulative exposure was adjusted for duration of exposure, it already contains per definition. Thus, the risk coefficient does not estimate the effect of cumulative exposure, but that of a concentration (although this is not an optimal approach to estimating the concentration effect). The authors responded to the criticism as follows: "Morfeld suggests that adjusting cumulative exposure by duration of employment time reduces cumulative exposure to an estimate of long-term average concentration. We agree that if exposure in our workers was relatively constant, cumulative exposure would be the simple product of duration and average exposure. However, exposure varies considerably over time and between and within jobs." We emphasize that this note does not justify the procedure, as the data was evaluated using time-dependent methods in the Cox analyses performed. So the following applies for every point in time and in every person: cumulative exposure = duration of exposure × average

Table 1 Input data on the primary analysis in Vermeulen et al. [1]

Study	lag/a	Exposure category	Average dose	Lower dose	Upper dose	RR	95 % CI		Number of persons	Number of cases
							Lower	Upper		
Steenland et al. 1998	5	Reference	0.0	0.0	0.0	1.00	1.00	1.00		
	5	Cat 1	84.5	0.0	<169.0	1.08	0.72	1.63		
	5	Cat 2	231.0	169.0	257.0	1.10	0.74	1.65		
	5	Cat 3	294.0	257.0	331.0	1.36	0.90	2.04		
	5	Cat 4	551.7	≥331.0		1.64	1.09	2.49		
Garshick et al. 2012[a]	5	Reference	15.5	0.0	<30.9	1.00	1.00	1.00	105513	122
	5	Cat 1	51.3	30.9	71.7	1.31	1.01	1.71	104909	191
	5	Cat 2	111.0	71.7	150.3	1.38	1.02	1.87	102496	202
	5	Cat 3	250.5	≥150.3		1.48	1.05	2.10	87397	226
Silverman et al. 2012	15	Reference	1.5	0.0	<3.0	1.00	1.00	1.00	207	49
	15	Cat 1	37.5	3.0	72.0	0.74	0.40	1.38	278	50
	15	Cat 2	204.0	72.0	536.0	1.54	0.74	3.20	206	49
	15	Cat 3	1036.0	≥536.0		2.83	1.28	6.26	173	50

Dose refers to the cumulative exposure to DEE in μg/m^3-years. For every category (Reference, Cat 1, Cat 2, Cat 3 and Cat 4), "averages" and the lower and upper limits of the dose are specified. Estimates of the relative risk RR with 95 % confidence interval (95 % CI) per category are given. Study size and number of lung cancer deaths are reported

[a]Garshick et al. [3] do not include mechanics as an employee group, and the risk estimates are adjusted for duration of exposure. For Garshick et al. [3], the number of person years is stated instead of the number of persons, as it is a cohort study. Steenland et al. [2] specify neither the number of persons nor the number of cases per exposure category

concentration. Adjusting for duration of exposure changes the analysis such that time-dependent average concentration is analysed, not the cumulative exposure. The authors justify the exposure duration adjustment they made in spite of this by claiming that it controls for the healthy worker survivor effect. However, other methods are required for this [9].

Neither of the other studies [2, 4] made adjustments of this type to the cumulative exposure. Another aspect of the Garshick study, which also affects the model specification, is covered in the discussion section.

Garshick et al. [3] offered coefficients of cumulative exposure without adjustment for duration of exposure. In order to give the coefficients their usual meaning, and to facilitate comparison with the other two studies, these coefficients were also included in this analysis. The data are shown in Table 2 and will be referred to as Garshick et al. [3] (modified) below.

The risk estimates are not only lower than in Table 1, but also do not exhibit a positive trend with increasing exposure levels.

Vermeulen et al. [1] also performed sensitivity analyses with data deviating from Garshick et al. [3] as reported in Table 1. However, these variations only involved the lag of the exposure variables and the inclusion/exclusion of the data from mechanics. By contrast, the authors do not take the problem of the cumulative exposure coefficients incorrectly adjusted for duration of exposure into consideration.

Re-analysis of the DEMS case/control study: Crump et al. 2015

Crump et al. [14] re-analysed the DEMS case–control study by Silverman et al. [4] and largely managed to reproduce its results: "We were able to replicate the findings reported by Silverman et al. (18) when we used the same analytical methods. This gave us confidence that we were using the same basic data set as Silverman et al.". Crump et al. investigated the influence of covariables which Silverman et al. [4] did not include in their final models. The radon exposure underground proved to be a main confounder, a result which did not match the statements by Silverman et al. [4]. On the cumulative exposure to radon, Silverman et al. [4] wrote "estimated cumulative exposure to radon ... were evaluated but not included in the final models because they had little or no impact on odds ratios (i.e., inclusion of these factors in the final models changed point estimates for diesel exposure by ≤10 %)". Crump et al. [14] noted the following on this: "However, when we reproduced the Silverman et al. analysis, we could not verify this statement." As a result, the present sensitivity meta-analysis only uses the estimates by Crump et al. [14] after an additional adjustment for cumulative radon exposure.

Crump et al. [14] also developed six new DEE exposure metrics, as an alternative to the estimates used in Attfield et al. [12] and Silverman et al. [4]: "We proceeded to apply six alternative REC metrics, five of which depended, as did the DEMS metrics, on extrapolations involving assumed relationships between CO and REC. A sixth REC metric, REC6, was used that did not involve any assumptions concerning the relationship between CO and REC, and was based on Adj_HP [adjusted horse power] and ventilation rates for each of the mines. Of the several REC metrics, we view REC6 as having some superior qualities because it avoids using the highly uncertain assumptions concerning the relationship between CO and REC." Therefore, we use REC6 as a primary alternative to the Silverman exposure data.

In their supplementary evaluations for the exposure estimates, Crump and van Landingham [15] determined $\beta = 0.3$ as the best estimate in the $REC \sim CO^{\beta}$ conversion model, as compared with the value of $\beta = 0.58$ according to Stewart et al. [16] or $\beta = 1.0$, which Silverman et al. [4] assumed in their analyses. The alternative exposure metric REC4 of Crump et al. [14] contains this best estimate, $\beta = 0.3$. REC4 is also directly based on the work by Crump and van Landingham [15] to estimate an alternative exposure, and takes several other aspects into consideration (see the detailed description of REC1 to REC4 in Crump et al. [14]). As a result, we also used the exposure metric REC4 as a second variation according to Crump et al. [14]. Table 3 gives an overview of the results of the re-analysis with REC4 and REC6 according to Crump et al. [14]. For the sake of clarity we emphasize that we only used results based on REC4 and REC6 after adjustment for radon exposure.

Table 2 Results from Garshick et al. [3] without adjustment for duration of exposure, referred to as Garshick et al. [3] (modified)

Exposure category	Average dose	Lower dose	Upper dose	RR	95 % CI		Person years	Number of cases
					Lower	Upper		
Reference	15.5	0.0	<30.9	1.00	1.00	1.00	105513	122
Cat 1	51.3	30.9	71.7	1.18	0.92	1.52	104909	191
Cat 2	111.0	71.7	150.3	1.17	0.88	1.55	102496	202
Cat 3	250.5	≥150.3		1.19	0.86	1.63	87397	226

Dose refers to the cumulative exposure to DEE in μg/m^3-years. For every category (Reference, Cat 1, Cat 2, Cat 3), averages and the lower and upper limits of the dose are specified. Odds ratio OR with 95 % confidence intervals (95 % CI) and the number of person years and the number of observed lung cancer deaths per dose category are reported

Table 3 Re-analysis of Silverman et al. [4] with adjustment for radon exposure (Crump et al. [14], Table 3)

Exposure category	Average dose	Lower dose	Upper dose	OR	95 % CI		Number of persons	Number of cases
					Lower	Upper		
Crump et al. [14], REC4								
Reference	0.71	0	<4.9	1	1	1	217	49
Cat 1	26.65	4.9	<70.4	0.80	0.41	1.55	266	50
Cat 2	243.43	70.4	<498.4	1.67	0.73	3.81	192	49
Cat 3	1522.10	-	≥498.4	1.50	0.54	4.17	189	50
Crump et al. [14], REC6								
Reference	0.61	0	<2.8	1	1	1	230	49
Cat 1	20.47	2.8	<50.6	1.07	0.57	2.00	247	50
Cat 2	158.27	50.6	<388.0	1.35	0.62	2.94	206	49
Cat 3	1156.89	-	≥388.0	1.43	0.52	3.94	181	50

The results are based on the exposure metrics REC4 and REC6 with a lag of 15 years (see text). Dose refers to the cumulative exposure to DEE in μg/m^3-years. For every category (Reference, Cat 1, Cat 2, Cat 3), averages and the lower and upper limits of the dose are specified. Odds ratio OR with 95 % confidence intervals (95 % CI) and the number of persons observed and the number of lung cancer deaths per dose category are reported

Re-categorised data: Möhner et al. 2013 (adapted)

Vermeulen et al. [1] omitted the German potash miner study of Möhner et al. [17] from their analysis, as they alleged the reference category defined was too high. Möhner et al. [17] was only used in two sensitivity analyses, however it was incorporated by Vermeulen et al. [1] either leaving the original RR estimates or correcting the risk estimates ad-hoc. Both approaches are less than ideal, which is why Vermeulen et al. [1] did not present either of the evaluations as part of their primary analysis, merely reporting on the results in the online appendix.

The German Potash miner study included 5,819 miners followed in mortality from 1970 through 2001. In 1991, exposure measurements of the concentration of total and elemental carbon (to a lesser extent) in the respirable dust fraction by coulometric analysis were undertaken. Because the mining technology and the mining equipment remained fairly stable since 1969, measurements from 1991 have been used for designing a job-exposure-matrix with three main job categories: production, maintenance, and workshop. Elemental carbon was the largest component of total carbon with a proportion of weight of about 63 %. Moreover, the two measures were highly correlated ($r = 0.89$). Cumulative exposure was determined as REC in μg/m^3-years.

In order to incorporate the German potash miner study as informatively as possible in this project, the data had to be used at a different scale to that published. We contacted the original authors for the information required to do so (the publication does not contain all relevant categorizations of exposure, and other detailed information was missing). On request, Dr. Möhner provided additional results from the Möhner et al. [17] study by e-mail on 03/07/2014. This included case numbers and odds ratio estimates with 95 % confidence intervals for a modified categorisation, referred to as "Möhner et al. [17] (adapted)" below.

The breakdown was adapted so that the reference category only consists of 5 cases, with the result that the exposure level of the reference category is far lower than in the original analysis (a criticism in Vermeulen et al. [1]). The other three categories were chosen in such a way that the case distribution is roughly equal. Table 4 shows the results of this re-categorisation of Möhner et al. [17].

Table 4 Additional results for the study by Möhner et al. [17] with changed (adapted) categorisation, referred to as Möhner et al. [17] (adapted)

Exposure category	Average dose	Lower dose	Upper dose	OR	95 % CI		Number of persons	Number of cases
					Lower	Upper		
Reference	263	0	≤380	1	1	1	29	5
Cat 1	728	380	1024	0.99	0.323	3.031	126	19
Cat 2	1386	1024	1840	1.69	0.53	5.403	126	25
Cat 3	2538	>1840		1.2	0.363	3.971	127	19

Dose refers to the cumulative exposure to DEE in μg/m^3-years. For every category (Reference, Cat 1, Cat 2, Cat 3), averages and the lower and upper limits of the dose are specified. Odds ratio OR with 95 % confidence intervals (95 % CI) and the number of persons observed and the number of lung cancer deaths per dose category are reported

Methods

Reproduction of the results and variation of modelling

The complex meta-analysis of Vermeulen et al. [1] of the categorised results of the individual studies was replicated. The exposure categorisation, which varied with the studies, and the potential differences in the design and size of the studies were a challenge. In addition to this, the results for the exposure categories are nested within the studies, creating a two-level structure (1st level: exposure groups, 2nd level: studies). In order to analyse this complex data situation appropriately, meta-regression analyses were performed on the results of the individual studies, both with fixed effects [18] and with random effects [19–21], to determine a shared exposure-response curve (see also [22]).

The analyses must be weighted by variances of the RR estimates per exposure category. This weighting is required as only aggregated data (i.e., no individual data on persons) are available in the evaluations, and the data points for the exposure categories differ substantially in a joint evaluation due to the varying number of cases within and between the studies. Different approaches were trialled for this:

- Linear regression with fixed effects for log RR with weights proportional to the inverse of the respective variance
  - Without adjustment by study
  - With adjustment by study. A global F-test on the heterogeneity of the risk levels (intercepts, offsets) between the studies was performed.
- Mixed linear regression for log RR with a random intercept incorporating the differences between the studies
  - With weights at the first level (exposure categories level) proportional to the inverse of the respective variance and with the totals of these weights as study weights at the second level (study level)
  - In a second evaluation approach, the weights of the first level were scaled effectively to the weights of the second level.
- Mixed linear regression for log RR with a random intercept and a random dose coefficient (slope) incorporating the differences between the studies
  - With weights at the first level (exposure categories level) proportional to the inverse of the respective variance and with the totals of these weights as study weights at the second level (study level)
  - In a second evaluation approach, the weights of the first level were scaled effectively to the weights of the second level.

The analyses do not take the reference points into account, as their weights are infinite, i.e., not a real number. That corresponds to the procedure in Vermeulen et al. [1]: Fig. 1 only contains 10 observation points, not 13.

Models with fixed effects are usually evaluated statistically via the Student's t-distribution [23]. As only a few

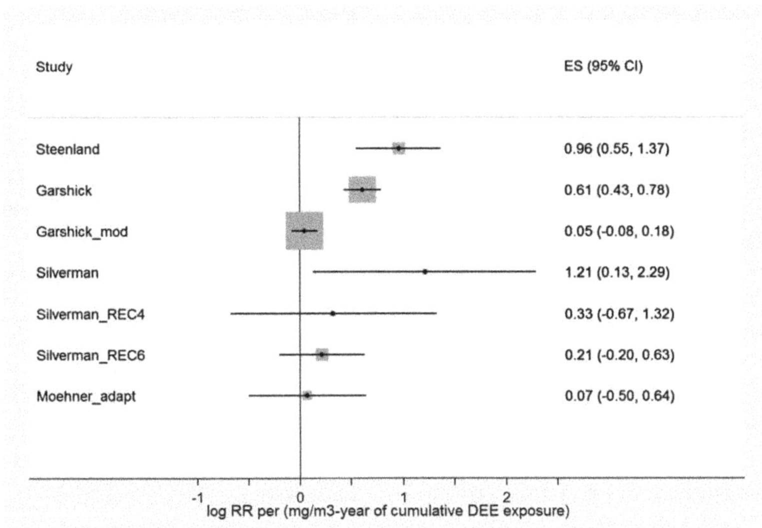

Fig. 1 Analysis of the individual studies. Linear regression with fixed effects for log RR with weights proportional to the inverse of the respective variance (represented by box size). Coefficients (effect size, ES) of the cumulative exposure (Dose) to DEE in mg/m^3-years with a 95 % confidence interval for the coefficient, calculated using the standard normal distribution. Steenland et al. [2] and Silverman et al. [4] were evaluated as used by Vermeulen et al. [1] as well as in accordance with the re-analysis by Crump et al. [14] with adjustment for the radon exposure (REC4, REC6, cf. Table 3), as was Garshick et al. [3] as used by Vermeulen et al. [1], and Garshick et al. [3] (modified) and the data based on Möhner et al. [17] (adapted)

data points are incorporated, which reflect groups rather than individuals (aggregated data), this tends to lead to over-estimations of P values and confidence interval widths. However, precision weightings only include the relative weighting differences between the data points in the analyses and, thus, does not solve this problem. Therefore, the models with fixed effects are evaluated based on the standard normal distribution as an alternative [23]. This tends to lead to P values and confidence intervals which are too narrow, in particular as the correlations between the groups within the studies are not taken into consideration. We note that all mixed regressions are always evaluated via the standard normal distribution.

However, the results reported in a study for the various exposure categories are not independent of one another, but correlate with one another, as they refer to a common reference category within this study. As a result, in addition to the evaluations described above, meta-regression methods including the correlations of the study results within the studies were attempted [24–26]. However, additional input is required to use this Greenland/Longnecker method: person years and case numbers or person numbers and case numbers per exposure category from the studies must be available. These data are not included in the supplement to Vermeulen et al. [1], and cannot be reconstructed in full from the original publications.

In their Methods section, Vermeulen et al. [1] mentioned almost all of these methods, but it remains unclear whether they always used the Greenland/Longnecker method, for instance, and which weighting structure was used in the mixed regressions. With different evaluation approaches, this research project aims to evaluate the extent to which and the method with which the results published by Vermeulen et al. [1] can be reproduced.

Vermeulen et al. [1] also used spline models, which permit a more flexible curve shape than log-linear models. However, these spline regressions did not result in a deviating curve for the estimated exposure-response relationship: "The linear model (Fig. 1) and the spline meta-regression model (data not shown) fit the data well, with virtually equivalent curves." That is why we did not use any spline functions or similar methods, instead following the main approach of Vermeulen et al., also to keep the number of parameters to be estimated as low as possible.

As the main modelling approach, a precision-weighted regression analysis with fixed effects and simultaneous adjustment for the individual studies was pursued, as it is more stable and easier to interpret. This approach also has other advantages over a regression with random effects (see the justifications in Allison [18], pp. 2, 3, and Cameron and Trivedi [19], p. 700). We examined whether the other approaches outlined above offer relevantly different results. If that is not the case, this method is used as the leading analytical strategy.

All analyses were calculated using Stata 12 [27].

Influence of the input data selected

One important aspect of data selection can be derived from the Letter to the Editor by Morfeld [13] regarding the Garshick et al. [3] paper, stating that the coefficients used by Vermeulen et al. [1] are incorrectly adjusted. Therefore, another analysis was performed to repeat the meta-analyses described above with the corrected coefficients per Garshick et al. [3] (modified) (cf. Table 2).

The results of the DEMS re-analysis were presented in an HEI (Health Effects Institute) webinar [28, 29] and published in detail afterwards [14, 30]. Crump et al. [14] contained revised OR estimates on Silverman et al. [4]; important alternative estimates from this paper are presented in Table 3. The "REC6" findings from this paper are incorporated in the meta-analysis after adjustment for the radon exposure instead of the data from Silverman et al. [4] (cf. Table 1). Variation in the results when using the "REC4" findings after adjustment for radon exposure was also investigated.

The German potash miner study [17] was also incorporated as part of a sensitivity analysis. We used the risk estimates from "Möhner et al. [17] (adapted)" (cf. Table 4).

As the paper by Steenland et al. [2] has significant limitations (see the "Material" section), meta-analyses were also performed without including this study.

Non-linearity: threshold search

We examined the data for non-linearities in the exposure-risk relationship. In particular, a systematic search was performed for cumulative exposure thresholds [31–33]. To do so, the algorithm presented in detail in Morfeld et al. [34] to determine a no-adverse effect level in the cumulative exposure was combined with the meta-regression methods. This analysis was restricted to the main modelling approach (precision-weighted regression analysis with fixed effects and simultaneous adjustment for individual studies).

10 $\mu g/m^3$-years was selected as the increment for threshold exploration (range: 0 $\mu g/m^3$-years to 500 $\mu g/m^3$-years). Accordingly, 51 models were calculated and compared per threshold search. The threshold analysis was made using special programs in Stata 12 [27].

Results

Reproduction of the results in Vermeulen et al. [1] and extended analyses

In Table 1 (primary analysis), Vermeulen et al. [1] reported on the three studies by Steenland et al. [2], Garshick et al. [3] and Silverman et al. [4]. The authors stated individual findings (risk coefficients calculated) and the result of the meta-analysis of the risk coefficients. We compare these findings with the results of the re-analysis below.

Analyses of the individual studies

All individual analyses were recalculated with fixed effects linear regression evaluating log RR (for methodological reasons, this analysis is identical to the mixed regression analysis if confined to a single study). Tables 5, 6, 7, 8 show the results for Steenland et al. [2], Garshick et al. [3], Silverman et al. [4] and Möhner et al. [17].

Table 1 in Vermeulen et al. [1] reports the following coefficient estimates for Steenland et al. [2]: dose = 0.00096 (95 % CI: 0.00033, 0.00159), constant = −0.032. The agreement in the coefficients is very good. The confidence interval is consistent when both calculation methods are taken into account (Student's t-distribution, normal distribution).

Table 1 in Vermeulen et al. [1] reported the following coefficient estimates for Garshick et al. [3]: dose = 0.00061 (95 % CI: −0.00088, 0.00210), constant = 0.24. This coefficient estimate is also very similar, and the interval estimate is a good match. The estimates differ clearly when we evaluate Garshick et al. [3] (modified): The dose coefficient is lower by more than an order of magnitude, and far from being significant ($P > 0.4$). A significant deviation of the constant (intercept) from the normal value zero is apparent. This normal value zero means a baseline level of the relative risk of 1, as is to be assumed for a DEE exposure of 0 μg/m^3-years.

Table 1 in Vermeulen et al. [1] reported the following coefficient estimates for Silverman et al. [4]: dose = 0.00120 (95 % CI: 0.00053, 0.00187), constant = −0.18. The coefficient estimates here also agree well (there is probably a typing error in Vermeulen et al. [1]: −0.18 instead of −0.148). The interval estimates are compatible too.

By contrast, the dose coefficients calculated using the Crump variations are far lower than the original values: They are only 27 % (REC4) or 18 % (REC6) of the Silverman coefficient. In these calculations, the t-test confidence intervals are largely symmetrical around zero, so that neither model reveals a trend. Even using the standard normal distribution, there is no indication of a significant influence of the DEE exposure on lung cancer mortality when REC4 or REC6 are used as the exposure metrics. We like to emphasize that REC4 and REC6 are both adjusted for radon exposure as a potential confounder.

Table 8 shows the results obtained by evaluating the study by Möhner et al. [17] with changed (adapted) exposure categorisation. The German study does not indicate an association between DEE exposure and lung cancer mortality.

Figure 1 gives an overview of the results of the regressions with fixed effects, assuming a normal distribution for statistical evaluation of all individual studies. Models with fixed effects are presented to prevent underestimation of the coefficients. We selected the normal distribution to rule out overestimation of the p-values (i.e., the confidence intervals presented are definitely not too wide). Deviating from Vermeulen et al. [1], we selected mg/m^3-years = 1000 × μg/m^3-years as the exposure unit, to keep the overview clearer. Each of the three data sets incorporated in the Vermeulen analysis [2–4] results in significantly elevated risk estimates, whereby Garshick et al. [3] paper has the greatest influence. When we analysed the results from Garshick et al. [3] without adjusting for exposure duration, i.e., Garshick et al. [3] (modified), the risk estimate drops considerably and is not significant. The Crump modifications (REC4, REC6) of the research in Silverman et al. [4] also result in considerably lower risk estimates than in the original Silverman et al. paper, and are not statistically significant. The study by Möhner et al. [17] does not give any indication of an association between DEE exposure and lung cancer mortality.

Joint analysis of the studies

According to Table 1 in Vermeulen et al. [1], the following values apply for "all studies combined" (i.e., [2–4]) as the coefficients of cumulative exposure (dose) to DEE in μg/m^3-years and the absolute term (constant): dose = 0.00098 (95 % CI: 0.00055, 0.00141) and constant = 0.088. Table 9 reports on the re-analysis of the three studies using a log-linear regression with fixed effects, without adjusting for the studies.

Table 9 shows relevant deviations from the results in Vermeulen et al. [1]. While the exposure-response

Table 5 Steenland et al. [2]: Linear regression with fixed effects for log RR with weights proportional to the inverse of the respective variance

Log RR	Coef.	Std. Err.	t	*P*	95 % CI	
Dose	0.00096	0.00021	4.55	0.045 (<0.001)	0.00005 (0.00055	0.00187 0.00137)
Constant	−0.031	0.070	−0.45	0.70	−0.33	0.27

Coefficient (Coef.) of the cumulative exposure (dose) to DEE in μg/m^3-years and absolute term (constant) with standard deviation (Std.Err.); t-test statistic for the coefficient with the corresponding P-value and a 95 % confidence interval for the coefficient, 95 % CI. The figures in parentheses are the results when using the standard normal distribution

Table 6 Garshick et al. [3]: Linear regression with fixed effects for log RR with weights proportional to the inverse of the respective variance

log RR	Coef.	Std. Err.	t	*P*	95 % CI	
Dose	0.00061	0.000091	6.6	0.095 (<0.001)	−0.00055 (0.00042	0.00177 0.00078)
Constant	0.244	0.013	18.6	0.034	0.078	0.411
Garshick (modified)						
Dose	0.00005	0.00007	0.75	0.59 (0.45)	−0.00077 (−0.00008	0.00087 0.00017)
Constant	0.159	0.009	16.87	0.038	0.039	0.279

Coefficient (Coef.) of the cumulative exposure (Dose) to DEE in μg/m^3-years and absolute term (Constant) with standard deviation (Std.Err.); t-test statistic for the coefficient with the corresponding P-value and a 95 % confidence interval for the coefficient, 95 % CI. The figures in parentheses are the results when using the standard normal distribution. Garshick et al. [3] as used by Vermeulen et al. [1], and Garshick et al. [3] (modified) were evaluated

association is statistically significant, the dose coefficient estimated without adjustment for the studies is approx. 20 % lower than that published by Vermeulen and colleagues (0.00076/0.00098 = 0.77). If the versions of the results according to Crump et al. [14] are incorporated in the evaluation, the meta-analysis does not indicate a significant association between DEE exposure and lung cancer mortality.

Table 10 also adjusts the coefficient estimates by studies.

Table 10 shows a good correlation for the dose coefficient and the corresponding confidence interval with the results reported in Vermeulen et al. [1] (dose = 0.00098, 95 %-CI: 0.00055, 0.00141; constant = 0.088). The recalculated coefficient exhibits minimal upward deviation. The two confidence interval calculations (Student's t-distribution, normal distribution) have largely matching results, so that the 10 data points are sufficient to permit a robust estimate, which also agrees to the results published by Vermeulen and his colleagues. The global F-test on the heterogeneity of the baseline risk levels between the studies, which was also calculated, results in $F(2, 6) = 5.5$, $P = 0.044$. Thus, the heterogeneity between the three studies is significant at a 5 % level. Heterogeneity refers to a systematic difference in the baseline risk of the three studies (i.e., setting exposure to zero). For a meaningful combination of the three studies, their base levels should match except for random deviations. However, the differences are statistically significant. The heterogeneity between the three studies results from a significant difference between Garshick et al. [3] and Steenland et al. [2], ΔConst1: p = 0.021. Accordingly, the Garshick study deviates significantly upwards in the baseline level of the risk from the other two studies, as was already indicated in the individual analysis (Table 6). Correcting the Garshick coefficients reduces the heterogeneity in the risk level considerably: $F(2, 6) = 0.50$, $P = 0.63$. This is not apparent from the individual analysis.

If we replace the original data per Silverman et al. [4] with the results from Crump et al. [14] (REC4 or REC6, both adjusted for radon exposure), the dose coefficients in the meta-regression are halved.

Table 11 shows results when a mixed linear regression for the three studies is fitted.

Table 11 results in a very good agreement to the finding published in Vermeulen et al. [1] (dose = 0.00098, 95 % CI: 0.00055, 0.00141; constant = 0.088). If the dose coefficient is also estimated as a random effect, the results do not change. The findings deviate slightly from Vermeulen et al. [1] without an effective scaling

Table 7 Silverman et al. [4]: Linear regression with fixed effects for log RR with weights proportional to the inverse of the respective variance

log RR	Coef.	Std. Err.	t	*P*	95 % CI	
Dose	0.00121	0.00055	2.20	0.27 (0.028)	−0.00579 (0.00013	0.00821 0.00229)
Constant	−0.148	0.299	−0.49	0.71	−3.95	3.65
Crump et al. [14], REC4						
Dose	0.00033	0.00051	0.64	0.63 (0.53)	−0.00615 (−0.00067	0.00680 0.00132)
Constant	0.00541	0.358	0.02	0.99	−4.54	4.55
Crump et al. [14], REC6						
Dose	0.00021	0.00021	1.01	0.50 (0.31)	−0.00247 (−0.00020	0.00289 0.00063)
Constant	0.137	0.108	1.27	0.42	−1.23	1.51

Coefficient (Coef.) of the cumulative exposure (Dose) to DEE in μg/m^3-years and absolute term (Constant) with standard deviation (Std.Err.); t-test statistic for the coefficient with the corresponding P-value and a 95 % confidence interval for the coefficient, 95 % CI. The figures in parentheses are the results when using the standard normal distribution. Silverman et al. [4] was evaluated as used by Vermeulen et al. [1], and in accordance with the re-analysis by Crump et al. [14] with adjustment for radon exposure (REC4, REC6, cf. Table 3)

Table 8 Möhner et al. [17] (adapted): Linear regression with fixed effects for log RR with weights proportional to the inverse of the respective variance

log RR	Coef.	Std. Err.	t	*P*	95 % CI	
Dose	0.00007	0.00029	0.24	0.85 (0.81)	−0.00364 (−0.00050	0.00378 0.00064)
Constant	0.119	0.492	0.24	0.85	−6.13	6.37

Coefficient (Coef.) of the cumulative exposure (Dose) to DEE in μg/m^3-years and absolute term (Constant) with standard deviation (Std.Err.); t-test statistic for the coefficient with the corresponding P-value and a 95 % confidence interval for the coefficient, 95 % CI. The figures in parentheses are the results when using the standard normal distribution

of the weights (result: dose coefficient = 0.00093, constant =0.096). If Garshick et al. [3] (modified) is included in the meta-analysis, the estimated meta-risk coefficient and the corresponding significance level decreases (test statistic changes from Z = 6.74 to Z = 4.58), however the positive dose–response association is always significant (see Table 11).

As in the models with fixed effects (Table 10), the dose coefficients in the meta-regression are halved in the mixed regression (Table 11) if the original data in accordance with Silverman et al. [4] is replaced with the findings from Crump et al. [14] (REC4 or REC6, both adjusted for radon exposure).

Crump [39] also recalculated some of the Vermeulen et al. [1] results using a mixed model, but did not see any way to obtain the data required to use the Greenland/Longnecker method (cf. our explanations in the Method section "Reproduction of the results and variation of modelling"). Crump wrote: "I ... reran the analysis of Vermeulen et al. [1], except that I did not model the dependence among the ORs from the same study. (I did not have access to data needed to model that dependence.) My analysis yielded a regression parameter [0.88; 95 % confidence interval (CI): 0.65, 1.11] similar to that obtained by Vermeulen et al. [1] (0.98; 95 % CI: 0.55, 1.41)." Crump [29] obviously selected a different unit of DEE exposure, at 1000 μg/m^3-years. The dose coefficient (0.88) he reported deviates more than the result of the recalculation performed in this paper (0.97), which corresponds very well with the Vermeulen result (0.98). It is not clear whether Crump scaled the weights, as even the recalculation in this report is slightly lower (0.93) without scaling, though not as pronounced as in Crump [29].

Variation of modelling

As Steenland et al. [2] did not provide details on the person years and case numbers per exposure category, this paper cannot be included in evaluations with the Greenland/Longnecker method. However, Garshick et al. [3], Silverman et al. [4] and Möhner et al. [17] (adapted) can be analysed jointly. Table 12 shows the results.

Table 12 shows that the linear regressions with fixed effects for log RR with weights proportional to the inverse of the respective variance and with adjustment for studies result in slightly more pronounced effect coefficients and somewhat lower P-values than models with random effects (that qualitatively matches the findings presented in the Results section: "Joint analysis of the studies"). However, if the dose coefficient is also calculated as a random effect, a similar value results (coefficient = 0.00059, P = 0.17) for the model with fixed effects. By contrast, the analyses with the Greenland/Longnecker method, recommended by methodologists and taking internal correlations into account, resulted in a lower coefficient than in the model with fixed effects, with a lower

Table 9 Linear regression with fixed effects for log RR with weighs proportional to the inverse of the respective variance, without adjustment for studies

log RR	Coef.	Std. Err.	t	*P*	95 % CI	
Dose	0.00076	0.00026	2.97	0.018 (0.003)	0.00017 (0.00026	0.00135 0.00126)
Constant	0.130	0.072	1.80	0.11	−0.0365	0.297
Crump et al. [14], REC4						
Dose	0.00033	0.00022	1.46	0.18 (0.15)	−0.00019 (−0.00011	0.00084 0.00076)
Constant	0.208	0.067	3.10	0.015	0.053	0.336
Crump et al. [14], REC6						
Dose	0.00034	0.00020	1.74	0.12 (0.083)	−0.00011 (−0.00004	0.00080 0.00073)
Constant	0.211	0.054	3.90	0.005	0.860	0.335

Coefficient (Coef.) of the cumulative exposure (dose) to DEE in μg/m^3-years and absolute term (Constant) with standard deviation (Std.Err.); t-test statistic for the coefficient with the corresponding P-value and a 95 % confidence interval for the coefficient, 95 % CI. The figures in parentheses are the results when using the standard normal distribution. Silverman et al. [4] was incorporated as used by Vermeulen et al. [1], and in accordance with the re-analysis by Crump et al. [14] with adjustment for radon exposure (REC4, REC6, cf. Table 3)

Table 10 Linear regression with fixed effects for log RR with weights proportional to the inverse of the respective variance, with adjustment for studies

log RR	Coef.	Std. Err.	t	P	95 % CI	
Dose	0.00106	0.00020	5.35	0.002 (<0.001)	0.00057 (0.00067	0.00154 0.00144)
ΔConst1	0.249	0.080	3.11	0.021	0.052	0.445
ΔConst2	−0.035	0.126	−0.28	0.79	−0.343	0.272
Constant	−0.059	0.079	−0.74	0.49	−0.252	0.135
Crump et al. [14], REC4						
Dose	0.00053	0.00021	2.49	0.047 (0.013)	0.00001 (0.00011	0.00105 0.00094)
ΔConst1	0.163	0.095	1.71	0.14	−0.070	0.396
ΔConst2	−0.167	0.169	−0.98	0.36	−0.581	0.248
Constant	0.091	0.091	1.01	0.35	−0.130	0.313
Crump et al. [14], REC6						
Dose	0.00054	0.00017	3.12	0.021 (0.0018)	0.00012 (0.00020	0.00096 0.00087)
ΔConst1	0.164	0.069	2.40	0.054	−0.003	0.332
ΔConst2	0.041	0.113	−0.37	0.73	−0.319	0.236
Constant	0.088	0.068	1.30	0.24	−0.079	0.255

Coefficient (Coef.) of the cumulative exposure (Dose) to DEE in µg/m^3-years and absolute term (Constant) with standard deviation (Std.Err.); t-test statistic for the coefficient with the corresponding P-value and a 95 % confidence interval for the coefficient, 95 % CI. The figures in parentheses are the results when using the standard normal distribution. Silverman et al. [4] was incorporated as used by Vermeulen et al. [1], and in accordance with the re-analysis by Crump et al. [14] with adjustment for radon exposure (REC4, REC6, cf. Table 3)
Constant: Steenland et al. [2] (reference study)
ΔConst1: Garshick et al. [3] - Steenland et al. [2]
ΔConst2: Silverman et al. [4] - Steenland et al. [2]

P-value = 0.035 (significant). In this joint analysis of Garshick et al. [3] (modified coefficients), Silverman et al. [4] and Möhner et al. [17] (adapted) using the Greenland/ Longnecker method, the dose coefficient is approximately a factor of 3 lower than the estimate in the primary analysis by Vermeulen et al. [1] (0.0032 vs. 0.00098).

The results reported by Vermeulen et al. [1] largely match the estimates in the models with random effects (cf. Results section on the "Joint analysis of the studies"). However, the Greenland/Longnecker method cannot be used in this case without access to further data. Vermeulen and his colleagues were obviously given access to these data from Steenland et al. [2], but did not disclose them in their paper, even in the supplement.

If we replace the original data per Silverman et al. [4] with the results from Crump et al. [14] (REC4 or REC6, after adjustment for radon exposure), the statements on the three analysis methods are qualitatively the same. Accordingly, the dose coefficients in the meta-regression are halved due to the data variation. In spite of the different models, the P-values are largely equivalent. One exception to this is regression with a random intercept for REC6, where the value is lower (P = 0.25). Like the deviating result of the Greenland/Longnecker regression on evaluation with the Silverman original data (P = 0.035), this indicates instabilities in the variance estimate.

In order to avoid discussions on a potential underestimation of the effect, all further analyses were made using adjusted regression models with fixed effects. In Tables 11 and 12, the dose coefficient estimates (fixed effects adjusted for studies and random effects) almost match, and are also almost identical with those in Vermeulen et al. [1]. A comparison of the interval estimates and P-values indicates a greater stability of the regression models with fixed effects. This justifies the decision to use adjusted regression models with fixed effects as a primary analysis method (main modelling approach) for this research project.

Influence of the input data selected

Regardless of the method selected, a simultaneous analysis of the three studies by Garshick et al. [3] (modified), Silverman et al. [4] and Möhner et al. [17] (adapted) results in a far lower effect coefficient in Table 12 than in the primary analysis by Vermeulen et al. [1]. Example: For the regression models with fixed effects and adjustment for studies, a reduction in the effect coefficient by approx. 50 % resulted, as the reproduced primary analysis in accordance with Vermeulen et al. [1] led to a coefficient of 0.0011 (per 1 µg/m^3-years), P = 0.002, and a 95 % CI of 0.00057 to 0.00154 (cf. Table 10).

An interesting finding to be noted is that a simultaneous analysis of the three studies by Garshick et al. [3] (modified), Silverman et al. 2012 and Möhner et al. [17] (adapted) only finds a significant dose–response relationship (Table 12) if the Greenland/Longnecker method

Table 11 Mixed linear regression for log RR with a random intercept with weights at the first level (exposure categories level) proportional to the inverse of the respective variance and with the totals of these weights as study weights at the second level (study level)

log RR	Coef.	Robust Std. Err.	Z	P	95 % CI	
Dose	0.00097	0.00014	6.74	<0.001	0.00069	0.00125
Constant	0.084	0.111	0.75	0.45	−0.134	0.300
Garshick (modified)						
Dose	0.00087	0.00019	4.58	<0.001	0.00050	0.00124
Constant	0.024	0.062	0.39	0.70	−0.097	0.145
Crump et al. [14], REC4						
Dose	0.00045	0.00021	2.10	0.035	0.00003	0.00086
Constant	0.178	0.094	1.90	0.057	−0.005	0.362
Crump et al. [14], REC4 and Garshick (modified)						
Dose	0.00048	0.00023	2.10	0.036	0.00003	0.00092
Constant	0.097	0.040	2.39	0.017	0.018	0.176
Crump et al. [14], REC6						
Dose	0.00053	0.00026	2.05	0.040	0.00002	0.00103
Constant	0.172	0.101	1.71	0.088	−0.025	0.369
Crump et al. [14], REC6 and Garshick (modified)						
Dose	0.00052	0.00025	2.09	0.036	0.00003	0.00101
Constant	0.095	0.051	1.87	0.061	−0.044	0.194

The weights of the first level are scaled effectively to the weights of the second level. Coefficient (Coef.) of the cumulative exposure (Dose) to DEE in μg/m^3-years and absolute term (Constant) with standard deviation (Std.Err.); Z-test statistic for the coefficient with the corresponding P-value and a 95 % confidence interval for the coefficient, 95 % CI. Silverman et al. [4] was incorporated as used by Vermeulen et al. [1], and in accordance to the re-analysis by Crump et al. [14] with adjustment for the radon exposure (REC4, REC6, cf. Table 3). Garshick et al. [3] as used by Vermeulen et al. [1], and Garshick et al. [3] (modified) were incorporated

is used. This could be due to instabilities in estimation in this complex procedure.

If the primary analysis in accordance with Vermeulen et al. [1] is performed with fixed effects and adjustment for studies and with modified Garshick coefficients, this results in a coefficient of 0.00098 (per 1 μg/m^3-year), $P = 0.006$, and a 95 % CI of 0.00041 to 0.00155, somewhat more pronounced but similar to the results of the regression calculation with random effects (cf. Table 11).

Thus, the modification of the Garshick coefficients only reduces the meta-coefficient by approx. 7 % and the statistical significance is maintained, although the P-value increases from 0.002 to 0.006. Correcting the Garshick coefficients reduces the heterogeneity in the base level of the risk considerably: $F(2, 6) = 0.50$, $P = 0.63$. Without correction we get: $F(2, 6) = 5.5$, $P = 0.044$.

Tables 10, 11, 12 are consistent in showing that replacing the original data from Silverman et al. [4] with the results from Crump et al. [14] (REC4 or REC6, both with adjustment for radon) reduces the dose coefficient by approximately half in the meta-regressions. If we analyse Steenland et al. [2], Crump et al. [14] and Garshick et al. [3] (modified) together, the dose–response relationship in adjusted regression models with fixed effects and evaluation with the standard normal distribution is significant (REC4: $P = 0.03$, REC6: $P = 0.01$), but clearly weaker than when analysing the original data used by Vermeulen et al. [1] ($P < 0.000001$). The lower confidence interval limits of the dose coefficient are correspondingly different: 0.00005, 0.00010 and 0.00067. They differ by a factor of at least 12 or 6.

Figure 2 gives an overview of the results of the meta-regressions with fixed effects for variations of the input data assuming a normal distribution for statistical evaluation. Models with fixed effects are presented to prevent

Table 12 Joint analysis of Garshick et al. [3] (modified coefficients), Silverman et al. [4] and Möhner et al. [17] (adapted)

	Coef.	P	95 % CI	
Fixed effects, adjusted	0.00054	0.14 (0.083)	−0.00026 (−0.00007	0.00133 0.00115)
Random intercept, scaled	0.00024	0.36	−0.00027	0.00074
Greenland/Longnecker method	0.00032	0.035	0.00002	0.00062
Crump et al. [14], REC4				
Fixed effects, adjusted	0.00020	0.35 (0.30)	−0.00029 (−0.00018	0.00069 0.00058)
Random intercept, scaled	0.00010	0.11	−0.00002	0.00022
Greenland/Longnecker method	0.00015	0.31	−0.00014	0.00044
Crump et al. [14], REC6				
Fixed effects, adjusted	0.00013	0.33 (0.28)	−0.00018 (−0.00010	0.00042 0.00035)
Random intercept, scaled	0.000073	0.025	0.00001	0.00014
Greenland/Longnecker method	0.00012	0.44	−0.00019	0.00043

Comparison of the estimated effect for the cumulative exposure to log RR, calculated with various regression methods. Coefficient (Coef.) of the cumulative exposure (Dose) to DEE in μg/m^3-years, corresponding P-value and 95 % confidence interval for the coefficient, 95 % CI. The figures in parentheses are the results when using the standard normal distribution in the model with fixed effects. Silverman et al. [4] was incorporated as used by Vermeulen et al. [1], and in accordance with the re-analysis by Crump et al. [14] with adjustment for radon exposure (REC4, REC6, cf. Table 3)

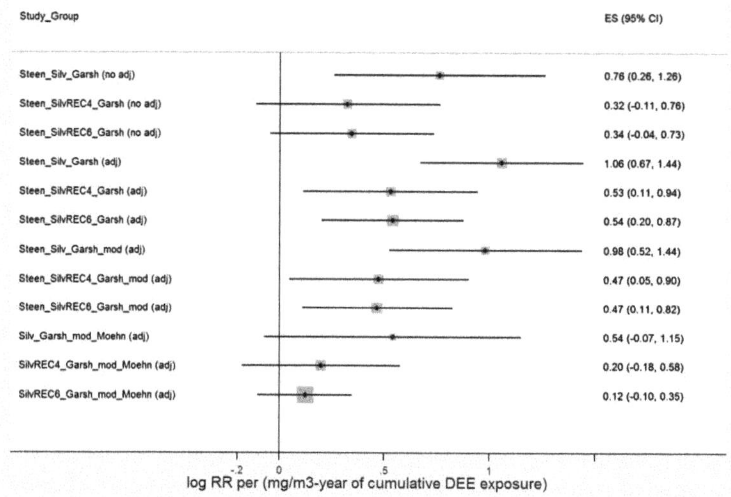

Fig. 2 Meta-analyses. Linear regression with fixed effects for log RR with weights proportional to the inverse of the respective variance (the box size illustrates the precision of the meta-estimate). Coefficients (effect size, ES) of the cumulative exposure (Dose) to DEE in mg/m^3-years with a 95 % confidence interval of the coefficient, calculated using the standard normal distribution. Steenland et al. [2] and Silverman et al. [4] were evaluated as used by Vermeulen et al. [1], as well as in accordance with the re-analysis by Crump et al. [14] with adjustment for the radon exposure (REC4, REC6, cf. Table 3), as was Garshick et al. [3] as used by Vermeulen et al. [1], and Garshick et al. [3] (modified) and the data based on Möhner et al. [17] (adapted)

underestimation of the coefficients. We selected the normal distribution to rule out overestimation of the p-values (i.e. the confidence intervals presented are definitely not too wide). Deviating from Vermeulen et al. [1], we selected mg/m^3-years = 1000 × μg/m^3-years as the exposure unit, to keep the overview clearer. Replicating the analysis as performed in Vermeulen et al. [1], i.e. Steen_Silv_Garsh (adj), results in the highest risk estimate of all data variations. If the modifications of the Silverman case–control study in accordance with Crump et al. 2015 (REC4, REC6, both adjusted for radon exposure) and Garshick et al. [3] are included in the analysis, the risk estimates are far lower (Steen_SilvREC4_Garsh_mod, Steen_SilvREC6_Garsh_mod: the coefficients are reduced roughly by half compared with the Vermeulen analysis). If the Steenland paper, which the authors believe is only exploratory in nature, is excluded, the modified risk estimates do not result in significant risk increases when incorporating Möhner et al. [17] (adapted) in the meta-analysis (SilvREC4_Garsh_mod_Moehn, SilvREC6_Garsh_mod_Moehn). The meta-coefficient is approx. 10 – 20 % of the value found in Vermeulen et al. [1] in the primary analysis.

Non-linearity: Threshold search

The primary analysis by Vermeulen et al. [1] was repeated (method: adjusted regression models, fixed effects), but taking a potential threshold into consideration. When evaluated with corrected coefficients in Garshick coefficients (cf. Table 2: Garshick et al. [3], modified), the analysis finds a threshold of 150 μg/m^3-years. However, the threshold does not differ statistically significantly from zero.

If we replace Silverman et al. [4] (Table 1) with the results from Crump et al. [14] (Table 4), the analysis also exhibits a threshold. However, this estimate is more difficult to express statistically due to the considerably weaker exposure-response relationship, and exhibits a broad uncertainty (threshold at 90 μg/m^3-years, 95 % CI: 0 μg/m^3-years to 361 μg/m^3-years).

Discussion

Vermeulen et al. [1] published a meta-regression analysis of three major epidemiological US studies [2–4] which analyzed the association between diesel engine exhaust (DEE), based on the cumulative exposure to elemental carbon (EC) in μg/m^3-years, and lung cancer mortality. In their meta-analysis, the authors described a statistically significant dose–response relationship and elevated cancer risks, even at very low exposures. The present reanalysis largely succeeded in reproducing the individual and main findings from the published study data. Of all the meta-analyses we performed, the evaluation of the data as used by Vermeulen et al. [1] resulted in the highest risk estimates. However, an investigation of the heterogeneity in the baseline level of risk – Vermeulen et al. [1] do not report on this – resulted in pronounced differences between the three studies (significant at the 5 % level). All three studies should exhibit a uniform baseline level of RR = 1 at a cumulative DEE exposure of 0 μg/m^3-years. A joint analysis of the three studies must therefore be viewed critically from a statistical point of view [34]. Other authors in other situations reject combinations of studies even with considerably less pronounced heterogeneity [35, 36]. This uncertainty in the baseline level renders the use of the analysis by Vermeulen et al. [1] a problem for risk estimates in the lower exposure region. Accordingly, the following statement by Vermeulen et al. [1] must be relativised: "Formal tests of heterogeneity of estimates among the studies were of limited value due to the small number of data points for each study."

Correcting the coefficients in Garshick et al. [3] [cf. 13] reduced the heterogeneity in the baseline relative risk levels between the three studies considerably ($P = 0.63$). This correction was indicated as the coefficients used by Vermeulen et al. [1] are incorrectly adjusted [13]: The cumulative exposure was adjusted for the exposure duration it already contains so that the risk coefficient does not estimate the effect of cumulative exposure. Our modification resulted in far lower risk estimates than reported on this study by Vermeulen et al. [1]: The corrected dose coefficient is lower by more than an order of magnitude, and far from being significant ($P = 0.6$). However, the correction of the Garshick coefficients only reduces the meta-coefficient by approx. 7 % and the statistical significance is maintained, although the P-value increases from 0.002 to 0.006.

Another aspect is important for correct evaluation of the Garshick study (see the Letter to the Editor by Morfeld [13], including the answer from the authors). Garshick et al. [3] made a double adjustment for the year of birth, though with different fineness, so that the models do not break down due to collinearity. However, over-adjustments of this type can distort the coefficient estimate. The authors responded that they incorporated the years twice to obtain meaningful results. That was the only way the proportional hazards assumption was fulfilled. However, this explanation does not change the double use of the year of birth information, and the potential over-adjustment it causes.

The highest exposure value included in the meta-study came from the DEMS case–control study by Silverman et al. [4]: 1036 μg/m^3-years with an OR = 2.83 (95 % CI: 1.28 to 6.26). Thus, the US mining study is particularly relevant for the meta-analysis. Critical comments and a list of open questions were published [37] on the DEMS publications [4, 12], to which the authors reacted with a letter to the editor [38]. However, many aspects remain open [see the author answer from Morfeld in 38]. Some of these open questions could be answered by additional analyses, which requires access to the original data. Access to the original data of the DEMS study has only been granted to a few researchers (working groups of S. Moolgavkar [30] and K. Crump [14]). It is currently unclear whether these authors had unrestricted access to all original data. However, aspects of the manner in which the Crump et al. [14] team was given access to the DEMS data is provided in the "Epilogue" section of their paper. The results of the DEMS re-analysis were presented in a HEI (Health Effects Institute) webinar [28, 29] and published in detail recently [14, 30].

In a Letter to the Editor on Vermeulen et al. [1], Crump [39] reported that an evaluation of the DEMS case–control study with an exposure lag of 5 years leads to far lower meta-risk coefficients than with the original value of 15 years. Crump also pointed out that the other two studies incorporated [2, 3] used a lag of 5 years. The authors qualitatively confirmed the Crump result, but did not consider it relevant, as the adjustment in the DEMS study using a lag of 15 years was better and there are inevitably differences in the exposures recorded in the different studies. Furthermore, Vermeulen et al. [1] referred to a sensitivity analyses they performed, in which they explored the influence a different lagging of the exposure has. However, the note by Crump [39] shows further uncertainties in the Vermeulen meta-analysis, which cannot be determined without access to the original DEMS data. Our re-analysis should be repeated applying different lags to the studies. Unfortunately, the necessary data are not publicly available.

Moolgavkar et al. [30] re-analysed, using both proportional hazard and biological based mechanistic models, the DEMS cohort study by Attfield et al. [12] and pointed out two important aspects:

1) Time-dependent factors are superimposed, so that model coefficients should not be estimated without considering the interaction with age. Accordingly, stating an isolated risk coefficient – as described in Attfield et al. [12] – does not make any sense according to Moolgavkar et al. [30].

2) One mine (limestone mine) is an outlier in the data. The DEE exposures in this mine are the lowest, but the risk estimates are the highest of all the mines. A Cox regression analysis of the data (without excluding the higher exposures as in Attfield et al. [12]) shows that a significant exposure-response association (P = 0.0014) was found in the limestone mine alone. If the limestone mine is excluded from the analyses, the P-value in the overall cohort increases from 0.02 to 0.18 [28], i.e., after excluding the limestone mine, no significant dose–response association results between the DEE exposure and lung cancer mortality in the DEMS cohort study. Although this special role of the limestone mine was not confirmed in the case–control re-analysis by Crump et al. [14], this observation about the limestone mine is a major interpretation problem for the cohort study and the

publication by Attfield et al. [12]. It is noteworthy that Moolgavkar et al. [30] described the ventilation in the limestone mine as follows: "All seven of these mines had substantial mechanical ventilation supplying large quantities of air to minimize airborne dust concentrations and, in the case of the trona mines, to minimize the build-up of methane, an explosive gas. The limestone mining operation was quite different from that in the seven other mines. The limestone mine primarily used natural ventilation, with air flowing up or down vertical shafts between the surface and the mining operations." In addition, the percentage of radon measurements above detection limit was 85 % in the limestone mine, the highest among all 8 mines; the average percentage among the other 7 mines was only 36 % (Roger O. McClellen, personal communication, 27 July 2015). This may explain why Crump and colleagues were unable to reproduce Moolgavkar's finding of the limestone mine being an outlier: "Moolgavkar et al. could not control for other covariables, including smoking and radon, because these data were not available" (Crump et al. [14]). Such a control for other covariables was done by Crump et al. [14].

Crump et al. [14] re-analysed the DEMS case–control study by Silverman et al. [4] and also investigated the influence of some covariables, which Silverman et al. [4] did not include in their final models. In the original paper, analysing the association of cumulative DEE exposure (lag = 15 years) and lung cancer mortality led to a trend *P*-value of $P = 0.001$ (Table 3, Silverman et al. [4]), which Crump et al. confirmed: $P = 0.0006$ in their re-analysis. Crump et al. [14] (Table 3) reported a trend P-value of $P = 0.02$, if adjustments are also made for radon exposure. This proves that the radon exposure has a considerable influence on the association, and weakens the statistical significance of the DEE variables after taking this covariable into account. Crump et al. [14] also developed six new DEE exposure metrics, as an alternative to the estimates used in Attfield et al. [12] and Silverman et al. [4]. If these alternative DEE exposure metrics are used, and also adjusted for the radon exposure, there is no significant association between the cumulative DEE exposure and lung cancer mortality in any constellation studied ($P \geq 0.17$ or the trend is negative). The analyses by Crump et al. [14] also did not reveal any significant association for the exposure metrics as used in Attfield et al. [12] and Silverman et al. [4], when the individual data in the analysis were used instead of the average values of the groups, and an adjustment was made for radon exposure: $P \geq 0.65$ or the trend is negative. The authors wrote: "Most importantly, we used the radon concentration data for the DEMS cohort provided by the DEMS investigators. When adjustment was made for radon, a known human lung carcinogen, the effect of REC on the association with lung cancer mortality was confined to only the three DEMS REC estimates. Most notably, there was no evidence of an association with any of the six alternate REC estimates, including REC6. When T2 trend tests were conducted, based on the use of individual worker REC estimates, the results were less statistically significant and in many cases the trends were negative. Indeed, for miners who always worked underground, five of the six REC metrics exhibited negative trends."

Moolgavkar et al. [30] and Crump et al. [14] concluded that the DEMS analyses by Attfield et al. [12] and Silverman et al. [4] are not suitable for use on their own in a quantitative risk analysis. The limitations of this DEMS data must also be taken into consideration for meta-analyses and derived limit values. The issue of Risk Analysis that contained the Moolgavkar et al. [30] and Crump et al. [14] papers contained a "note" by the Editors, Cox and Lowrie, on the use of results of analyses of the same data set using alternative models [40]. The Editors described that the reanalysed data set was influential in IARC's decision to classify DEE as a human carcinogen and concluded: "These findings can be viewed as raising important questions about the usefulness and reliability of expert judgements about the causal interpretation of model-dependent associations in general, and about whether DEE is in fact carcinogenic to humans in these studies in particular."

If the paper by Crump et al. [14] (REC4, REC6, both adjusted for radon exposure) is incorporated instead of Silverman et al. [4], our meta-re-analysis of Vermeulen et al. [1] results in a considerably weakened association between DEE exposure and lung cancer mortality. Tables 10, 11, 12 are consistent in showing that a corresponding replacement of the original data roughly halves the dose coefficient in the meta-regression. If we analyse Steenland et al. [2], Crump et al. [14] and Garshick et al. [3] (modified) together, the dose–response association in an adjusted regression model with fixed effects is just about significant ($P = 0.03$), i.e., less certain than in the original data analysis ($P < 0.000001$).

We were unable to apply the recommended Greenland/Longnecker method on the oldest study, that of Steenland et al. [2], as the publication lacks important additional information. However, we did perform meta-analyses of Garshick et al. [3], Silverman et al. [4] and Möhner et al. [17] with this statistical method. Regardless of the evaluation method (random, fixed, Greenland/Longnecker), a joint analysis of Garshick et al. [3] (modified), Silverman et al. [4] and Möhner et al. [17] (adapted) resulted in similar coefficient estimates, whereby the Greenland/Longnecker estimate was between the results from the model with random effects and the adjusted model with fixed effects. This justified focussing our analyses on the adjusted model with fixed effects, which made analyses possible in all data situations. After excluding the explorative study by Steenland et al. [2], the lowest risk estimate resulted in a meta-analysis of the three studies Garshick et al. [3] (modified), Silverman et al. [4] (modified in accordance with Crump et al. [14] and Möhner et al. [17] (adapted). In this evaluation, the meta-coefficient decreased to approx. 10 % to 20 % of the value published by Vermeulen et al. [1] as a result of their primary analysis. In addition to this, the association between the DEE exposure and lung cancer mortality in this analysis is no longer statistically significant.

Vermeulen et al. [1] noted: "We were not able to investigate other model forms in our meta-regression, beyond the linear and spline curves because of the limited number of data points. If nonlinear exposure-response curves were actually a better fit (e.g., attenuation at higher exposures, for which there is some evidence in Silverman et al. (2012), then this might change the estimate burden of disease due to DEE." If we supplement the meta-analysis of the three US studies [2–4]) with a threshold search, i.e., examine the dose–response relationship for non-linearity, and use the corrected Garshick coefficients it results in a threshold estimate for the cumulative DEE exposure at 150 $\mu g/m^3$-years. However, this estimate does not differ significantly from zero.

Sun et al. [41] created an overview of the results from 42 cohort studies and 32 case–control studies on the association between the DEE exposures and lung cancer. The authors concluded: "Overall, neither cohort nor case–control studies indicate a clear exposure-response relationship between DE exposure and lung cancer. Epidemiological studies published to date do not allow a valid quantification of the association between DE and lung cancer." Although this research does not reach the methodological level of the meta-analytical approach by Vermeulen et al. [1], the varying study results in Sun et al. [41] verify the uncertainty underlying epidemiological studies on the association between DEE and lung cancer.

Similarly to our analysis of the Vermeulen analysis, the re-analysis of the German potash miner study by Möhner et al. [17] led to a clearly weakened and different statement compared with the original research [42]: "Only for very high cumulative dose, corresponding to at least 20 years of exposure in the production area, some weak hints for a possible risk increase could be detected."

The meta-regression analysis performed in this paper has considerable restrictions. Major limitations result from the fact that neither DEE concentration values (only details on cumulative exposures) nor the individual data for this research project were available. Threshold analyses for dust should focus on a concentration threshold [see the discussion in 43]. Empirical findings on thresholds in quartz dust exposure, based on the German porcelain worker cohort, did not result in a threshold for the cumulative exposure, but did for the concentration [43]. Similarly, it is probable in this case that the restriction of the data to cumulative DEE exposure means that we can assume that the actual concentration threshold is underestimated. The statistical significance of the finding would be far clearer if the original studies were analysed incorporating concentration values in the meta-analysis. The data are only available in aggregated form (grouped data) (cf. Table 1), while the original data are individual. Analyses of this type are difficult when using data already collapsed into categories, as results can occur depending on how the cut points are chosen, and precision of estimates decreases with categorisation in comparison to continuous analyses. In general, categorisations result in information losses, potential distortions and decreases in power [44].

The limitations mentioned affect the analysis by Vermeulen et al. [1] and our re-analysis accordingly. Although all main authors of the individual studies are co-authors of the meta-analysis, Vermeulen et al. [1] did not pool and analyse the original data, but focused on grouped data from the result tables of the three publications. However, reliable analyses should refer to the individual data and consider the DEE concentration as a key variable in analyses. We note that a similar point was made by Crump [39]: "Vermeulen et al. used very crude exposure summaries (e.g., midpoints of exposure intervals)."

The meta-regressions performed here show significant variations in the results, depending on the study data incorporated or the analytical methods applied. The data used by Vermeulen and colleagues led to the highest risk estimates in our meta-analysis (statistically significant). After excluding the explorative study by Steenland et al. [2], the lowest risk estimate resulted in an analysis of the three studies Garshick et al. [3] (modified), Silverman et al. [4] (modified in accordance with [14]) and Möhner et al. [17] (adapted). In this evaluation, the meta-coefficient decreased to approx. 10–20 % of the value published by Vermeulen et al. [1] as the main result of their primary analysis. The association between DEE exposure and lung cancer mortality in this analysis is not statistically significant. The risk estimates derived from Vermeulen et al. [1] in the very low exposure range and the corresponding limit value proposals derived [6] are therefore less than convincing, as the data – after correction of the Garshick coefficients – are also generally compatible with a threshold.

Toxicological results of the current ACES study from controlled long-term experiments on rats with new technology diesel exhaust (NTDE) did not exhibit tumour growth or precancerous conditions [45], by contrast to earlier studies with traditional DEE (TDE) from diesel motors without particle reduction and without other forms of exhaust treatment. The summary of IARC workshop results for re-evaluation of DEE in 2012 revealed that only toxicological data with pre-2000 motors and fuel technologies were incorporated [5]. Accordingly, the IARC classification from 2012 referred only to possible carcinogenic potential from diesel engine exhaust without modern exhaust treatment (TDE), using the epidemiological data from Steenland et al. [2], Garshick et al. [3], Silverman et al. [4]. However, the new results from the animal experiments in the ACES study highlight the need to include engine and exhaust treatment technologies in the discussion on workplace limit values and possible lung cancer risks from DEE. McClellan et al. [46] also explicitly mentioned the qualitative and quantitative differences between TDE and NTDE and recommended that these differences should be considered when evaluating the carcinogenic risks. The authors reviewed the substantial changes made in diesel technology, and the resulting changes in diesel exhaust emissions from post-WW II to the present time. The changes in technology and emissions post-1990 have been particularly dramatic. This raises questions with regard to the use of the findings of any of the epidemiological studies analysed in this paper for projecting lung cancer risks of diesel exhaust exposures post-2000.

Regardless of the fundamental restrictions mentioned above, the present re-analysis also revealed that the results of the meta-regression study by Vermeulen et al. [1] should not be used in any quantitative lung cancer risk evaluation without reservations, as the results vary significantly depending on the input data selected and the statistical methods used. This is particularly true for the low exposure region.

Conclusions

- Vermeulen et al. [1] published a meta-regression analysis of three key epidemiological US studies on the association between diesel engine exhaust (DEE) and lung cancer. They found a statistically significant dose–response relationship and elevated cancer risks even for very low DEE exposures.
- The present re-analysis largely succeeded in reproducing the individual cohort results and main meta-findings of Vermeulen et al. [1] from the published study data. Our meta-regressions, however, show significant variations of the results, depending on the study data incorporated or the analytical methods applied.
- Therefore, the results of the meta-regression analysis by Vermeulen et al. [1] should not be used in a risk assessment without reservation, especially not in the low-DEE exposure range.

Competing interests

PD Dr. Peter Morfeld is a member of the Research Advisory Board of the European Research Group on Environment and Health in the Transport Sector (EUGT e.V., www.eugt.org), PD Dr. Spallek is managing director of EUGT e.V. The authors (PM and MS) have not testified during the last 5 years in any regulatory or legal proceedings concerning the contents of this paper.

Authors' contribution

PM conducted the analysis. MS drafted the introduction and discussion sections. Both authors read, revised and approved the final manuscript.

Acknowledgements

The research by PD Dr. Peter Morfeld was supported by the European Research Group on Environment and Health in the Transport Sector (EUGT, www.eugt.org). EUGT's goal is to study the effects and interaction of emissions, immissions and health. We wish to thank two unknown reviewers for helpful comments on the manuscript.

Author details

[1]Institute and Policlinic for Occupational Medicine, Environmental Medicine and Prevention Research of Cologne University, Kerpener Str. 62, 50937 Köln, Germany. [2]Institute for Occupational Epidemiology and Risk Assessment (IERA) of Evonik Industries AG, Rellinghauser Str. 1-11, D-45128 Essen, Germany. [3]Institute for Occupational, Social and Environmental Medicine of the Goethe University Frankfurt/Main, Theodor-Stern-Kai 7, 60590 Frankfurt am Main, Germany. [4]European Research Group on Environment and Health in the Transport Sector (EUGT e.V.), Fritschestr. 35, 10627 Berlin, Germany.

References

1. Vermeulen R, Silverman DT, Garshick E, Vlaanderen J, Portengen L, Steenland K. Exposure-response estimates for diesel engine exhaust and lung cancer mortality based on data from three occupational cohorts. Environ Health Perspect. 2014;122(2):172–7.
2. Steenland K, Deddens J, Stayner L. Diesel exhaust and lung cancer in the trucking industry: exposure-response analyses and risk assessment. Am J Ind Med. 1998;34(3):220–8.
3. Garshick E, Laden F, Hart JE, Davis ME, Eisen EA, Smith TJ. Lung cancer and elemental carbon exposure in trucking industry workers. Environ Health Perspect. 2012;120(9):1301–6.
4. Silverman DT, Samanic CM, Lubin JH, Blair AE, Stewart PA, Vermeulen R, et al. The diesel exhaust in miners study: a nested case–control study of lung cancer and diesel exhaust. J Natl Cancer Inst. 2012;104(11):855–68.
5. Benbrahim-Tallaa L, Baan RA, Grosse Y, Lauby-Secretan B, El Ghissassi F, Bouvard V, et al. Carcinogenicity of diesel-engine and gasoline-engine exhausts and some nitroarenes. Lancet Oncol. 2012;13(7):663–4.
6. Park RM. Diesel engine emissions and risk assessment at NIOSH. In: Presentation at the workshop "Diesel Exhaust, Lung Cancer and Quantitative Risk Assessment". Boston, MA: Health Effects Institute; 2014.
7. The Advisory Committee on Safety and Health at Work: Supplementary opinion on the approach and content of an envisaged proposal by the Commission on the amendment of Directive 2004/37/EC on Carcinogens and Mutagens at the workplace. Supplementary opinion Doc. 727/13. Adopted on 30/05/2013. European Commission, DG Employment, Social Affairs and Inclusion Employment and Social Legislation, Social Dialogue, Health, Safety and Hygiene at Work. 2013. Available from: https://circabc.europa.eu/d/d/workspace/SpacesStore/85739c10-4b49-42ac-8982-aafc9a38f0eb/Doc%20%20727-13-%20EN%20Supplementary%20CMD%20Opinion_FINAL.pdf. Accessed June 10, 2015
8. Cherrie JW, Gorman M, Shafrir A, van Tongeren M, Mistry R, Sobey M, Corden C, Rushton L, Hutchings S: Health, socio-economic and environmental aspects of possible amendments to the EU directive on the protection of workers from the risk related to exposure to carcinogens and mutagens or work. 2011. Available from: http://ec.europa.eu/social/main.jsp?catId=716&langId=de&moreDocuments=yes. Accessed June 15, 2015
9. Rothman KJ, Greenland S, Lash TL. Modern Epidemiology. 3rd ed. Philadelphia: Lippincott Williams & Wilkins; 2008.

10. Steenland NK, Silverman DT, Hornung RW. Case–control study of lung cancer and truck driving in the Teamsters Union. Am J Public Health. 1990;80(6):670–4.
11. Zaebst DD, Clapp DE, Blade LM, Marlow DA, Steenland K, Hornung RW, et al. Quantitative determination of trucking industry workers' exposures to diesel exhaust particles. Am Ind Hyg Assoc J. 1991;52(12):529–41.
12. Attfield MD, Schleiff PL, Lubin JH, Blair A, Stewart PA, Vermeulen R, et al. The diesel exhaust in miners study: a cohort mortality study with emphasis on lung cancer. J Natl Cancer Inst. 2012;104(11):869–83.
13. Morfeld P. Letter to Garshick et al. 2012: Cox model setup may lead to erroneous conclusions. Environ Health Perspect. 2012;120(10):A382 (Author response A382-A383).
14. Crump KS, Van Landingham C, Moolgavkar SH, McClellan R. Reanalysis of the DEMS nested case–control study of lung cancer and diesel exhaust: Suitability for quantitative risk assessment. Risk Anal. 2015;35(4):676–700.
15. Crump K, Van Landingham C. Evaluation of an exposure assessment used in epidemiological studies of diesel exhaust and lung cancer in underground mines. Crit Rev Toxicol. 2012;42(7):599–612.
16. Stewart PA, Coble JB, Vermeulen R, Schleiff P, Blair A, Lubin J, et al. The diesel exhaust in miners study: I. Overview of the exposure assessment process. Ann Occup Hyg. 2010;54(7):728–46.
17. Möhner M, Kersten N, Gellissen J. Diesel motor exhaust and lung cancer mortality: reanalysis of a cohort study in potash miners. Eur J Epidemiol. 2013;28(2):159–68.
18. Allison PD. Fixed effects regression models. Los Angeles: SAGE; 2009.
19. Cameron AC, Trivedi PK. Microeconometrics. Methods and applications. Cambridge: University Press; 2005.
20. Cameron AC, Trivedi PK. Microeconometrics using stata. revisedth ed. Texas: StataCorp LP, College Station; 2010.
21. Diggle PJ, Heagerty PJ, Liang K-Y, Zeger SL. Analysis of longitudinal data. 2nd ed. New York: Oxford University Press Inc.; 2002.
22. Berlin JA, Longnecker MP, Greenland S. Meta-analysis of epidemiologic dose–response data. Epidemiol. 1993;4(3):218–28.
23. Neter J, Wasserman W, Kutner MH. Applied linear statistical models. Regression, Analysis of variance and experimental designs. 2nd ed. Homewood, Illinois: Richard Dr. Irwin; 1985.
24. Greenland S, Longnecker MP. Methods for trend estimation from summarized dose–response data, with applications to meta-analysis. Am J Epidemiol. 1992;135(11):1301–9.
25. Orsini N, Bellocco R, Greenland S. Generalized least squares for trend estimation of summarized dose–response data. The Stata Journal. 2006;6:40–57.
26. Orsini N, Li R, Wolk A, Khudyakov P, Spiegelman D. Meta-analysis for linear and nonlinear dose–response relations: examples, an evaluation of approximations, and software. Am J Epidemiol. 2012;175(1):66–73.
27. StataCorp. Release 12. Statistical Software. TX: College Station, StataCorp LP; 2013.
28. Crump K, van Landingham C, Moolgavkar S, Mc-Clellan R (2014) Reanalysis of the DEMS nested case-control study of lung cancer and diesel exhaust: suitability for quantitative risk assessment. Health Effects Institute, Boston (Webinar September, 2014)
29. Moolgavkar S (2014) Diesel engine exhaust and lung cancer mortality – temporal factors in exposure and risk. Health Effects Institute, Boston (Webinar September, 2014).
30. Moolgavkar SH, Chang ET, Luebeck G, Lau EC, Watson HM, Crump KS, et al. Diesel engine exhaust and lung cancer mortality: Time-related factors in exposure and risk. Risk Anal. 2015;35(4):663–75.
31. Hudson DJ. Fitting segmented curves whose join points have to be estimated. J Am Stat Assoc. 1966;61(316):1097–129.
32. Jones RH, Molitoris BA. A statistical method for determining the breakpoint of two lines. Anal Biochem. 1984;141(1):287–90.
33. Ulm K. A statistical method for assessing a threshold in epidemiological studies. Stat Med. 1991;10(3):341–9.
34. Morfeld P. Letter to the editor: formaldehyde and leukemia: missing evidence! Cancer Causes Control. 2013;24(1):203–4.
35. Al Khalaf MM, Thalib L, Doi SAR. Combining heterogenous studies using the random-effects model is a mistake and leads to inconclusive meta-analyses. J Clin Epidemiol. 2011;64(2):119–23.
36. Checkoway H, Boffetta P, Mundt DJ, Mundt KA. Critical review and synthesis of the epidemiologic evidence on formaldehyde exposure and risk of leukemia and other lymphohematopoietic malignancies. Cancer Causes Control. 2012;23(11):1747–66.
37. Morfeld P. Diesel exhaust in miners study: how to understand the findings? Journal of Occupational Medicine and Toxicology 2012;7(1):Available from: http://www.occup-med.com/content/7/1/10. Accessed August 10, 2015.
38. 38.Silverman DT, Attfield MD. RE: "Diesel exhaust in miners study: how to understand the findings?" by Peter Morfeld. J Occup Med Toxicol 2013:http://www.occup-med.com/content/7/1/10/comments. Accessed June 15, 2015.
39. Crump K. Meta-analysis of lung cancer risk from exposure to diesel exhaust: study limitations. Environmental Health Perspectives 2014;122(9):A230 (author´s reply: 230-231). http://dx.doi.org/10.1289/ehp.1408482.
40. Cox T, Lowrie K. Editorial: what do we really know about effects of diesel exhaust on lung cancer risk? Risk Anal. 2015;35(4):556.
41. Sun Y, Bochmann F, Nold A, Mattenklott M. Diesel exhaust exposure and the risk of lung cancer-a review of the epidemiological evidence. Int J Environ Res Public Health. 2014;11(2):1312–40.
42. Neumeyer-Gromen A, Razum O, Kersten N, Seidler A, Zeeb H. Diesel motor emissions and lung cancer mortality–results of the second follow-up of a cohort study in potash miners. Int J Cancer. 2009;124(8):1900–6.
43. Morfeld P, Mundt KA, Taeger D, Guldner K, Steinig O, Miller BG. Threshold value estimation for respirable quartz dust exposure and silicosis incidence among workers in the German porcelain industry. J Occup Environ Med. 2013;55(9):1027–34.
44. Royston P, Altman DG, Sauerbrei W. Dichotomizing continuous predictors in multiple regression: a bad idea. Stat Med. 2006;25(1):127–41.
45. HEI Advanced collaborative emissions study (ACES): Lifetime cancer and non-cancer assessment in rats exposed to new-technology diesel exhaust. Health Effects Institute. Boston: MA; 2015. Available from: http://pubs.healtheffects.org/view.php?id=430. Accessed June 15, 2015.
46. McClellan RO, Hesterberg TW, Wall JC. Evaluation of carcinogenic hazard of diesel engine exhaust needs to consider revolutionary changes in diesel technology. Regul Toxicol Pharmacol. 2012;63(2):225–58.

4

Sickness absenteeism and associated factors among horticulture employees in Lume district, southeast Ethiopia

Sebsibe Tadesse[1*], Kamil Ebrahim[2] and Zemichael Gizaw[1]

Abstract

Background: Sickness absenteeism is the major occupational health problem in developing countries where the majority of working population are engaged in hazardous sectors, such as agriculture. However, there is a dearth of studies clarifying the situation in most of Subsaharan African countries, like Ethiopia. The present study determined the magnitude of sickness absenteeism and associated factors among horticulture employees in Lume District, southeast Ethiopia.

Methods: An institutional-based cross-sectional study was conducted among horticulture employees in Lume District, southeast Ethiopia from March to May 2014. Stratified sampling followed by simple random sampling techniques was used to select the study participants. A pre-tested and structured questionnaire was used to collect data. Multivariable analyses were employed to see the effect of explanatory variables on dependent variable.

Results: The magnitude of sickness absenteeism was 58.8 % [95 % CI: (54.9, 62.5)] in the past three months. Absence of periodic medical checkup, working for more than 48 h per week, working overtime, job dissatisfaction, and job stress were factors significantly associated with sickness absenteeism.

Conclusions: In this study a relatively higher rate of sickness absenteeism was reported compared to other studies. Interventions to reduce sickness absenteeism should focus on areas, such as periodic medical checkup, monitoring work schedules, improving employees' job satisfaction, and managing job stress.

Keywords: Employees, Horticulture, Sickness absenteeism, Ethiopia

Background

Sickness absenteeism is the major occupational health problem in developing countries where the majority of working population are engaged in hazardous sectors, such as agriculture; causing loss of work-hours, reduced productivity and workplace disputes [1–5]. According to International Labor Organization 2008, more than 317 million accidents and diseases occurred on the job annually; and about two-thirds of them caused employees away from work for four working days resulting in economic effects and loss of labor time in both developing and developed countries [6]. In Subsaharan Africa, 42 million work-related accidents caused at least three days absence from work in which agriculture plays the major role [2]. About half million accidents caused at least four days off work in Ethiopia [7].

Horticulture investment is the most growing agriculture sector in East Africa, especially in the lowland regions of Ethiopia [8]. The industry uses many hazardous chemicals that may affect the health of employees if proper safety procedures are not followed [2, 5]. However, there is limited evidence on the magnitude, nature and role of different factors associated with sickness absenteeism among horticulture employees in Ethiopia. Moreover, many organizations do not have proper data recording and reporting systems to generate statistics that shows how cosmic the problem is at local and national levels [9]. Therefore, this study aimed to determine the magnitude of sickness absenteeism and associated factors among horticulture employees in Lume District, southeast Ethiopia. The findings of the study

* Correspondence: sbsbtadesse90@gmail.com
[1]Institute of Public Health, The University of Gondar, Gondar, Ethiopia

could provide information for safety officers, employers and policy makers to design strategies that aid to prevent the different health and safety hazards and improve employees' attendance.

Methods

Study area, design and period

An institutional-based cross-sectional study was conducted to assess the magnitude of sickness absenteeism and associated factors among horticulture employees in Lume District, southeast Ethiopia, from March to May 2014. The district is located at 75 km East of Addis Ababa, the capital city of Ethiopia. According to the 2007 Ethiopian population statistics, the district has a total of 117,080 populations. Of whom, 51.4 % were males and 33 % were urban dwellers [10]. The study covered eight horticulture industries employing more than 80 % of all employed workers in the district. During the investigation, there are 5900 employees working in the industries; 62.9 % of whom were females [11].

Participants and data collection

All horticulture employees who have worked for at least three months prior to the study period were included in the study until the required sample size was obtained. Women on maternity leave during the time of data collection were excluded from the study. Data were collected using structured interview questionnaire comprising of *workplace stress scale* developed by Marlin Company and the American Institute of Stress [12] and *generic job satisfaction scale* developed by Scott Macdonald and Peter Macintyre [13] with some modification. The questionnaire also contained detailed information on socio-demographic, behavioral and other workplace conditions.

Sample size calculation

Epi info version 7 was used to determine the sample size required for this study by taking 5900 total population, 50 % expected proportion of sickness absenteeism, 4 % confidence limit, and 95 % confidence level. By adding 10 % non-response rate, the total sample size was 600.

Sampling procedure

Stratified sampling followed by simple random sampling techniques was used to select the study participants. That is, the industries were stratified into three departments, namely production, technical and management department. Then, the total of 600 samples was proportionally allocated to each department. The participants were drawn from the factory's list of workers using simple random sampling.

Data quality control

The training of data collectors and supervisors emphasized issues such as data collection instrument, field methods, inclusion–exclusion criteria, time of interview, and record keeping. The completed questionnaires were spot-checked and reviewed on a daily basis to ensure the completeness and consistency of the data collected. The interview questionnaire was pre-tested on 40 respondents who had characteristics nearly similar to employees in Lume district in order to identify potential problem areas, unanticipated interpretations, and cultural objections to any of the questions. Based on the pre-test results, the questionnaire was adjusted contextually.

Data management and statistical analyses

Data entered and cleaned using Epi info version 7 statistical software were analyzed on SPSS version 20. Frequency distribution, mean, standard deviation, and percentage, were employed for most variables. All independent variables were fitted separately into bivariate logistic model to evaluate the degree of association with sickness absenteeism. Then, variables with a p-value < 0.20 were exported to multivariable logistic regression model to control confounders. The odds ratio (OR) with a 95 % confidence interval (CI) was used to test the statistical significance of variables.

Operational definitions

Horticulture

Organization that produces fruits, vegetables and flowers and avail on level of local and global market [8].

Sickness absenteeism

Self-reported employees' absence from their normal duty for the reasons stemming from health problem in the past three months.

Job stress

The employee was considered as stressed with work when his/her sum of workplace stress scale score was 21 or above [12].

Satisfied with job

The employee was considered as satisfied with job when his/her sum of generic job satisfaction scale score was 32 or above [13].

Permanent employee

Any contract of employment between employee and employer concluded for an indefinite period [14].

Temporary employee

Any employment contract between employee and employer made for definite period [14].

Overtime work

An employee was considered as worked overtime when she/he had worked on average greater than or equal to 2 h more than the standard working hours per week within the past 3 months [14].

Cigarette smoker

An employee who was smoking one cigarette a day for at least one year [3].

Alcohol drinker

An employee who drink at least five drinks per week for men and two drinks per week for women for at least one year [3].

Khat chewer

An employee chewing Khat three times a week for at least one year [3].

Attendance-based incentive

An incentive provided for employee for his/her being only present at work.

Ethical considerations

The study protocol was reviewed and approved by the Institutional Review Board of the University of Gondar via the Institute of Public Health. Permission was obtained from Lume District Labor and Social Affairs Office prior to data collection. Study participants were interviewed after informed written consent was obtained. They were also informed that their participation was voluntary and that they could withdraw from the interview at any time without consequences. The participants were assured that their responses would be treated confidentially through the use of strict coding measures.

Literature search strategy

PubMed, Medline, and Scopus were the main databases searched for literature and bibliographic alerts were set up for additional papers to be identified whenever they cited key articles. Keywords for the literature search were identified by means of Medical Subject Headings (MeSH) thesaurus which is available through PubMed online (http://www.ncbi.nlm.nih.gov/pubmed). Some MeSH terms used were 'horticulture', 'horticulture employees', 'horticulture workers', 'sickness absenteeism', and 'workplace factors'. Although the bibliographic search was meant to find the most up-to-date information, some old but highly influential papers were also reviewed. EndNote software (http://www.endnote.com/) was used to store citations together with their respective articles in pdf format, so that an annotated bibliography could be built and eventually cited and referenced.

Results

Socio-demographic characteristics

A total of 590 employees completed the questionnaire making response rate 98.3 %. Of whom 71.9 % were females. The mean age with a standard deviation of the employees was 26.9 ± 7.1. More than two-thirds, 70.8 %, of them belonged to the age group of 19–29 years. Those who attended primary education were 32.9 %. More than two-thirds, 70.5 %, served for less than five years. Regarding religion 74.9 % of the employees were Christian. The married were 44.6 %. Nearly half, 48.3 %, had a monthly salary of less than or equal to Birr 700 (Table 1).

Workplace characteristics

The majority, 89.2 %, of the respondents were permanent employees. Regarding hours spent on work 88.6 % of

Table 1 Socio-demographic characteristics of horticulture employees in Lume district, southeast Ethiopia, 2014

Variables	Number	Percent
Sex		
Male	166	28.1
Female	424	71.9
Age (in years)		
≤18	23	3.9
19-29	418	70.8
30-40	114	19.3
>40	35	5.9
Marital Status		
Single	252	42.7
Married	263	44.6
Widowed/divorced	75	12.7
Educational status		
Illiterate	186	31.5
Primary education	194	32.9
Secondary education	153	25.9
Above secondary education	57	9.7
Religion		
Christian	442	74.9
Muslim	148	25.1
Monthly salary (in Birr)		
≤700	285	48.3
701-1500	245	41.5
>1500	60	10.2
Work experiences (in years)		
<5	416	70.5
≥5	174	29.5

the employees had worked for ≤48 h per week. Two-thirds, 66.8 %, of them worked overtime. About three-fourths (71.7 %) were dissatisfied with their current job, and 62.7 % were stressed. The majority, 89.3 % and 85.4 %, of them had no pre-employment screening and periodic medical checkup, respectively. More than two-thirds, 69.0 %, of them didn't receive attendance-based incentive (Table 2).

Magnitude of sickness absenteeism

The magnitude of sickness absenteeism among horticulture employees was observed to be 58.8 % [95 % CI: (54.9, 62.5)] in the past three months. Of whom 73.5 % were females. The majority, 72.6 % and 69.7 %, of them belonged to the age group of 19 to 29 years and attended primary and below education, respectively. The average frequency of absence was 1.73 [95 % CI: (1.63, 1.84)]. The mean number of lost working days per absentee was 6.63. The total of 2302 working days was lost.

Table 2 Workplace characteristics of horticulture employees in Lume district, southeast Ethiopia, 2014

Variables	Number	Percent
Employment type		
Permanent	526	89.2
Temporary	64	10.8
Working hours per week		
≤48	523	88.6
>48	67	11.4
Work overtime		
Yes	394	66.8
No	196	33.2
Job satisfaction		
Satisfied	167	28.3
Dissatisfied	423	71.7
Workplace stress		
Not stressed	220	37.3
Stressed	370	62.7
Pre-employment medical		
Screening		
Yes	63	10.7
No	527	89.3
Periodic medical checkup		
Yes	86	14.6
No	504	85.4
Received attendance-based incentive		
Yes	183	31.0
No	407	69.0

Perceived causes of sick absenteeism

The most common health problems that lead employees away from their work were 48.7 % minor illness, 36.6 % typhoid, 35.7 % diarrhea, 32.3 % Musculo-Skeletal Disorders (MSDs) (Fig. 1).

Factors associated with sickness absenteeism

Table 3 presents factors which remained statistically significant in the bivariate and multivariable logistic regression analyses. In this study, the independent predictors of sickness absenteeism on the multivariable analysis include absence of periodic medical checkup [AOR: 3.6, 95 % CI: (2.1, 6.1)], working for >48 h per week [AOR: 1.9, 95 % CI: (1.0, 3.5)], working overtime [AOR: 2.8, 95 % CI: (1.9, 4.2)], job dissatisfaction [AOR: 1.8, 95 % CI: (1.2, 2.7)], and job stress [AOR: 2.0, 95 % CI: (1.4, 2.9)], (Table 3).

Discussion

Sickness absenteeism remains to be the major occupational health problem among horticulture employees. In this study the magnitude of sickness absenteeism among horticulture employees was 58.8 % [95 % CI: (54.9, 62.5)]. This finding is higher than that of studies from Ethiopia (53.9 %) [15], Nigeria (15.8-25.0 %) [16, 17] and Denmark (12.0 %) [18]. The difference could be due to methodological differences, like study population and methods of data collection, and workplace conditions, like employees' level of awareness on hazard control and disease prevention and accessibility to health care services [15–18].

This study identified important predictors influencing sickness absenteeism. Employees who didn't undergo periodic medical checkup were more likely to experience sickness absenteeism than those who did so. Timely medical examination helps as a preventive medicine for detecting and treating early initiation of health problems on regular basis before it goes to hard step. Thus, it is a moral imperative for the employers to know health status of their employees periodically and take the necessary interventions to protect them from further harming.

In this and other studies employees who worked for greater than 48 h per week were more likely to experience sickness absenteeism than those who did not [5, 19]. This is true for employees who engaged in overtime work [20]. The reason could be that working above normal working hours would affect muscular activities and caused mental fatigue which might lead employees to increased risk of accidents. It could be recommended that assignment of employees should take into account the implementation of shiftwork scheduling. Moreover, recruiting additional employees could also improve the situation.

Job dissatisfaction and stress were also found significantly associated with sickness absenteeism. Other studies support these findings [21–24]. Existing research has

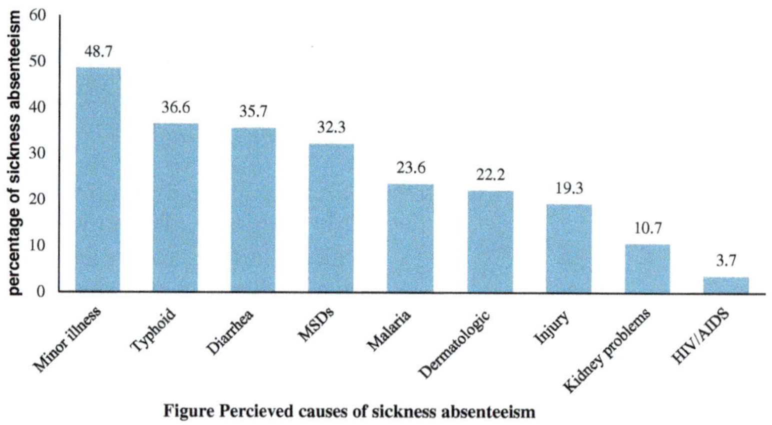

Fig. 1 Percieved causes of sickness absenteeism

recognized heavy workload, insufficient resources, work relationships, lack of professional respect, and lack of promotion opportunities as possibly the most salient job stressors [25–27]. Chronic exposure to stress may be harmful to the health of employees and may also affect productivity of organization through employee dissatisfaction, burnout, poor performance, high turnover, and increased absence from work [28–32].

Social desirability bias is a potential limitation in self-reported studies like this one, in that employees might report more socially acceptable responses than their actual day to day practice. As this is a cross-sectional study, the limitations that come with this type of design need to be taken into consideration when interpreting the findings.

Table 3 Factors associated with sickness absenteeism among horticulture employees in Lume District, southeast Ethiopia, 2014

Variables	Sickness absenteeism		Crude OR (95 % CI)	Adjusted OR (95 % CI)
	Yes	No		
Periodic medical checkup				
Yes	36	50	1	1
No	311	193	2.2(1.4, 3.6)	3.6(2.1, 6.1)
Working hours per week				
≤48	302	221	1	1
>48	45	22	1.5(0.9, 2.6)	1.9(1.0, 3.5)
Worked overtime				
No	88	108	1	1
Yes	259	135	2.4(1.7, 3.3)	2.8(1.9, 4.2)
Job satisfaction				
Satisfied	84	83	1	1
Dissatisfied	263	160	1.6(1.1, 2.3)	1.8(1.2, 2.7)
Workplace stress				
Not stressed	106	114	1	1
Stressed	241	129	2.0(1.4, 2.8)	2.0(1.4, 2.9)

Conclusions

In this study a relatively higher rate of sickness absenteeism was reported compared to other studies. Interventions to reduce sickness absenteeism should focus on areas, such as periodic medical checkup, monitoring work schedules, improving employees' job satisfaction, and reducing workplace stress.

Competing interests

The authors declare that they have no competing interest.

Authors' contribution

Author 1. ST: Involved in write up of the research proposal, the data analyses, and wrote the manuscript, Author 2. KE: Involved in write up of the research proposal, the data analyses, and manuscript writingt, Author 3. ZG: Involved in write up of the research proposal, the data analyses, and manuscript writing. All authors read and approved the final manuscript.

Acknowledgments

The authors wish to thank the Oromia Labor and Social Affairs Bureau for logistic and administrative support, and data collectors for their support in making this study possible. They also extend their deepest gratitude to the study participants.

Author details

[1]Institute of Public Health, The University of Gondar, Gondar, Ethiopia.
[2]Labour and social affairs, Oromia Regional State, Addis Ababa, Ethiopia.

References

1. Royal Australasian College of Physicians. Workplace Attendance and Absenteeism. Sydney: Australasian Faculty of Occupational Medicine; 1999.
2. Finnish Institute of Occupational Health. Social determinants of health and the workplace. African Newsletter on Occupational Health and Safety. 2013;23(3):3.
3. Melchior M, Niedhammer I, Berkman LF, Goldberg M. Do psychosocial work factors and social relations exert independent effects on sickness absence? A six year prospective study of the GAZEL cohort. J Epidemiol Community Health. 2003;57:285–93.
4. Essy C, Omorogbe V, Orji I, Oyovwe L. Self-reported absenteeism among hospital workers in benin city, nigeria. Ghana Med J. 2008;42:1.

5. International Labour Organization. Decent Work in Agriculture. International Workers' Symposium on Decent Work in Agriculture; Geneva: Bureau for Workers' Activities; 2009.
6. International Labour Organization. LABORSTA database. Geneva: Statistics Do; 2008.
7. International Labour Organization. Occupational accident report by region. Geneva: International labour conference; 2008.
8. Ahmed A. Horticultural Marketing in Ethiopia. Addis Ababa University; Ethiopia. 2007.
9. World Health Organization/International Labour Organization. Occupational Health and safety in Africa. Addis Ababa: Meeting report. 2010.
10. Central Statistical Authority. Population and Housing Census of Ethiopia: Results for Amhara Regional State. Addis Ababa, Ethiopia: Central Statistical Authority; 2007.
11. Lume District Labour and Social Affairs Office. Second quarter work report. Modjo: Ethiopia. 2014.
12. The Marlin Company and the American Institute of Stress. The Workplace Stress Scale. Yonkers, NY. Accessed on: 02/05/2014, Available at: http://www.executivestresscoach.com/JOBSTRESS.html.
13. Macdonald S, MacIntyre P. The generic job satisfaction scale: Scale development and its correlates. Employee Assistance Quarterly. 1997;13(2):1–16.
14. Ministry of Labour and Social Affairs. Labour proclamation No.377/2003. Ministry of Labour and Social Affairs, Addis Ababa, Ethiopia; 2003.
15. Tadesse T, Kumie A. Prevalence and factors affecting work-related injury among workers engaged in Small and Medium-Scale Industries in Gondar wereda, north Gondar zone, Amhara Regional State, Ethiopia. Ethiop J Health Dev. 2007;21(1):25–34.
16. Erinoso AO, Bamgboye E. Sickness absenteeism in a Nigerian polytechnic. Afr J Med Med Sci. 1988;17(1):57–61.
17. Bamgboye EA, Al A. Sickness absenteeism in a Nigerian teaching hospital. East Afr Med J. 1992;69(8):450.
18. Ballebye M. Nielsen HO. Oxford Research Institute: Factors influencing sickness absence; 2008.
19. Viswanathan R, Sridharan P, Thiyagarajan S. Absenteeism-a menace to indian BPO industry. SMART J of Business Mgt Studies. 2013;9(1):43–50.
20. Taylor P, Pocock S, Sergean R. Absenteeism of shift and day workers: a study of six types of shift system in 29 organizations. British J of Industrial Medicine. 2000;29(2):208–13.
21. Nakata A, Takahashi M, Irie M, Ray T, Swanson NG. Job satisfaction, common cold, and sickness absence among white-collar employees: a cross-sectional survey. Ind Health. 2011;49(1):116–21.
22. Estryn BM, Kaminski M. Rates of sickness absenteeism among employees of a modern hospital: the role of demographic and occupational factors. British J of Industrial Medicine. 1985;42(11):787–8.
23. Aaviksoo E, Baburin A, Kiivet RA. Risk factors for sickness absence among Estonian employees. Occup Med. 2013;63(2):156–9.
24. Beyamin MS, Azar K, Esmaiel R, Mohammad FK, Zolaykha A, Bagherian FE, et al. Prevalence and causes of medical absenteeism among staff (Case study at Mazandaran University of Medical Sciences: 2009–2010). Mater Sociomed. 2013;25(4):233–7.
25. Kim HJ. Work stress and job satisfaction of community mental health nurses in South Korea: a qualitative content analysis. J Korean Acad Psychiatr Ment Health Nurs. 2013;22:295–306.
26. Johnson SJ, O'Connor EM, Jacobs S, Hassell K, Ashcroft DM. The relationships among work stress, strain and self-reported errors in UK community pharmacy. Res Social Adm Pharm. 2014;10(6):885–95.
27. Qu NQ, Zhou H, Fan LH. Analysis on work stress and occupational burnout among community health service staff in Harbin. Med Soc. 2013;26:87–9.
28. Chen XJ, Tan XR, Li LP. Health problem and occupational stress among Chinese doctors. Chin Med. 2013;4:1–6.
29. Nabirye RC, Brown KC, Pryor ER, Maples EH. Occupational stress, job satisfaction and job performance among hospital nurses in Kampala, Uganda. J Nurs Manage. 2011;19:760–8.
30. Voltmer E, Rosta J, Siegrist J, Aasland OG. Job stress and job satisfaction of physicians in private practice: comparison of German and Norwegian physicians. Int Arch Occ Env Health. 2012;85:819–28.
31. Saijo Y, Chiba S, Yoshioka E, Nakagi Y, Ito T, Sugioka Y, et al. Job stress and burnout among urban and rural hospital physicians in Japan. Aust J Rural Health. 2013;21:225–31.
32. Sun Y, Luo ZN, Fang PQ. Factors influencing the turnover intention of Chinese community health service workers based on the investigation results of five provinces. J Commun Health. 2013;38:1058–66.

5

Telemedicine – a scientometric and density equalizing analysis

David A. Groneberg[1*], Shaghayegh Rahimian[2], Matthias Bundschuh[1], Mario Schwarzer[1], Alexander Gerber[1] and Beatrix Kloft[3]

Abstract

Background: As a result of the various telemedicine projects in the past years a large number of studies were recently published in this field. However, a precise bibliometric analysis of telemedicine publications does not exist so far.

Methods: The present study was conducted to establish a data base of the existing approaches. Density-equalizing algorithms were used and data was retrieved from the Thomson Reuters database Web of Science.

Results: During the period from 1900 to 2006 a number of 3290 filed items were connected to telemedicine, with the first being published in 1964. The studies originate from 101 countries, with the USA, Great Britain and Canada being the most productive suppliers participating in 56.08 % of all published items. Analyzing the average citation per item for countries with more than 10 publications, Ireland ranked first (10.19/item), New Zealand ranked second (9.5/item) followed by Finland (9.04/item). The citation rate can be assumed as an indicator for research quality. The ten most productive journals include three journals with the main focus telemedicine and another five with the main focus "Information/Informatics". In all subject categories examined for published items related to telemedicine, "Health Care Sciences & Services" ranked first by far. More than 36 % of all publications are assigned to this category, followed by "Medical Informatics" with 9.72 % and "Medicine, General & Internal" with 8.84 % of all publications.

Conclusion: In summary it can be concluded that the data shows clearly a strong increase in research productivity. Using science citation analysis it can be assumed that there is a large rise in the interest in telemedicine studies.

Keywords: Telemedicine, Bibliometry, Scientometry, Density equalizing map, Citation

Introduction

Telemedicine and telemetrics are increasingly important for occupational and environmental medicine and many routine and research approaches use technology of this field for different purposes [1]. One definition is that "Telemedicine is the use of electronic information and communication technologies to provide and support health care when distance separates the participants" [2]. The first telemedical activities were documented in 1897, when the telephone was used to confirm a diagnosis [3], and there are reports from 1922 which certify the exchange of medical information between ships and coast guards [4]. Since then telemedicine plays an important role for all aspects of public health. Especially in areas, which are not densely populated, telemedicine may serve as a powerful tool to implement improvements of the public health system.

The invention of television induced the first wave of telemedicine projects. In 1959 Jutras succeeded to interconnect several hospitals via a cable supported TV system. This system enabled the transmission of roentgenograms over a distance of up to five miles [5]. With the development of new telecommunication technologies such as UMTS, infrared or Bluetooth telemedicine is today a growth market with high potentials and great opportunities for global health care. Telemedicine is most beneficial for populations living in isolated communities and remote regions and is currently being applied in virtually all medical domains. This new technology has mostly been used as a communication and consultation tool between a general practitioner

* Correspondence: ArbSozMed@uni-frankfurt.de
[1]Department of Health Economics, The Institute of Occupational Medicine, Social Medicine and Environmental Medicine, Goethe University Frankfurt, Theodor-Stern-Kai 7, 60590 Frankfurt, Germany
Full list of author information is available at the end of the article

and a specialist available at a remote location. In recent years, the focus has also been on monitoring a patient at home using known devices like blood pressure monitors and transferring the information to a caregiver. These telemonitoring solutions have a focus on current high morbidity chronic diseases, such as chronic heart failure or diabetes mellitus. Telemedicine holds big promises to solving major health care problems; hence, in the last years various studies were concluded. However, there is no in-depth bibliometric analysis of the current state of research regarding telemedicine available. Due to the importance of telemedicine for public health, the NewQIS project (New Quality and Quantity Indices in Science) [6–8] elected the topic of telemedicine as a primary research focus and established an in depth scientometric study. Large-scale data analysis and bibliometric approaches including density-equalizing mapping were performed.

Methods

Data source

The project is embedded in the NewQIS platform which already addressed numerous topics with importance to the field of public health Data [6, 9] was retrieved from the database Web of Science from the former Institute for Scientific Information of Thomson Reuters [10].

Search strategies

For the different searches the keyword telemedicine was used. The search included all document types (e.g. original articles, reviews, letters, editorials and news reports).

Time span

The initially analyzed time span included the period from 1900 to 2006. The last seven years were not analyzed since the evaluability of the number of citations is not given and it hardly allows to draw conclusions. Thus, the half live of citations has confined the period of investigation so far. To examine particular aspects of the retrieved data in depth, the time span was partly restricted to a period between 1976 and 2006.

Citation quantities

Published items were further analyzed [6, 11, 12] by using the function "citation report" of the Web of Science database. This method was used to examine the number of citations per citation year, the number of citations per publishing year and the average number of citations per item.

Data categorization

In accordance with the NewQIS platform [6, 9, 13], all data files were analyzed regarding a variety of different aspects, e.g. the publishing countries and languages, the publication years, the source titles and subject categories. Subsequently, the data was transferred to charts, analyzed and the findings visualized.

Density-equalizing mapping was used according to a method of Gastner and Newman [14]. With the application of this technique, territories were resized depending on a particular variable, e.g. the number of published items. For the resizing procedure the area of each country was scaled in proportion to its total number of published items regarding telemedicine.

Results

Total number of published items

The number of published items was used as an indication of research productivity. During the period 1900–2006 3290 items with the keyword telemedicine were identified. The first studies were published in the year 1964, but till the early 1990ies the total quantity of publications was

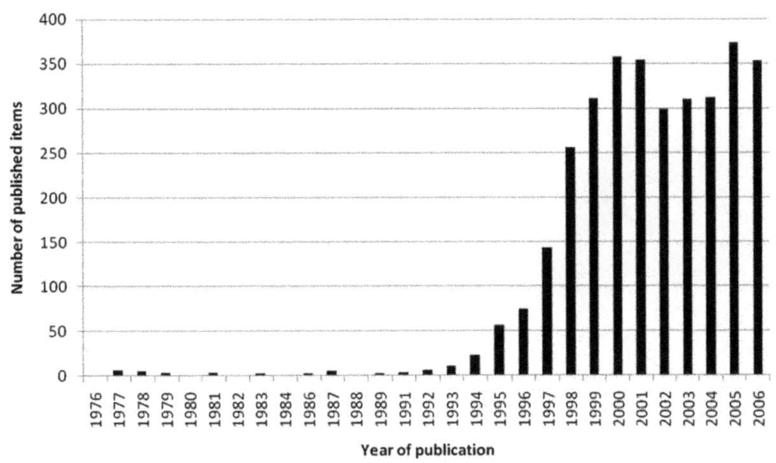

Fig. 1 Published items related to telemedicine in the Web of Science database 1900–2006

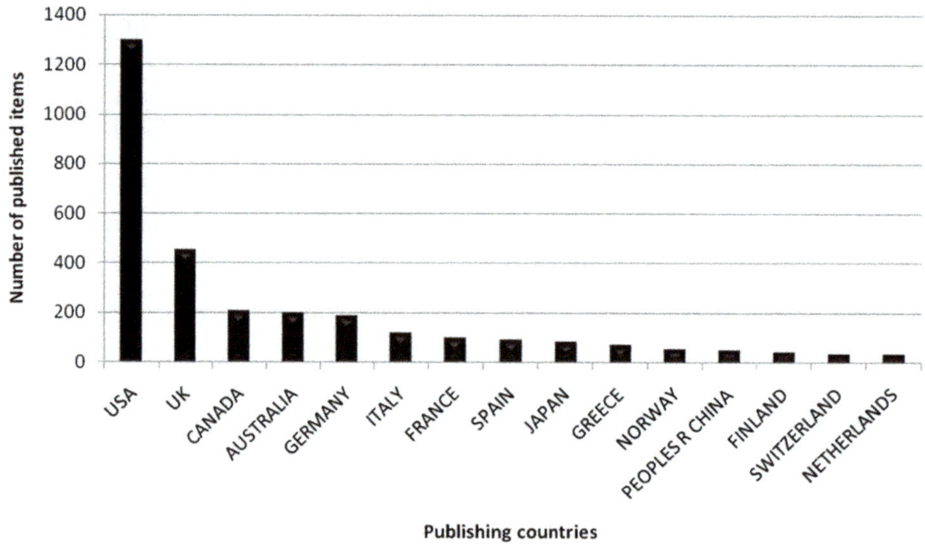

Fig. 2 Ranking of country total numbers of published items related to telemedicine

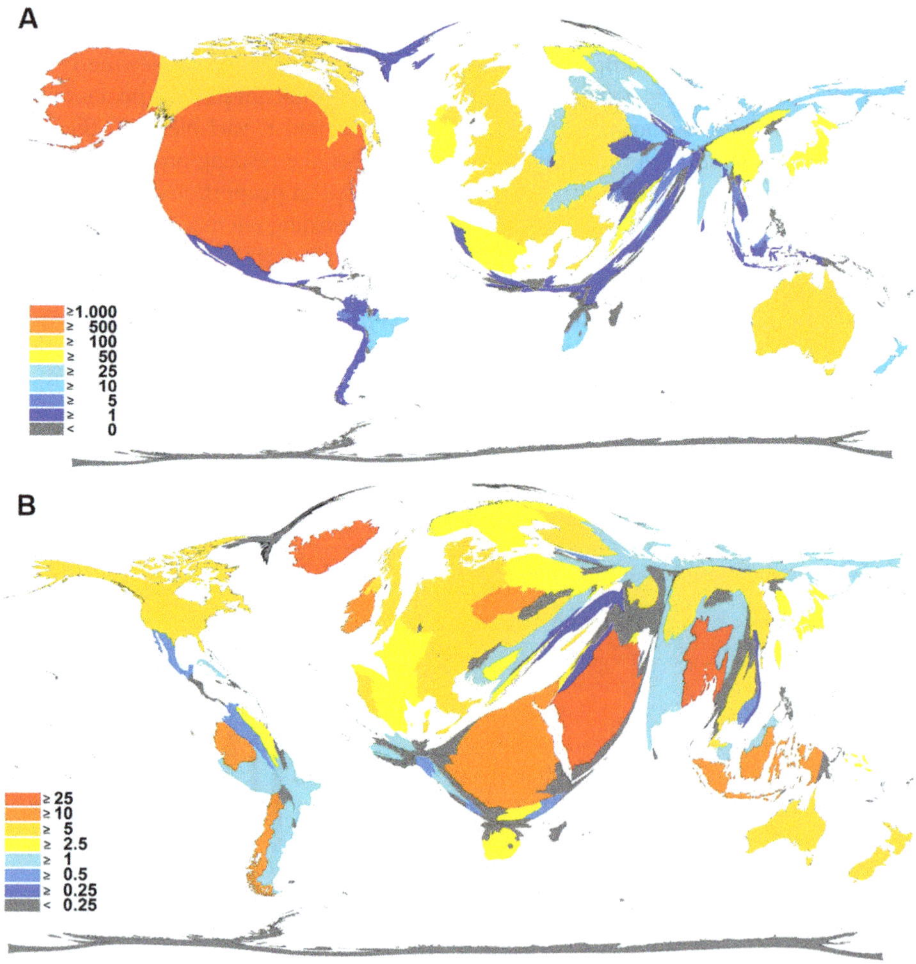

Fig. 3 a Density-equalizing map illustrating the number of publications in each particular country. The area of each country was scaled in proportion to its total number of publications regarding telemedicine. **b** Density-equalizing map showing the average citations per item of each particular country. The area of each country was scaled in proportion to its average number of citations per item regarding telemedicine

insignificant. However, numbers increase highly in the middle of the 1990ies. The number of published items jumps from 23 in the year 1994 up to 143 in 1997 and 357 in the year 2000. This is a considerable increase of 1450 % in a period of 6 years (Fig. 1).

Analysis of origin

The 3290 identified publications were originated from 101 countries, with the USA, Great Britain and Canada being the most productive ones (Fig. 2) participating in 56.08 % of all published items. Australia and Germany are also among the top five countries with the highest number of studies regarding telemedicine. The positions five to ten go to Italy, France, Spain, Japan and Greece. The cumulated publications of the top ten publishing countries encompassed 82.26 % of all published items. Density-equalizing mapping of this set of data demonstrates that a relatively small number of countries is responsible for the majority of research efforts (Fig. 3a).

Citation parameters

The average citation per item was used as an indicator for research quality, and differences were found in relation to research quantity figures: when analyzing all 3290 published items regarding the average citation of each item in a country-specific manner, Bangladesh has the highest average citation rate (35/item), with Iceland ranking second (31/item) and Saudi Arabia ranking third (25/item) (Fig. 4, Table 1). Differences to output quantity (Fig. 3a) can be visualized by the use of a density-equalizing calculation to provide a global scheme of the average citations per item of each country (Fig. 3b). When a threshold of at least ten publications is set up, Bangladesh (1 publication), Iceland (1 publication) and Saudi Arabia (1 publication) are no longer ranked in the top ten, and Ireland (80 publications) moves into first position, with an average citation rate of 10.19/item. Additionally New Zealand with 9.5 citations per item and Finland with 9.04 citations per item enter the top three (Table 2). To assess the reception of the subject matter over the time, the number of citations per citation year was recorded from 1976 to 2006 (Fig. 5) and a trend of increasing citations was present since 1976 (Fig. 6), which parallels the increase in published articles.

Table 1 Average citation per item of each particular country and total number of publications

Country	Average citation per Item	Number of publications
Bangladesh	35	1
Iceland	31	1
Saudi Arabia	25	1
Sudan	21	1
Indonesia	15	1
Czech Republic	11.25	4
Ecuador	10.2	5
Ireland	10.19	80
Chile	10	3
Egypt	10	1

Publishing journals

The ten most productive journals include three journals with the main focus telemedicine, such as "Journal of Telemedicine and Telecare", "Telemedicine Journal and E-Health" and "Telemedicine Journal". Another five have the main focus Information/Informatics, which are the "Journal of the American Medical Informatics Association", the

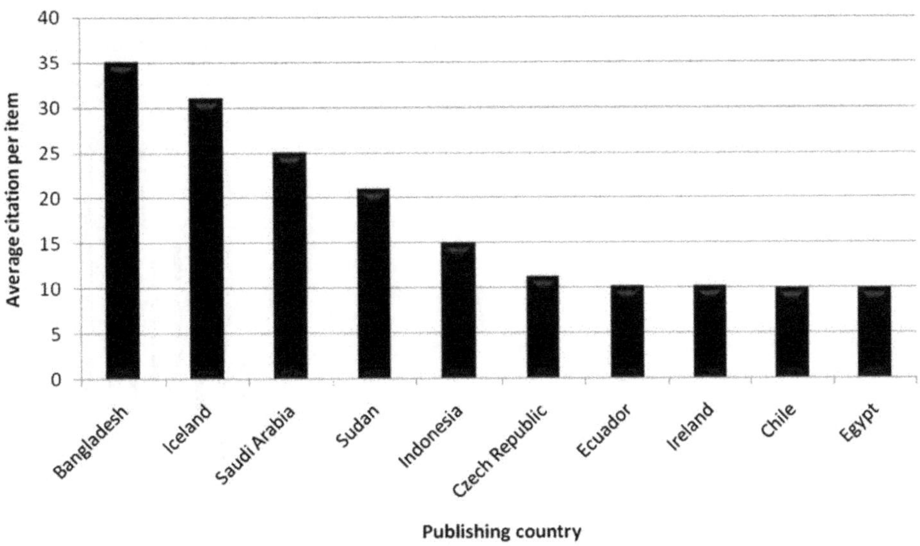

Fig. 4 Average citation per item of each particular country

Table 2 Average citation per item of each particular country and the total number of publications (threshold excludes countries with < 10 publications)

Country	Average citation per Item	Number of publications
Ireland	10.19	80
New Zealand	9.5	12
Finland	9.04	46
Denmark	8.72	25
USA	7.41	1,297
Austria	7.26	34
Belgium	7.24	17
China	7.05	56
Switzerland	6.87	39
Italy	6.72	120

"International Journal of Medical Informatics", the "IEEE Transactions of Information Technology in Biomedicine", the "Computer Methods and Programs in Biomedicine" and the "Methods of Information in Medicine" (Fig. 7).

Analysis of assigned subject categories

In all subject categories examined for published items related to telemedicine, "Health Care Sciences & Services" ranked first by far, followed by the categories "Medical Informatics" and "Medicine, General & Internal" (Fig. 8). While the numbers of publications in most categories show a less steep growth, the category "Health Care Sciences & Services" has increased remarkably since 1997. All categories showed a temporary increasing of publication numbers in 2001 (Fig. 9).

Discussion

The NewQIS platform decided to assess telemedicine on a scientometric level due to its increasing importance for public health and occupational and environmental medicine. Especially in countries in which the health systems are not area-wide, or occupational offshore settings, telemedical inventions may be of utmost importance. The present study provides a first precise international bibliometric evaluation of telemedicine-related research in a closed an defined time period which was set between 1900 and 2006. The methodology is based on internationally established databases, such as the Web of Science [10], and novel bibliometric tools including density-equalizing mapping [14]. The time span in some search routines was restricted to the period between 1976 and 2006. This period was chosen because the worldwide number of published items before 1976 was relatively low. Generally, there is a constant increase of interest in this field since the middle of the 1990ies. The main reason for this is the rapid progress and development in the field of communication technologies in this era. New methods of digitizing images and compressing data, as well as video coverage via low bandwidth enabled new telemedical options [15]. This strong progress in the area of computer and network technologies mainly initiated the development of telemedicine.

Data analysis of productivity parameters shows that research groups from the US maintain a leadership position in research productivity concerning telemedicine, along with Great Britain and Canada. More than 56 % of all publications are originated from these three countries.

By bringing the number of publications in relation to the respective population it can be seen that the USA with a ratio of approx. 4.3 publication/1 m residents do have a significantly lower output than the UK with 7.8 publication/1 m residents. Making the same calculation for Australia, Norway and Finland, a comparatively high ratio of approx. 10 publication/1 m for Australia, 12.4 publication/1 m for Norway and 9.2 publication/1 m for Finland can be found.

The reason for these results might be that territorial states such as Australia or Scandinavia do have special

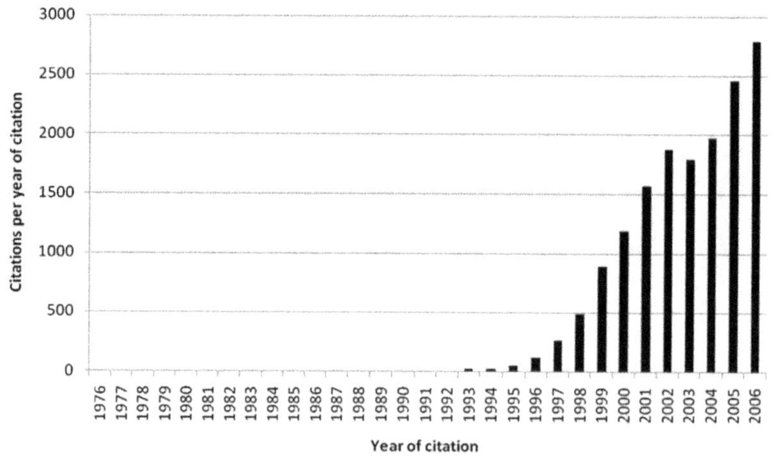

Fig. 5 Citations per year of citation

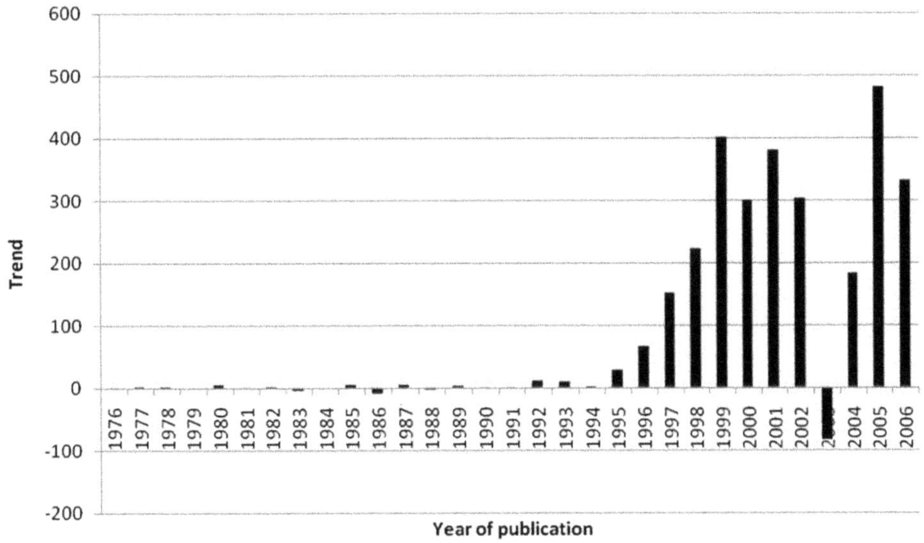

Fig. 6 Increase and decrease of citations per year of citation

requirements regarding medical care, which accelerate the development of telemedicine in these countries [16]. Therefore, telemedicine is very advanced in those countries where medical specialists are not available in most of the regions, or where climate issues cause serious transportation issues, as is the case in wide territories of Scandinavia.

While telemedicine is highly accepted and used in countries such as Scandinavia, Australia or the USA, Germany still struggles with this new technology [17]. In Germany only 2.3 published items per 1 m residents could be found. One of the main reasons for this is the unregulated compensation situation, together with the high physician concentration. Medical professionals in Germany are still very conservative regarding telemedicine, because they are afraid of possible staff savings and quality losses caused by this new technology [18].

Whereas the number of published items was considered as an indicator for research productivity, the average citation per item was used as a sign for research quality as generally accepted. Therefore all articles were analyzed regarding the average citation of items published in each particular country. Using this average citation per item index without thresholds, Bangladesh appears to have the highest rank, followed by Iceland and Saudi Arabia. It has to be annotated that the results for those countries with a very small amount of published items appear disproportionately high. To objectify these outliers, a threshold of ten published items was introduced and, as a result, Bangladesh (1 publication), Iceland (1 publication) and Saudi Arabia (1 publication) are no longer included in the ranking. Ireland (10.19 citations/item and 80 publications) moves up to first position, followed by New Zealand and Finland (Table 2).

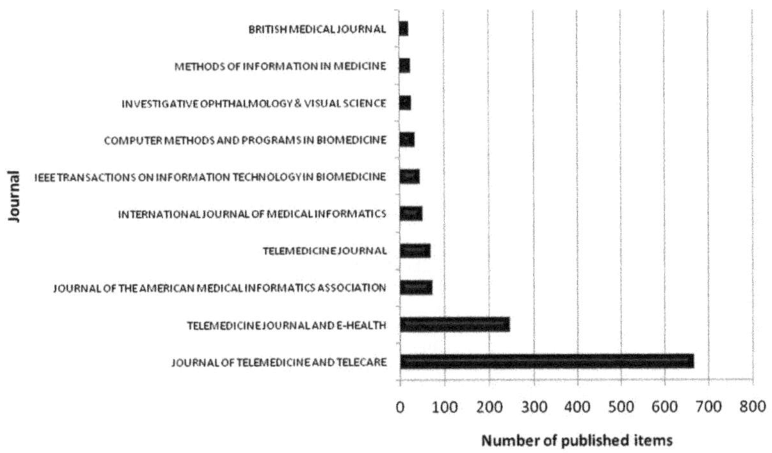

Fig. 7 Top 10 ranking of sources by the number of published items during the period from 1900 to 2006

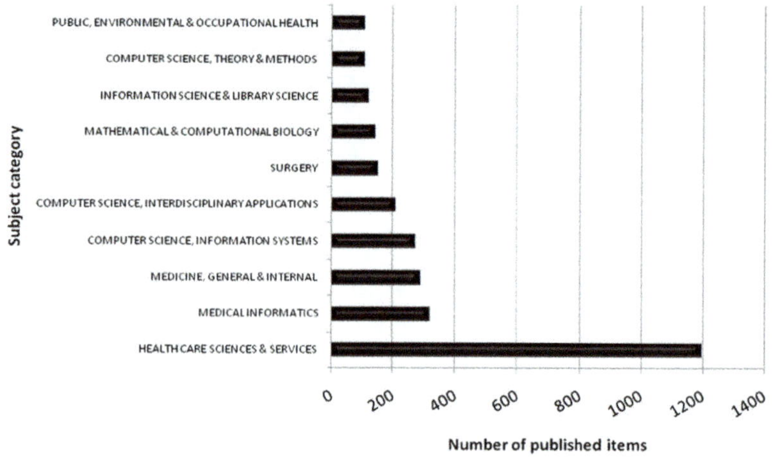

Fig. 8 Top10 list of assigned subject categories of published items related to telemedicine; study period from 1900 to 2006

This result once again underlines the importance of telemedicine in territorial countries, such as New Zealand or Finland. Because of Finland being highly developed in matters of telecommunications, numerous telemedicine projects could successfully be established in this region [19]. Today telemedicine is very well implemented in the Finish health care system, so that necessary waiting time shortenings for seeing a medical specialist could be achieved [20].

When focusing on assigned categories in the Web of Science database related to telemedicine, the field "Health Care Sciences & Services"plays a leading role, with a steep increase of published items since 1997. More than 36 % of all publications are assigned to this category, followed by "Medical Informatics" with 9.72 % and "Medicine, General & Internal" with 8.84 % of all publications. This trend confirms the high impact of telemedicine for the health care system. Telemedicine is no longer only a vision which is

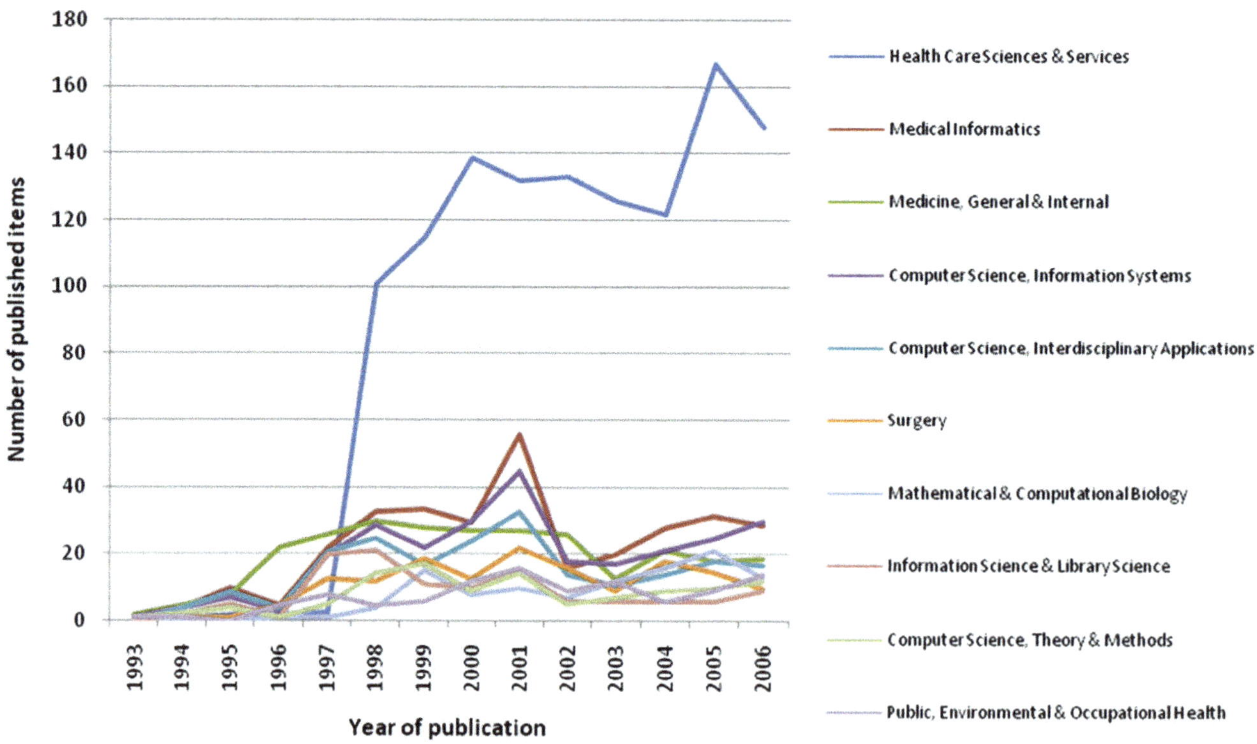

Fig. 9 Time dynamics of top 10 assigned subject categories; study period from 1900 to 2006

covered in theoretical or technical fields, such as "Computer Science, Theory & Methods" or "Computer Science, Information Systems". Today telemedicine is reality and successfully applied in a high number of medical fields [21]. Hence, more and more publications deal with the application of telemedicine in order to optimize the health care system. It is also an interesting aspect that the number of publications in the category "Health Care Sciences & Services" was insignificantly low till the mid 1990ies and then abruptly took a turn to become the most important field (Fig. 9). This change can be explained with the improvement of telecommunication technologies in that time, which eventually enabled the development of telemedicine.

Conclusion

The present study represents the first detailed scientometric analysis of the research regarding telemedicine. The data shows clearly a strong increase in research productivity. Using science citation analysis it can be assumed that there is a large increase of interest in telemedicine studies. While the majority of data originates from the USA, smaller countries such as Ireland and New Zealand take a lead in citation per item rankings. Future studies should address the development of the field after 2006.

Competing interests

The authors declare that they have no competing interests.

Authors' contributions

DAG, SR, MB, MS, AG and BK have made substantial contributions to the conception and design of the study, acquisition of the data and interpretation. They have been involved in drafting and revising the manuscript. All authors have read and approved the final manuscript.

Acknowledgement

We thank Dr Christian Scutaru for the establishment of the analysis unit and helpful comments. This study is part of a MD thesis project.

Funding acknowledgement statement

This research received no specific grant from any funding agency in the public, commercial, or not-for-profit sectors.

Author details

[1]Department of Health Economics, The Institute of Occupational Medicine, Social Medicine and Environmental Medicine, Goethe University Frankfurt, Theodor-Stern-Kai 7, 60590 Frankfurt, Germany. [2]Institute of Occupational Medicine, Charité School of Medicine, Thielallee 73, 14195 Berlin, Germany. [3]Health Economics, Department of Gynecology and Obstetrics, Goethe University Frankfurt, Theodor-Stern-Kai 7, 60590 Frankfurt, Germany.

References

1. Uibel S, Scutaru C, Mueller D, et al. Mobile air quality studies (MAQS) in inner cities: particulate matter PM10 levels related to different vehicle driving modes and integration of data into a geographical information program. J Occup Med Toxicol. Oct 2012;7.
2. Field MJ. Telemedicine: A Guide to Assessing Telecommunications in Health Care. Washington (DC)1996.
3. Spencer DC, Daugird AJ. The nature and content of telephone prescribing habits in a community practice. Fam Med. 1990;22(3):205–9.
4. Squibb NJ. Video transmission for telemedicine. J Telemed Telecare. 1999;5(1):1–10.
5. Jutras A. Teleroentgen diagnosis by means of video-tape recording. Am J Roentgenol Radium Ther Nucl Med. 1959;82:1099–102.
6. Groneberg-Kloft B, Fischer TC, Quarcoo D, Scutaru C. New quality and quantity indices in science (NewQIS): the study protocol of an international project. J Occup Med Toxicol. 2009;4:16.
7. Borger JA, Neye N, Scutaru C, et al. Models of asthma: density-equalizing mapping and output benchmarking. J Occup Med Toxicol. 2008;3 Suppl 1:S7. Feb 27.
8. Scutaru C, Quarcoo D, Sakr M, et al. Density-equalizing mapping and scientometric benchmarking of European allergy research. J Occup Med Toxicol. 2010;5:2.
9. Vitzthum K, Mache S, Quarcoo D, Scutaru C, Groneberg DA, Schoffel N. Scoliosis: density-equalizing mapping and scientometric analysis. Scoliosis. 2009;4:15.
10. Sevinc A. Web of science: a unique method of cited reference searching. J Natl Med Assoc. 2004;96(7):980–3.
11. Schoffel N, Mache S, Quarcoo D, et al. Rheumatoid arthritis: scientific development from a critical point of view. Rheumatol Int. 2010;30(4):505–13.
12. van Mark A, Vitzthum K, Hondorf F, Kloss L, Quarcoo D, Groneberg DA. Shift- and Nightwork - a scientometric analysis. Wien Med Wochenschr. 2011;161(7-8):209–16.
13. Vitzthum K, Scutaru C, Musial-Bright L, et al. Scientometric analysis and combined density-equalizing mapping of environmental tobacco smoke (ETS) research. PLoS One. 2010;5(6):e11254.
14. Gastner MT, Newman ME. From The Cover: Diffusion-based method for producing density-equalizing maps. Proc Natl Acad Sci U S A. 2004;101(20):7499–504.
15. Oeser R. Technologieunabhängige Systembetrachtung zur Umsetzung telemedizinischer Konzepte: Dissertation, Technische Universität Wien2001.
16. Dietzel G. Gesundheitstelematik, Telemedizin und eHealth - Deutsche und Europäische Perspektiven. Vol 2001: Telemedizinführer Deutschland; 2001.
17. Stranzinger E, Treumann TC, Dreier D. Teleradiologie bei notfallmäßigen Schädel-CT-Untersuchungen. Fortschr Röntgenstr. 2003;175(05):646–53.
18. Walz M, Klose, K.J., Wein, B. Bericht zu Teleradiologie-Aktivitäten und -Ergebnissen der ANARAD-Studie und AGIT. 1999; http://www.unimedizin-mainz.de/radiologie/agit/berichte/frameset_berichte.htm, aktualisiert 1.11.1999.
19. Bässler M. Andere Länder - andere Telemedizin?: Seminararbeit. 2006.
20. Ärzteblatt.de. Finnland: Sinkende Wartezeiten, 28.06.206. 2006; Online article. Available at: http://www.aerzteblatt.de/nachrichten/24728/Finnland-Sinkende-Wartezeiten. Accessed 28.06.2006, 2006.
21. W. MG. Telemedizin und Integrierte Versorgung, 26.10.2006, 3. DGIV Jahreskongress Forum Telemedizin. 2006; http://www.dgtelemed.de/downloads/dgiv-forum-6-meyer.pdf.

6

Chronic low back pain among French healthcare workers and prognostic factors of return to work (RTW)

B. Cougot[1,2], A. Petit[3], C. Paget[3], C. Roedlich[1], G. Fleury-Bahi[2], M. Fouquet[1], P. Menu[4], C. Dubois[4], C. Geraut[1], Y. Roquelaure[3] and D. Tripodi[1,2*]

Abstract

Background: Many factors influence the return to work of workers with chronic low back pain (CLBP). They have been said to vary according to socio-professional group. This study first aimed to compare prognostic factors influencing the return to work of CLBP healthcare workers (HCWs) and other workers (non-HCWs) after rehabilitation coupled with an occupational intervention. The second objective was to improve the evolution of indicators such as clinical examination, psychosocial impact and pain impact.

Methods: Between 2007 and 2012, a cohort of 217 CLBP workers (54.8 %-women; mean age = 41.3 ± 9.5 years, 118 non-HCWs; 99 HCWs mainly from the public sector) was included in an ambulatory rehabilitation program (standard physiotherapy or intensive network physiotherapy) coupled with an occupational intervention. Workers completed a questionnaire and had a clinical examination at baseline and after 24 months' follow up. Physical, social and occupational data was collected at the same time. Statistical analyses were performed to evaluate prognostic factors for return to work and compare the two worker populations.

Results: There was no difference between groups for the rate of OP (occupational physician) intervention or type of physiotherapy. 77.3 % of workers returned to work after 2 years following inclusion. To be an HCW (OR 0.1; 95 % CI [0.03–0.34]), to have less than 112 sick- leave days (OR 1.00; 95 % CI [0.93–1.00]), a small fingertip-floor distance (OR 0.96; 95 % CI [0.93–0.99]), a low anxiety/depression score (OR 0.97; 95 % CI [0.95–1.00]), a low impact of CLBP on daily life (OR 0.96; 95 % CI [0.93–1.00]), and on quality of life (OR 0.98; 95 % CI [0.95–1.00]) at baseline were statistically associated with return to work after 2 years of follow up. Only the profession (workplace) was statistically associated with return to work after 2 years of follow up using multivariate analysis.

Conclusion: To our knowledge, this is the first cohort study concerning predictive factors of RTW among CLBP workers after 2 years of follow up. Interventions in the work environment did not seem to predict job retention significantly. But only 50 % of the employees in both groups (HCW and non-HCW) had one intervention at their workplace after 2 years. This study underlined the fact that the type of physiotherapy with a well-trained physiotherapist used to take care of CLBP could not impact on the RTW forecast. To develop these initial results, it might be interesting to study the comparison between private and public sectors and to randomize the physiotherapeutic intervention.

* Correspondence: dominique.tripodi@chu-nantes.fr
[1]External Consultation on Occupational and Environmental Health, Department of Occupational and Environmental Health, Nantes University Hospital, 5 rue du Doyen Boquien, Nantes F 44 093, France
[2]Laboratory of Psychology of Pays de la Loire (LPPL - UPRES EA 4638), Nantes University - Faculty of Psychology, Nantes F 44 312, France
Full list of author information is available at the end of the article

Background

Chronic low back pain (CLBP) and identification of risk factors in evolution toward chronicity has been the subject of numerous controversial works [1]. This is a chronic pain syndrome (recurrent or continuous) in the lower back region, lasting for at least 3 months (with or without radiculalgia). In the USA, the prevalence of LBP is from 15 to 45 % according to cross-sectional studies. Data from Western countries is similar. UK estimates place LBP as the biggest single cause of absence from work in 1988–89, when it was responsible for about 12.5 % of all days of sickness absence [1]. The "low back pain triangle" (organic factor, socioprofessional factor and psychological factor) makes the need for multidisciplinary care obvious. Recent studies show: the need for networked care for the patient, including health actors as well as interlocutors within the company, to enhance diagnosis and care quality [2]; the effectiveness at 6 months of 3 weeks' multidisciplinary care on pain repercussions, disability and quality of life [3]; the slightly better impact of a functional restoration programme than of individual physiotherapy on absenteeism [4]; and the importance of educational and informational components in physical care (physical training) to improve patients' self confidence [5].

It is important to note that the feasibility of the care content needs scientific backing for better efficiency [6]. Moreover, it seems that a rigorous theoretical approach along with patient-centered listening would make it possible to remove obstacles linked to professional constraints [7]. In France, in 2008, the HAS Haute, Autorité de Santé (French National Authority for Health), recommended the following modalities for chronic pain care: ambulatory outpatient identification, assessment, and treatment setting, or a request for an opinion from specialized structures and guidance to the attending physician. We note that the occupational physician is not included in these recommendations (Circulaire DGOS/DH n°98–47, 12). To date, few studies have investigated the factors of continued employment in the public sector, including care services. Therefore, those studies pay little attention to organizational context or intervention in the workplace before the decision to return to work.

Aims of the study

The aim of this study was first to investigate prognosis factors for return to work at 2 years of a population of CLBP employees after care in a specialized occupational pathology consultancy with two main areas of intervention: conventional care in ambulatory functional rehabilitation and intervention by the OP in the company, comparing a population of healthcare workers (HCW) and a population of non-healthcare workers (non-HCW control group). The secondary objective was to analyze the overall effectiveness of the programme and the evolution of indicators such as clinical examination, psychosocial and pain impact.

Methods study design

A prospective cohort study, monitoring changes for a period of two years. Potential predictors for staying at work were initially recorded at baseline (T1), and their evolution after a physiotherapeutic and occupational approach was recorded at each follow-up visit, that is at 6 months, one year and two years.

Population

The workforce followed up by OPs in the department of Loire Atlantique (West of France) consisted of 472,483 employees in 2009. An information letter on the establishment of a Specialized Professional Pathology Consultancy for management of CLBP, based on the biopsychosocial model, along with the establishment of a link with the occupational physician or the company during sick-leave was sent out in 2006. The letter to General Practitioners (GPs) ($n = 800$) and OP ($n = 120$), explained the rules for inclusion in the programme. The initial multidisciplinary consultation was carried out by an OP, a rehabilitation physician and an occupational psychologist. This first meeting was to explore the factors involved in the LBP issue in a multidimensional perspective. If indications were raised, the patient was included in the protocol. Inclusion criteria were: to be between 18 and 65 years old, to be an employee in the care sector or outside the care sector, and to have suffered from LBP for more than three months. Exclusion criteria were: surgical indications, inflammatory disease (rheumatoid arthritis, ankylosing spondylitis...), or scalable lower back sciatica, fibromyalgia, being unemployed or self-employed.

Under a protocol of exploratory research, consultation was open to care staff in the public sector for 2 years (HCW reference group), and then to the private industrial and commercial sectors for 2 years (control group).

The intervention approach comprised two dimensions:

1. During the visit to decide on inclusion (T1) and after clinical examination by the rehabilitation physician and the OP, the principle of ambulatory physiotherapy was outlined to the patient: it was either a standard rehabilitation program with the patient's usual physiotherapist, or a more intensive program with a physiotherapist of the Regional CLBP network. The choice was determined by the distance between home and the physiotherapist's practice. A typical prescription was issued to the patient at the end of the consultation, explaining the principle and requesting a signed consent. Care by the patient's usual physiotherapist (MKH) comprised three sessions of 30 min per week for 5 weeks. Care

by the network physiotherapist included three one-hour sessions per week for 5 weeks. It was an active treatment excluding the use of any kind of passive technique, massage or acupuncture. The exercises were intended to promote flexibility, training, stretching, muscular strengthening, endurance working and proprioception exercises. The program also included an educational component, with learning exercises to be performed only at home. To minimize the risks associated with the resumption of sustained physical activity in the deconditioned subject, attention focused on the progressive nature of the program and on adapting techniques to the person. In addition to the 15 initial sessions, the patient might also receive five additional booster sessions during the following year.

2. During the inclusion visit (T1), a review of the curriculum and the link between pain and work was recorded by the OP and the occupational psychologist. This involved noting the patient's speech, his feelings in specific work situations, and the constraints perceived in the description of his work. The psychic balance involved in work is connected with the meaning of work, investment of personality in work, identity investment materialized in gesture. What, in the encounter between the organization of work and investment of the subject, could develop or worsen the subject's health?

This was a specific and single qualitative analysis of the situation. It included identifying (– if this had not already been done during the clinical interview with the doctor) satisfaction at work, historical items relating to the company and to the professional background, the quality of relationships with superiors and colleagues, pathogenic organizational practices, organizational changes, the arrival of a new manager, and new working techniques.

The various biomechanical and psychosocial risk factors were explained, as well as the interest in linking GP, OP and employer from a staying-at-work perspective. This second session took 60 min per patient on average. At the end of the consultation, a summary and a letter were dictated to the patient and sent to the principal correspondents, that is OPs and other doctors looking after the case, such as rheumatologists, physiotherapists, surgeons, pain specialists etc. The patient was sent a copy. At the end of the letter, appointments were proposed at six months (T2), twelve months (T3) and 24 months (T4). There was no interim relaunch. Follow-up consultations were carried out by the OP, who recorded the follow-up indicators.

Follow-up

Variables recorded during the medical visit for inclusion were: the number of days' sick leave (declarative data) before inclusion, clinical examination data, i.e. history of back pain or sciatica, smoking, comorbidity (psychiatric illness, chronic disease), level of pain intensity (visual analogic scale), weight, height, Schober index (10-cm Schober test), fingertip-floor distance, evaluation of the psychological impact of pain on social and professional life: Hamilton Anxiety Depression (HAD, Fear Avoidance Belief Questionnaire (FABQ), Dallas, and Quebec scales [8–11]. Work questionnaire: job description, employee's satisfaction at the workplace, vision of his future career, development training, and ways to improve on his job.

Variables collected during the follow-up were: employee satisfaction at the workplace, the job maintenance of the employee at the workplace or at an adapted one, termination, sick leave absence, clinical examination data: level of pain intensity (visual analogic pain scale), weight, height, Schober index (10-cm Schober test), fingertip-floor distance, evaluation of the psychological impact of pain on social and professional life (HAD, FABQ), Dallas, and Quebec questionnaires. The work questionnaire mentioned the intervention of the OP in the subject's company, the way toward a return to the work, the individual's desire to keep his job or desire for a change of career.

Confronted with a large number of lost follow-up participants at two years, a recovery program was implemented from September to December 2012. A systematic callback of lost follow-up patients was organized by means of a standardized guided interview and operating engaging techniques. Patients were offered a consultation and/or the opportunity to respond to a questionnaire or to answer a few telephone questions. The primary objective here was to collect "staying at work" outcomes. The secondary objective was to improve the evolution of other indicators (clinical, psychosocial and impact of pain). The local Ethic Committee (Groupe Nantais d'Etudes Cliniques) approved the study.

Statistical analysis

Descriptive raw data of our two "HCW" and "control" groups are presented. Comparisons of means by student test or Wilcoxon test well modeled by a normal distribution were performed, and comparisons of percentages by chi-2 or Fisher test. A 5 % degree of significance was found. Univariate and multivariate regression models were used to evaluate prognostic factors for return to work. SAS (R) software Version 9.3 was used for data analysis.

Results

Description of the sample: 217 patients were included between January 2007 and December 2012. Among them, 21 were excluded on the basis of clinical criteria and 42 because they had less than 2 years' follow up. Consequently, 154 patients were included between January 2007 and December 2011, allowing a 2-year follow-up period.

Confronted with a large number ($n = 97$) of lost follow-up participants with two years' follow-up, a recovery program was implemented from September to December 2012. We were unable to contact 34 of the subjects at 2 years, so a total of 120 patients were included in the statistical analysis with complete data (Fig. 1). Both the two initial groups and the final group were comparable for each descriptive variable (no statistical difference due to lost follow-up patients).

Our initial cohort thus included a group of 99 carers mainly from the public sector (2/3 of them nursing assistants, 1/3 nurses and logistics services workers) and a group of 118 non-carers from the industrial or commercial sector and the private sector (drivers of heavy construction machinery, agricultural machinery drivers, construction workers and public works masons, painters, plumbers, electricians, cable installers of telecommunications agents, commercial agents' vehicle drivers, delivery drivers, mechanics, janitors, industrial cleaning agents).

Sociodemographic data: the mean age of our population was 41.3 +/− 9.5 years with no significant difference between the two groups; there was a total of 55 % women but the carer group included 88 % women. For other variables such as: marital and social status, there

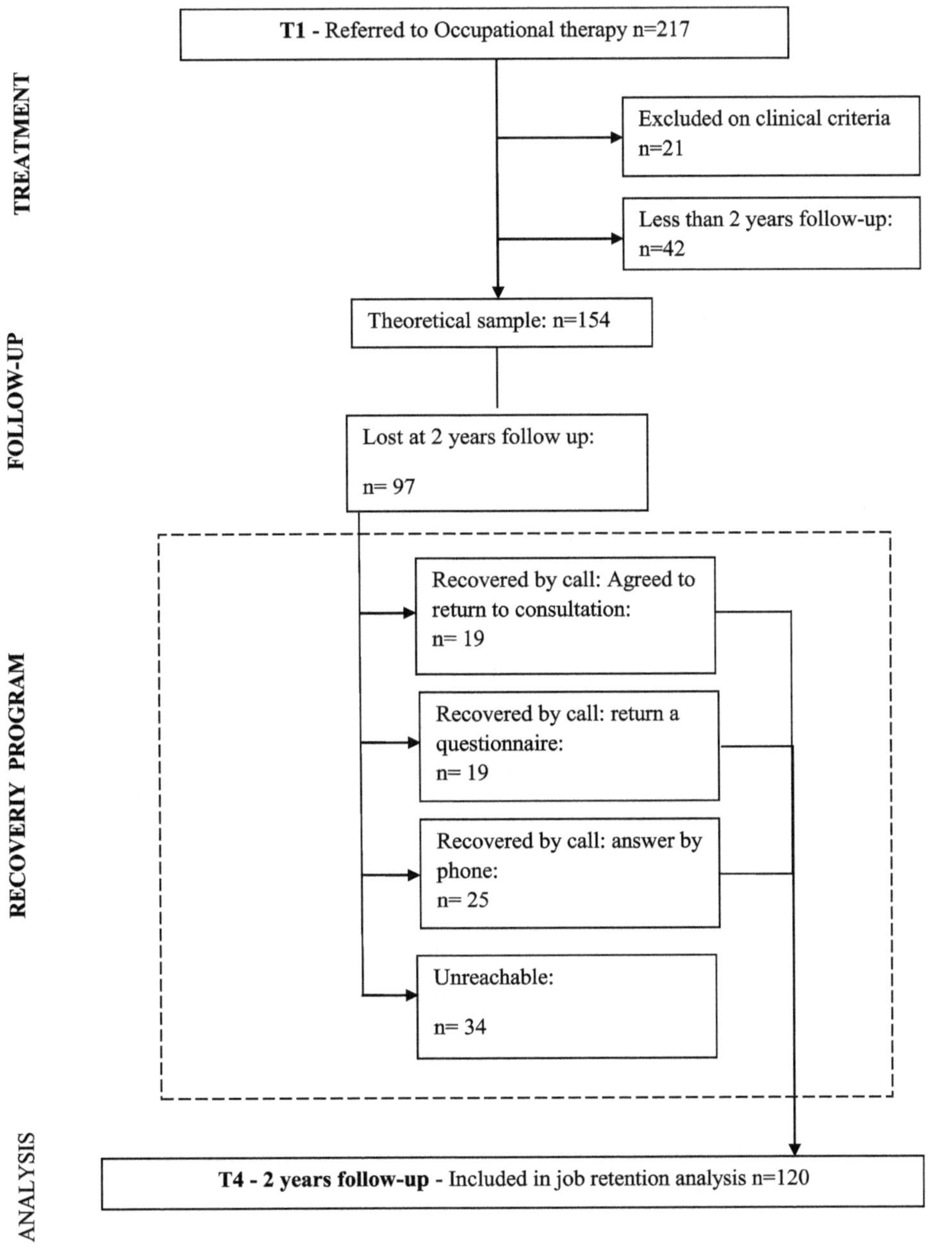

Fig. 1 Patients flow chart through the study

was no significant difference between the two groups (Table 1).

Professional Data: Job satisfaction: 78 % of patients reported job satisfaction with no significant difference between the two groups, but the number of days' sickness leave absence before inclusion was significantly higher in the non-HCW group (mean of 174.1 days versus 93.5 days; $p = 0.0002$).

Data relating to intervention: intervention in the workplace by the OP or guidance to change the job was involved in 49.5 % of cases in both groups. However the type of interventions were different for the two groups. In the HCW group, most interventions involved reclassification to "soft" jobs such as reception, admissions for nursing aides, technicians, or clinical research assistants for nurses. In the control group, there were most adjustments in the working conditions, such as modification of schedules, temporary part-time work, temporary drop loads to be handled, or ergonomic design of seats for drivers. The type of rehabilitation program did not differ between the two groups in terms of numbers of interventions, but differed according to the group in terms of orientation: carers more often consulted network physiotherapists, while employees in the private sector consulted their usual physiotherapist more frequently ($p = 0.0125$).

- Clinical and morphological data: weight and size were lower in the HCW group but the mean BMI was the same.
- Concerning pain before inclusion in the program: The pain level was lower in the HCW group (3.33 versus 4.53). Duration of pain was not significantly different between the two groups (HCW/92 days - non HCW/72 days, $p = 0.0001$). As regards the history of lumbago, radiculopathy, or the presence of comorbidity, including of psychiatric origin, there was no significant difference between the two groups.
- Psychosocial variables and impact of pain assessed by psychometric tests: scores for depression and anxiety (HAD) were slightly higher in the non-HCW group (depression = 7.62 versus 6.07; $p = 0.034$) but the mean scores remained within the thresholds of risk (10/20). Scores for avoidance of fear (FABQ) in the face of pain were similar in both groups at baseline. The impact of pain on the level of anxiety/depression, on daily activities and sociability (DALLAS) were significantly higher in the non-HCW group (daily activity = 60.5 versus 52.6; $p = 0.009$) (Table 1).

When analyzing the overall effectiveness of the program, effectiveness had been maintained at two years in terms of functional criteria (fingertip-floor distance), psychological factors including reduced apprehension and avoidance in relation to pain, decreased impact of pain on professional activities, daily activities and recreation (Table 2).

- The overall "staying at work" rate was 77 % at two years (Table 3).

The favorable prognostic factors at baseline for staying at work were, in our study, to be a carer, to have fewer than 112 days' sick leave, a small initial fingertip-floor distance, and low scores for the impact of anxiety, depression and daily discomfort. Satisfaction at work was a good predictor of staying at work after 2 years. (Tables 3 and 4).

Univariate analysis showed some positive prognostic factors for those included in the study for returning to or staying at work : being a carer (OR 0.1; 95 % CI [0.03–0.34]), a low fingertip-floor distance (OR 0.96; 95 %o CI [0.93; 0.99]), a low anxiety/depression score (OR 0.97; 95 %o CI [0.95; 1.00]), the functional impact of the pain (OR 0.96; 95 % CI [0.93–1.00]), and the impact of the pain on social relationships (OR 0.98; 95 % CI [0.95–1.00]) (Table 5).

Intervention by the physiotherapist seemed to show its effectiveness particularly when designed to support the chronic LBP with longer sessions (one hour) focusing on stretching and not on massage or focusing on self-rehabilitation at home; the effect was maintained over time. Intervention at the workplace did not seem to affect staying at work at this stage of the analysis. After multivariate analysis, only occupation remained a good prognosis factor for job retention at two years follow up (Table 6).

Discussion

To our knowledge, this is the first study that analyses RTW prognosis factors of workers with CLBP at 2 years' follow-up. The studies proposed in the scientific literature are based first on RTW rates and second on the method of CLBP management (individual = AIT or multidisciplinary = RFP). In our study, we found 77.3 % of RTW after 2 years of follow up. To date, we found in the literature only 5 weeks to 1 year of follow-up studies with very different return-to-work rates : 86 % at 5 weeks follow-up and 60 % at 3 months (12) [12], 70 % at one year [13], and 72 % completely recovered at 1 year [14]. One study compared FRP versus AIT at 6 months and demonstrated 69 % RTW with FRP versus 66.7 % RTW with AIT [15]; another showed 22 % RTW with only a brief vocationally oriented intervention, but there was no statistical difference from the control group [16]. Our study, with two years of follow up, highlighted predictive factors for staying at work before inclusion in the rehabilitation program, such as being a healthcare worker, a low rate of absenteeism, and care by a well-trained physiotherapist (physiotherapist of the Regional Network). Regarding the impact of physiotherapy, we compared

Table 1 Individual patient characteristics (T1) and "caring" procedure

Individual patient characteristics	Non-HCW	HCW	Total	*p*-value
	N = 118	*N* = 99	*N* = 217	
Sociodemographic factors				
Age [y, mean (SD)]	42.03 (9.32)	40.49 (9.72)	41,33 (9.51)	0.2361
Age (classes) (%)				
20–29	11.02 %	18.18 %	14.29 %	/
30–39	27.12 %	25.25 %	26.27 %	
40–49	41.53 %	37.37 %	39.63 %	
50–59	19.49 %	18.18 %	18.89 %	
60–69	0.85 %	1.01 %	0.92 %	
Sex (%)				
Female	27.12 %	87.88 %	54.84 %	*< 0.001*
Male	72.88 %	12.12 %	45.16 %	
Conjugal relationship with or without child (%)				
Yes	48.18 %	40.91 %	44.95 %	0.3067
No	51.82 %	59.09 %	55.05 %	
Socio-occupational factors				
Sick leave before inclusion on the study [days, mean (SD)]	174.13 (185)	93.45 (132)	136.93(168)	*0.0002*
Work Satisfaction (%)				
Yes	74.44 %	82.89 %	78.31 %	0.1881
No	25.56 %	17.11 %	21.69 %	
Clinical factors				
BMI [kg/m^2, mean (SD)]	24.67 (4.58)	24.04 (4.62)	24.39 (4.60)	0.3365
Weight [kg, mean (SD)]	73,95 (15.90)	66,61 (13.64)	70,63 (15.33)	*0.0005*
Height [cm, mean (SD)]	172.48 (9.53)	166.30 (8.40)	169.75 (9.54)	*<0.0001*
Cigarette Smoking [packs years, mean (SD)]	5.91 (9.70)	1.86 (4.54)	4.06 (8.01)	*0.0009*
Visual Analogic Pain Scale VAPS [mean (SD)]	4.53 (2.04)	3.33 (2.35)	3.99 (2.26)	*0.0001*
Duration of Pain [months, mean (SD)]	91.83 (93.04)	71.92 (82.66)	82.80 (88.84)	0.1011
Finger-Tip Score [cm, mean (SD)]	20.45 (14.73)	15.73 (17.40)	18.31 (16.13)	*0.0054*
Schober Index [cm, mean (SD)]	3.23 (1.42)	3.24 (1.15)	3.23 (1.30)	0.6855
Comorbidity (%)				
No-one	47.66(%)	60.00(%)	53.13(%)	0.1756
Others (cardiovascular, musculoskeletal…)	32.71(%)	28.24(%)	30.73(%)	
Phsychiatric Disorders	19.63(%)	11.76(%)	16.15(%)	
History of lumbago (%)				
Yes	53.10 %	56.38 %	54.59 %	0.6364
No	46.90 %	43.62 %	45.41 %	
History of sciatica (%)				
Yes	38.94 %	48.39 %	43.20 %	0.1731
No	61.06 %	51.61 %	56.80 %	
Psychosocial factors and impact of pain				
FABQ Activity [mean (SD)]	16.48 (6.13)	14.29 (7.49)	15.49 (6.85)	0.0517
FABQ Work [mean (SD)]	27.96 (11.88)	24.56 (10.64)	26.41 (11.42)	0.0698
QUEBEC [mean (SD)]	37.35 (15.67)	31.97 (19.53)	34.91 (17.67)	0.0615

Table 1 Individual patient characteristics (T1) and "caring" procedure *(Continued)*

HAD Anxiety Scale [mean (SD)]	10.08 (4.26)	9.01 (4.48)	9.60 (4.38)	0.1266
HAD Depression Scale [mean (SD)]	7.62 (5.33)	6.07 (3.82)	6.92 (4.75)	*0.0345*
DALLAS Anxiety/Depression [mean (SD)]	42.47 (26.77)	33.92 (26.13)	38.61 (26.74)	*0.0412*
DALLAS Work and Leisure [mean (SD)]	58.28 (20.42)	51.68 (24.85)	55.30 (22.70)	0.0637
DALLAS Daily Activities [mean (SD)]	60.54 (16.62)	52.58 (21.38)	56.95 (19.27)	*0.0098*
DALLAS Sociability [mean (SD)]	33.89 (26.47)	24.26 (20.25)	29.54 (24.28)	*0.0110*
Interventions				
Workplace interventions				
Yes	49.5 % (58)	49.5 %(49)	55,36 %	
No	50.5 % (60)	50.5 % (50)	44,64 %	
Physiotherapy				
None	6.06 %	5.13 %	5.65 %	*0.0125*
Trained Physiotherapist	54.55 %	33.33 %	45.20 %	
Not Trained Physiotherapist	39.39 %	61.54 %	49.15 %	
Physiotherapy [number of sessions, mean (SD)]	24.30 (31.94)	20.55 (12.11)	22.68 (25.36)	0.8205

Comparison of means by Student' test or Wilcoxon' test. Comparison of % by X^2 test or fisher' test

"standard care" by the physiotherapist (private financing), with treatment by a physiotherapist of the regional network which is more active, with stretching, muscular strengthening, and for longer sessions (private rehabilitation center with additional public financing). Our results showed that intervention by a trained physiotherapist to take care of CLBP might have very good results as regards preservation of the employment (univariate analysis). That would show the specificity of this type of rehabilitation and the need to train more physiotherapists to understand reconditioning during strain the education of patients through lifestyle advice and advice on good movements and postures for carrying loads or repetitive movements, to adapt exercises to each patient, including enabling auto-rehabilitation at home. In our study, HCWs had less often trained physiotherapists (Table 1), however they returned more often to work (Table 3). This may be explained by the fact that we have included in the study HCWs working in large public-sector organizations.

Similarly, 17 out of 19 HCWs with classic physiotherapy returned to work, 31 out of 31 with trained physiotherapists returned to work and the *p*-value for the HCW is $p = 0.0177$ (Table 4) : this is the test for trend including the no therapy group; this *p*-value is based on two successful observations only and therefore is not robust.

In addition, our study highlights predictors of job retention with a two-year follow-up, with a positive effect of the occupational factor (56.52 % versus 43.48 %; $p < 0.0001$). That was confirmed by multivariate analysis. This better level of RTW for HCW can be potentially explained by a better method of reintegrating public healthcare employees in France. Rehabilitation shows an overall positive effect on physical parameters but both

Table 2 Analysis of two year effectiveness of the rehabilitation program (T1 = start of the study, T4 = end of the study); only variables with a statistically significant effect ($p < 0.05$) after two years are reported in the table

Variables	N	T1	T4	T4 - T1	*p*-value
◊ Clinical factors					
Fingertip-floor distance [cm, mean (SD)]	64	21.96 (18,12)	13.88 (13,36)	- 8.09 (17,40)	<0.0001
◊ Psychosocial factors					
FABQ activity [mean (SD)]	54	15.85 (7,11)	13.35 (7,20)	−2.50 (7,60)	0.0191
FABQ work [mean (SD)]	54	27.24 (12,46)	23.57 (12,02)	−3.67 (11,46)	0.0225
QUEBEC [mean (SD)]	55	38.05 (20,24)	31.56 (21,44)	−6.49 (18,03)	0.0100
DALLAS work and leisure [mean (SD)]	60	57.00 (26,62)	48.95 (28,41)	−8.05 (26,74)	0.0231
DALLAS daily activities [mean (SD)]	60	58.13 (28,48)	48.98 (25,99)	−9.15 (22,62)	0.0027

Table 3 Potential predictive factors of return to work (RTW) at baseline (T1)

Predictive factors at T1		RTW = No	RTW = Yes	Total RTW	*p*-value
		N = 27	*N* = 92	*N* = 119	
Sociodemographic factors					
Age	Mean (SD)	42.07 (8.69)	39.83 (9.65)	40.42 (10.19)	0.3177
Sex (%)	Female	37.4	58.70	53.78	0.0472
	Male	62.9	41.3	46.22	
Conjugal relationship (%)	Yes	42.31	44.44	43.97	0.8467
	No	57.69	55.56	56.03	
Pain level					
Duration of pain (months)	Mean (SD)	99.48 (87.58)	85.07 (88.93)	84.34 (88.47)	0.2793
VAS (Visual Analogue Scale 1–10)	Mean (SD)	4.34 (2.29)	3.74 (2.23)	3.87 (2.25)	0.2976
Repetitive Lumbago history	Yes	66.67	57.61	59.66	0.3989
	No	33.33	42.39	40.34	
Recurrent Lombosciatica	Yes	48.15	45.65	46.22	0.8191
	No	51.85	54.35	53.78	
Comorbidity	0	34.62	58.43	53.04	0.0913
(0 = none; 1 = cardiovascular, others…; 2 = psychiatric)	1	42.31	29.21	32.17	
	2	23.08	13.36	14.78	
Tobacco (packs.years)	Mean (SD)	5.90 (11.50)	3.06 (6.39)	3.65 (7.74)	0.3137
Clinical examination data					
Weight (Kg)	Mean (SD)	72.37 (16.30)	68.61 (14.39)	69.47 (14.86)	0.2868
Height (cm)	Mean (SD)	170.58 (9.40)	169.33 (9.18)	169.61 (9.20)	0.5218
Body Mass Index (kg/m2)	Mean (SD)	24.96 (5.85)	23.81 (4.20)	24.07 (4.62)	0.4924
Fingertip-floor distance (cm)	Mean (SD)	26.65 (15.63)	17.03 (14.23)	19.15 (15.02)	0.0053
Schober index (10-cm Schober test)	Mean (SD)	2.94 (1.08)	3.22 (1.07)	3.16 (1.07)	0.4908
Occupational factors					
Absenteeism before inclusion (days)	Mean (SD)	196 (177)	111 (131)	129 (145)	0.0151
Work Satisfaction (%)	Yes	60.00	80.50	76.50	0.076
	No	40.00	19.50	23.50	
Occupation (%)	HCWs	11.11	56.52	46.22	<0.0001
	No Hcws	88.89	43.48	53.78	
Psychosocial factors and impact of the pain					
FABQ activity	Mean (SD)	16.67 (6.04)	14.56 (7.54)	14.96 (7.29)	0.1466
FABQ work	Mean (SD)	30.50 (9.47)	25.97 (12.44)	26.78 (12.04)	0.2795
QUEBEC scale	Mean (SD)	46.73 (17.14)	33.84 (19.40)	36.35 (19.56)	0.0272
HAD scale anxiety	Mean (SD)	10.25 (4.60)	9.00 (4.33)	9.24 (4.38)	0.3724
HAD scale Depression	Mean (SD)	7.69 (4.06)	6.33 (4.09)	6.59 (4.10)	0.1901
DALLAS Anxiety/Depression	Mean (SD)	57.19 (27.63)	37.64 (27.31)	41.32 (28.26)	0.0156
DALLAS Work and leisure	Mean (SD)	68.13 (18.98)	54.71 (24.59)	57.24 (24.12)	0.0610
DALLAS Daily activities	Mean (SD)	66.47 (14.98)	55.33 (20.89)	57.42 (20.31)	0.0644
DALLAS Sociability	Mean (SD)	44.84 (27.33)	29.17 (23.66)	32.12 (24.99)	0.0467
Intervention factors					

Table 4 Potential predictive factors for Return to Work: Healthcare Workers versus Non-Healthcare Workers

Predictive factors for RTW		« Healthcare Worker » group				« Non-Healthare Worker » group			
		RTW = No $N = 3$	RTW = Yes $N = 52$	Total $N = 55$	*p*-value	RTW = No $N = 24$	RTW = Yes $N = 40$	Total $N = 64$	*p*-value
Sociodemographic factors									
Age	Mean (SD)	43.67 (6.51)	40.06 (10.37)	40.25 (10.19)	0.5927	41.88(9.02)	39.78(8.48)	40.56(8.68)	0.3452
Sex	Female	3 (100.0 %)	45 (86.54 %)	48 (87.27 %)	1.0000	7 (29.17 %)	9 (22.50 %)	16 (25.00 %)	0.5510
	Male	0 (0.00 %)	7 (13.46 %)	7 (12.73 %)		17 (70.83 %)	31 (77.50 %)	48 (75.00 %)	
Conjugal relationship	Yes	1 (33.33 %)	23 (46.00 %)	24 (45.28 %)	1.0000	10 (43.48 %)	17 (42.50 %)	27 (42.86 %)	0.9398
	No	2 (66.67 %)	27 (54.00 %)	29 (54.72 %)		13 (56.52 %)	23 (57.50 %)	36 (57.14 %)	
Pain level									
Duration of pain (months)	Min-Max	[12.00,'72.00]	[2.00,384.00]	[2.00,384.00]	0.5547	[5.00,336.00]	[5.00,324.00]	[5.00,336.00]	0.2882
	Mean (SD)	35.33 (32.15)	83.38(90.69)	80.76(89.04)		107.50(89.31)	87.25(87.69)	94.84(88.15)	
	Median	22.00	36.00	36.00		102.00	60.00	66.00	
VAS Visual Analogue Scale TO	Min-Max	[2.00,3.00]	[0.00,9.00]	[0.00,9.00]	0.7343	[0.50,8.00]	[0.00,8.00]	[0.00,8.00]	0.9824
	Mean (SD)	2.50 (0.71)	3.14 (2.26)	3.11 (2.22)		4.51 (2.32)	4.48 (1.99)	4.49 (2.09)	
	Median value	2.50	3.00	3.00		4.55	5.00	5.00	
Repetitive Lumbago history	Yes	3 (100.0 %)	30 (57.69 %)	33 (60.00 %)	0.2667	15 (62.50 %)	23 (57.50 %)	38 (59.38 %)	0.6934
	No	0 (0.00 %)	22 (42.31 %)	22 (40.00 %)		9 (37.50 %)	17 (42.50 %)	26 (40.63 %)	
Recurrent Lumbosciatica	Yes	2 (66.67 %)	27 (51.92 %)	29 (52.73 %)	1.0000	11 (45.83 %)	15 (37.50 %)	26 (40.63 %)	0.5111
	No	1 (33.33 %)	25 (48.08 %)	26 (47.27 %)		13 (54.17 %)	25 (62.50 %)	38 (59.38 %)	
Comorbidity (0 = none; 1 = cardiovascular,	0	1 (33.33 %)	33 (66.00 %)	34 (64.15 %)	0.3853	8 (34.78 %)	19 (48.72 %)	27 (43.55 %)	0.5871
	1	2 (66.67 %)	13 (26.00 %)	15 (28.30 %)		9 (39.13 %)	13 (33.33 %)	22 (35.48 %)	
others…;2 = psychiatric)	2	0 (0.00 %)	4 (8.00 %)	4 (7.55 %)		6 (26.09 %)	7 (17.95 %)	13 (20.97 %)	
Tobacco (packs.years)	Min-Max Mean (SD)	[0.00,0.00]	[0.00,15.00]	[0.00,15.00]	0.5277	[0.00,45.00]	[0.00,30.00]	[0.00,45.00]	0.7779
		0.00 (0)	1.64	1.57		6.53	5.03	5.57	
Clinical examination data									
Weight (Kg)	Min-Max Mean (SD)	[62.00,70.00]	[42.00,90.00]	[42.00,90.00]	0.5799	[43.00,118.00]	[43.00,117.00]	[43.00,118.00]	0.7507
		66.17 (4.01)	64.55	64.64		73.15	73.90	73.62	
Height (cm)	Min-Max Mean (SD)	[160.00,160.00]	[150.00,187.00]	[150.00,187.00]	0.1520	[153.00,190.00]	[150.00,190.00]	[150.00,190.00]	0.4942
		160.00 (0)	166.58 (7.60)	166.33 (7.56)		171.46 (9.25)	172.85 (9.90)	172.32 (9.61)	
BMI	Mean	25.78 (2.21)	23.25 (4.40)	23.35 (4.35)	0.2491	24.89 (6.07)	24.53 (3.87)	24.67 (4.78)	0.7247
Fingertip-floor distance (cm)	Min-Max	[10.00,37.00]	[−5.00,90.00]	[−5.00,90.00]	0.6308	[0.00,57.00]	[0.00,45.00]	[0.00,57.00]	0.0289
	Mean (SD)	19.67 (15.04)	16.47 (15.96)	16.65 (15.79)		27.57 (15.79)	17.76 (11.76)	21.34 (14.07)	
	Median	12.00	16.50	16.00		25.00	19.00	22.00	

Table 4 Potential predictive factors for Return to Work: Healthcare Workers versus Non-Healthcare Workers *(Continued)*

	value								
Schober index (cm)	Min-Max	[2.00,4.00]	[1.00,7.00]	[1.00,7.00]		[0.00,5.00]	[1.50,5.00]	[0.00,5.00]	0.5258
	Mean (SD)	3.00 (1.00)	3.23 (1.16)	3.22 (1.14)		2.93 (1.11)	3.22 (0.94)	3.10 (1.01)	
	Median value	3.00	3.00	3.00		3.00	3.00	3.00	
Socio-occupational factors									
Absenteeism	Min-Max	[0.00,365.00]	[0.00,570.00]	[0.00,570.00]	0.7976	[0.00,720.00]	[0.00,540.00]	[0.00,720.00]	0.1189
Before inclusion (days)	Mean (SD)	142 (196)	91 (120)	94 (123)		204 (178)	134 (142)	161 (158)	
	Median value	60.00	47.00	53.50		140.00	83.50	110.00	
Job Satisfaction	Yes	1 (50.00 %)	36 (78.26 %)	37 (77.08 %)	0.4096	11 (61.11 %)	30 (83.33 %)	41 (75.93 %)	0.0961
	NO	1 (50.00 %)	10 (21.74 %)	11 (22.92 %)		7 (38.89 %)	6 (16.67 %)	13 (24.07 %)	
Psychosocial factors and impact of pain									
FABQ activity	Min-Max	[14.00,'24.00]	[0.00,42.00]	[0.00,42.00]	0.2288	[3.00,24.00]	[0.00,24.00]	[0.00,24.00]	0.3785
	Mean (SD)	18.67 5.03)	14.34 (8.56)	14.68 (8.37)		16.17 (6.37)	14.83 (6.22)	15.22 (6.21)	
	Median value	18.00	13.00	13.50		18.00	15.00	16.00	
FABQ work	Min-Max	[30.00,40.00]	[0.00,42.00]	[0.00,42.00]	0.1124	[14.00,42.00]	[2.00,42.00]	[2.00,42.00]	0.8801
	Mean (SD)	34.33 (5.13)	23.31 (12.36)	24.18 (12.28)		29.45 (10.28)	29.17 (11.98)	29.25 (11.41)	
	Median value	33.00	23.00	25.50		32.00	33.00	33.00	
QUEBEC scale	Min-Max	[34.00,71.00]	[5.00,72.00]	[5.00,72.00]	0.2717	[16.00,80.00]	[3.00,65.00]	[3.00,80.00]	0.0855
	Mean (SD)	46.67 (21.08)	32.58 (21.35)	33.75 (21.40)		46.7 (17.12)	35.28 (17.16)	38.63(17.74)	
	Median value	35.00	28.00	33.50		48.50	33.00	38.00	
HAD scale anxiety	Min-Max	[4.00,15.00]	[1.00,19.00]	[1.00,19.00]	0.2726	[3.00,18.00]	[3.00,17.00]	[3.00,18.00]	0.7932
	Mean (SD)	11.00 (6.08)	7.86 (4.31)	8.11 (4.45)		10.08 (4.48)	10.25 (4.05)	10.20 (4.13)	
	Median value	14.00	8.00	8.00		10.00	10.00	10.00	
HAD scale Depression	Min-Max	[5.00,10.00]	[0.00,14.00]	[0.00,14.00]	0.2182	[1.00,13.00]	[1.00,18.00]	[1.00,18.00]	0.6710
	Mean (SD)	8.00(2.65)	5.54(4.00)	5.74 (3.94)		7.62 (4.41)	7.19 (4.08)	7.31 (4.13)	
	Median value	9.00	4.00	5.00		9.00	7.00	7.00	
DALLAS Anxiety/ Depression	Min-Max	[50.00,80.00]	[0.00,85.00]	[0.00,85.00]	0.0785	[0.00,100.00]	[0.00,90.00]	[0.00,100.00]	0.1862
	Mean (SD)	60.00 (17.32)	31.28 (26.18)	33.44 (26.59)		56.54 (30.03)	45.00 (27.11)	48.33 (28.14)	
	Median value	50.00	25.00	30.00		65.00	48.75	55.00	
DALLAS Work and leisure	Min-Max	[35.00,85.00]	[2.50,90.00]	[2.50,90.00]	0.6099	[40.00,95.00]	[5.00,90.00]	[5.00,95.00]	0.1294
	Mean (SD)	61.67 (25.17)	51.88 (26.72)	52.61 (26.43)		69.62 (18.22)	57.98 (21.82)	61.34 (21.32)	
	Median value	65.00	57.50	60.00		70.00	60.00	65.00	

Table 4 Potential predictive factors for Return to Work: Healthcare Workers versus Non-Healthcare Workers *(Continued)*

DALLAS	Min-Max	[42.00,90.00]	[0.00,81.00]	[0.00,90.00]	0.3219	[45.00,87.00]	[24.00,93.00]	[24.00,93.00]	0.3713
Daily activities	Mean (SD)	66.00 (24.00)	49.86 (21.61)	51.08 (21.89)		66.58 (13.58)	61.64 (18.38)	63.07 (17.13)	
	Median value	66.00	54.00	55.50		69.00	64.50	66.00	
DALLAS	Min-Max	[35.00,45.00]	[0.00,75.00]	[0.00,75.00]	0.1345	[10.00,85.00]	[0.00,90.00]	[0.00,90.00]	0.5172
Sociability	Mean (SD)	40.00 (5.00)	22.70 (20.80)	24.00 (20.54)		45.96 (30.37)	36.64 (24.86)	39.33 (26.56)	
	Median value	40.00	20.00	20.00		50.00	35.00	35.00	
Intervention factors									
Ergonomic and OP intervention	Yes	0 (0.00 %)	24 (47.06 %)	24 (45.28 %)	0.4949	12 (54.55 %)	26 (70.27 %)	38 (64.41 %)	0.2225
	No	2 (100.0 %)	27 (52.94 %)	29 (54.72 %)		10 (45.45 %)	11 (29.73 %)	21 (35.59 %)	
Physiotherapy 0 = none 1 = classic	0	1 (33.33 %)	1 (2.04 %)	2 (3.85 %)	0.0177	2 (8.70 %)	2 (5.56 %)	4 (6.78 %)	0.7026
	1	2 (66.67 %)	17 (34.69 %)	19 (36.54 %)		13 (56.52 %)	18 (50.00 %)	31 (52.54 %)	
2 = trained physiotherapist	2	0 (0.00 %)	31 (63.27 %)	31 (59.62 %)		8 (34.78 %)	16 (44.44 %)	24 (40.68 %)	
Physiotherapy	Yes	1 (33.33 %)	1 (2.00 %)	2 (3.77 %)	0.1110	2 (8.33 %)	2 (5.41 %)	4 (6.56 %)	0.6427
	No	2 (66.67 %)	49 (98.00 %)	51 (96.23 %)		22 (91.67 %)	35 (94.59 %)	57 (93.44 %)	
	Min-Max	[0.00,'20.00]	[0.00,100.00]	[0.00,100.00]	0.5231	[0.00,300.00]	[0.00,60.00]	[0.00,300.00]	0.2150
Physiotherapy (number of training sessions)	Mean (SD)	13.33 (11.55)	20.70 (13.53)	20.28 (13.44)		41.13 (62.31)	20.32 (12.30)	28.51 (41.04)	

Table 5 Odds ratios (OR) and confidence interval for keeping job after 2 years

Pronostic factors	N	OR	IC 95 %	*p*-value
Carer: no vs yes	119	0.10	[0.03; 0.34]	*0.0003*
Fingertip-floor distance	118	0.96	[0.93; 0.99]	*0.0079*
DALLAS Anxiety/Depression	85	0.97	[0.95; 1.00]	*0.0164*
Sick leave	108	1.00	[0.99; 1.00]	*0.0190*
QUEBEC	77	0.96	[0.93; 1.00]	*0.0267*
DALLAS Social comportment	85	0.98	[0.95; 1.00]	*0.0282*
Gender : female vs male	119	2.42	[1.00; 5.85]	0.0506
DALLAS work and leisure	85	0.97	[0.94; 1.00]	0.0523
DALLAS daily activities	85	0.97	[0.94; 1.00]	0.0523
Work satisfaction: no vs yes	102	0.36	[0.13; 1.04]	0.0585
Physiotherapy (0 = none; 1 = liberal; 2 = trained physiotherapy) 0 vs 2	111	0.17	[0.03; 1.00]	0.0621
Physiotherapy (0 = none; 1 = liberal; 2 = trained physiotherapy) 1 vs 2	111	0.40	[0.15; 1.04]	.
Comorbidity (0 = none; 1 = other; 2 = psy) 0 vs 2	115	3.15	[0.93; 10.68]	0.1006
Comorbidity (0 = none; 1 = other; 2 = psy) 1 vs 2	115	1.29	[0.38; 4.36]	.
Physiotherapy (n sessions): 0 vs >0	114	0.29	[0.05; 1.51]	0.1399
FABQ work	78	0.97	[0.91; 1.02]	0.2060
HAD Depression	83	0.92	[0.81; 1.05]	0.2351
Pain intensity	113	0.89	[0.72; 1.09]	0.2465
Weight	119	0.98	[0.96; 1.01]	0.2495
Schober index	106	1.30	[0.83; 2.02]	0.2507
Body mass index	115	0.95	[0.87; 1.04]	0.2731
Age	119	0.97	[0.93; 1.02]	0.2972
HAD scale anxiety	83	0.94	[0.82; 1.06]	0.3055
FABQ activity	79	0.96	[0.89; 1.04]	0.3160
Cigarette smoking : 0 vs >0	102	1.65	[0.60; 4.52]	0.3296
Lumbago history : no vs yes	119	1.47	[0.60; 3.62]	0.4005
Pain duration	119	1.00	[0.99; 1.00]	0.4562
Height	115	0.99	[0.94; 1.03]	0.5410
Sciatalgia history : no vs yes	119	1.11	[0.47; 2.61]	0.8191
Maried : no vs yes	116	0.92	[0.38; 2.21]	0.8467

Level of significance based on logistic regression analysis. $p < 0.05$ in italics.

rehabilitation programme and intervention in the workplace does not seem to predict job retention. The studies published so far about the healthcare sector show a strong link between CLBP and biomechanical risk factors, CLBP and psychosocial risk factors as evidenced by numerous cohort studies [6, 17–22] and recent case–control studies [23–27]. There is no study in the literature to date showing the effectiveness of dual management involving both functional rehabilitation and action at the workplace. Nonetheless, further research is needed on possible interactions between the effect of intervention at the workplace and the effect of the physiotherapy factor.

On the level of absenteeism, people who have been on long-term sickness leave seem to have greater difficulty in returning to work. This variable was highlighted in some studies but only after 6 or 12 months [13]. Concerning the clinical criteria, a low fingertip-floor distance seems to be a factor for good prognosis; the initial severity of the pain and RTW are not linked as evidenced by other authors who highlighted chronicity factors such as the intensity of the initial pain, apprehension, psychosocial factors and the intensity of the work [17, 19]. Physiotherapeutic care with education of the patients could decrease this "phobia" of movement and apprehension of pain that probably play a role in the delayed resumption of activities. We also highlighted a significant improvement in the scores estimating the perception of the pain and the psychosocial data, the decrease in apprehension of

Table 6 Potential predictive factors of RTW: multivariate analysis, only variables with $p < 0.15$ were selected

Potential predictive factors	N	OR	IC	*p*-value
Absenteeism	71	1.00	[0.99; 1.01]	0.6562
Comorbidity : 0 vs 2		1.95	[0.12; 32.08]	0.2061
Comorbidity : 1 vs 2		0.23	[0.02; 3.38]	
Physiotherapy		0.95	[0.87; 1.04]	0.2629
Satisfaction at work: no vs yes		0.13	[0.01; 1.52]	0.1045
HCW : no vs yes		0.02	[0.00; 0.62]	0.0249
DALLAS anxiety/depression		0.96	[0.90; 1.02]	0.1577
DALLAS work and leisure		0.99	[0.92; 1.06]	0.7587
DALLAS daily activities		1.04	[0.94; 1.14]	0.4413
Fingertip-floor distance		0.98	[0.89; 1.09]	0.7639
FABQ work		1.07	[0.95; 1.21]	0.2340
Quebec		0.97	[0.89; 1.06]	0.5185
Sex: female vs male		0.08	[0.00; 1.45]	0.0878
Sociability		1.00	[0.95; 1.06]	0.9445

the pain between T1 and T4 (Table 2). Initial pain is thus a variable important to consider, but we should not neglect the psychosocial aspects, being able to be at the origin of a resumption of work pushed away that we were able to highlight in our study through the analysis of the QUEBEC and DALLAS questionnaires.

In our study, interventions in the work environment did not seem to predict significantly job retention. However only 50 % of the employees in the both groups (HCW and non-HCW) had one intervention at their workplace after 2 years. These were most often implemented by the OP of the company, the supervisor, or on the employee's initiative. The difference between the HCW group and the non-HCW group could be due to the various interventions and the proposals made in every group, as for example: in the hospital sector, professional reassignment usually takes place in admission consultation, outpatient services, telephone reception, post office consultation; while in the industrial or commercial private sector, it especially involves ergonomic arrangements, set-up of workstations with purchase of an adapted seat, change of desk, or ample room to move, ergonomic arrangement of the controls or modification of the traveled distance for the commercial workers. In France, another by no means obvious element to consider, is the possibility of a therapeutic or part-time/half-time resumption of work in the General Healthcare Insurance System for the private sector; while for public workers part-time or half-time resumption of work is possible only after at least 6 months of sick leave, which is most probably a brake on an early return to work. The best way to intervene would thus be to identify patients with a high risk of chronic pain and introduce preventive measures to reduce the risk of delayed healing. Interventions in the work environment and physiotherapy seem to be obvious ways to achieve this, thereby enabling a resumption of activities in the best possible conditions. This is what we tried to set up in this study over 2 years, with 6 months, 1 and 2 year follow-up consultations. The repetition of those consultations allowed us to adjust the care before the end of the program, for example by proposing new physiotherapy sessions and/or adjustments to work stations or schedules. They also made it possible to safeguard a professional activity that would not have been possible with a more intensive program requiring work schedule arrangements or hospitalization as in the most intensive programmes. To date, we find no study in the literature showing the efficiency of double coverage involving both simultaneous intervention by a trained physiotherapist and action at the workplace. However, our study needs to follow up its investigations by quantifying more exactly the types of job design and the modalities of resumption of work in the private and public sector.

Our study has some limitations

An insufficient number of trained therapists, the low number of subjects ($N = 120$) and a large number of variables, the number of lost participants (67 % at two years, reduced to 22 % thanks to the program of phone call reminders and emails), the absence of randomization, so it is not really a RCT. The two groups are non-comparable in terms of sex, professional sector (public-private), but comparable in terms of number of interventions in the workplace and number of sessions of physiotherapy. At this stage, our multivariate analysis should be approached with cautions.

Our rehabilitation programme with trained physiotherapists, and interventions in the workplace did not show statistically significant effectiveness probably because of lack of power of the study; indeed, our cohort should be developped.

Interventions in the workplace are not of the same type in hospitals and in the "control area", especially in the industrial sector: in the first case, the employees especially benefited from professional outplacement to suitable posts such "advice", phone reception, courier in the second case, it was mainly ergonomic improvements with purchase of ergonomic seats, changes of work tables, modifying career path for businessmen. Our study therefore requires further investigation involving quantifying more precisely the types of work adjustments by sector. Another area to investigate would be the return to work modalities, which vary between the public and the private sector in France. In the private sector, employees are affiliated to the General Regime of Social Security and physicians may ask for any person who has stopped work a "therapeutic half-time" or a "therapeutic part-time" return to work. In the public sector, French legislation prescribes a period of six months off work before allowing a half-time or part-time return to work, which is probably an obstacle to an early return to work. Overall, these considerations deserve to be supported by a further study.

Competing interests
The authors declare they have no competing interests.

Authors' contributions
The research reported in this article was supported by the Nantes University Hospital, the Pays de Loire Regional Health Agency (ARS des Pays de Loire). DT, MD, PhD, contributed significantly to the development of this research project, the inclusion of the patients helped by CD, AP, and PM; they all contributed significantly to the development the project and testing of patients. BC, Master 2 grade research from the Psychology Laboratory of Pays de Loire, elaborated the recovery program, and actively participated in editing of the paper. MF, occupational psychologist, participated in the workers' interviews when included in the study. AP, postgraduate researcher from at the LEEST (Laboratory of Ergonomic Epidemiology and Occupational Health, Angers, France) took part in the regional development of the project, including the clinical examination of patients, and in the critical analysis of the study. CP, medical intern from the department of Occupational and Environmental Health, participated in the clinical examination of the patients and wrote up the discussion of the paper. MF contributed to the clinical and psychological approach. All authors read and approved the final manuscript. We gratefully acknowledge professor Yves Roquelaure, director of the LEEST (Laboratory of Ergonomic Epidemiology and Occupational Health, Angers, France), Professor Christian Geraut, Professor Emeritus, member of the French National Academy of Medicine, and Professor Ghozlane Fleury Bahi, director of the LPPL (Psychology Laboratory of Pays de la Loire), who so generously support this study. We particularly thank Christèle Volteau of the Department of Biostatistics (Plateforme de Biométrie, CHU Nantes) for the data analysis. Furthermore, we would like to thank all occupational and health practitioners, physiotherapists and trained physiotherapists who took part in the study. We thank them for their helpful comments and suggestions on this paper and all participating patients, health practitioners and occupational health practitioners for their time and effort.

Author details
[1]External Consultation on Occupational and Environmental Health, Department of Occupational and Environmental Health, Nantes University Hospital, 5 rue du Doyen Boquien, Nantes F 44 093, France. [2]Laboratory of Psychology of Pays de la Loire (LPPL - UPRES EA 4638), Nantes University - Faculty of Psychology, Nantes F 44 312, France. [3]Laboratory of Ergonomics & Epidemiology in Occupational Health, LEEST, UA-InVS - IFR 132, UPRES EA 4336 Faculty of Medicine, University of Angers, Angers F 49 000, France. [4]Physical Medicine Rehabilitation Department, Nantes University Hospital, 85 rue Saint Jacques, Nantes F 44 093, France.

References
1. Ramond A, Bouton C, Richard I, Roquelaure Y, Baufreton C, Legrand E, et al. Psychosocial risk factors for chronic low back pain in primary care–a systematic review. Fam Pract. 2011;28(1):12–21.
2. Andersson GB. Epidemiological features of chronic low-back pain. Lancet. 1999;354(9178):581–5.
3. Ammendolia C, Cassidy D, Steensta I, Soklaridis S, Boyle E, Eng S, et al. Designing a workplace return-to-work program for occupational low back pain: an intervention mapping approach. BMC Musculoskelet Disord. 2009;10:65.
4. Moradi B, Hagmann S, Zahlten-Hinguranage A, Caldeira F, Putz C, Rosshirt N, et al. Efficacy of multidisciplinary treatment for patients with chronic low back pain: a prospective clinical study in 395 patients. J Clin Rheumatol Pract Rep Rheum Musculoskelet Dis. 2012;18(2):76–82.
5. Roche-Leboucher G, Petit-Lemanac'h A, Bontoux L, Dubus-Bausière V, Parot-Shinkel E, Fanello S, et al. Multidisciplinary intensive functional restoration versus outpatient active physiotherapy in chronic low back pain: a randomized controlled trial. Spine. 2011;36(26):2235–42.
6. Sorensen PH, Bendix T, Manniche C, Korsholm L, Lemvigh D, Indahl A. An educational approach based on a non-injury model compared with individual symptom-based physical training in chronic LBP. A pragmatic, randomised trial with a one-year follow-up. BMC Musculoskelet Disord. 2010;11:212.
7. Kamioka H, Okuizumi H, Okada S, Takahashi R, Handa S, Kitayuguchi J, et al. Effectiveness of intervention for low back pain in female caregivers in nursing homes: a pilot trial based on multicenter randomization. Environ Health Prev Med. 2011;16(2):97–105.
8. Scott NA, Moga C, Harstall C. Managing low back pain in the primary care setting: the know-do gap. Pain Res Manag J Can Pain Soc J Société Can Pour Trait Douleur. 2010;15(6):392–400.
9. Friedman S, Samuelian JC, Lancrenon S, Even C, Chiarelli P. Three-dimensional structure of the Hospital Anxiety and Depression Scale in a large French primary care population suffering from major depression. Psychiatry Res. 2001;104(3):247–57.
10. Chaory K, Fayad F, Rannou F, Lefèvre-Colau M-M, Fermanian J, Revel M, et al. Validation of the French version of the fear avoidance belief questionnaire. Spine. 2004;29(8):908–13.
11. Yvanes-Thomas M, Calmels P, Béthoux F, Richard A, Nayme P, Payre D, et al. Validity of the French-language version of the Quebec back pain disability scale in low back pain patients in France. Jt Bone Spine Rev Rhum. 2002;69(4):397–405.
12. Marty M, Blotman F, Avouac B, Rozenberg S, Valat JP. Validation of the French version of the Dallas Pain Questionnaire in chronic low back pain patients. Rev Rhum Engl. 1998;65(2):126–34.
13. Roche G, Ponthieux A, Parot-Shinkel E, Jousset N, Bontoux L, Dubus V, et al. Comparison of a functional restoration program with active individual physical therapy for patients with chronic low back pain: a randomized controlled trial. Arch Phys Med Rehabil. 2007;88(10):1229–35.
14. Oyeflaten I, Hysing M, Eriksen HR. Prognostic factors associated with return to work following multidisciplinary vocational rehabilitation. J Rehabil Med. 2008;40(7):548–54.
15. Henschke N, Maher CG, Refshauge KM, Herbert RD, Cumming RG, Bleasel J, et al. Prognosis in patients with recent onset low back pain in Australian primary care: inception cohort study. BMJ. 2008;337:a171.
16. Jousset N, Fanello S, Bontoux L, Dubus V, Billabert C, Vielle B, et al. Effects of functional restoration versus 3 h per week physical therapy: a randomized controlled study. Spine. 2004;29(5):487–93. discussion 494.
17. Magnussen L, Strand LI, Skouen JS, Eriksen HR. Motivating disability pensioners with back pain to return to work–a randomized controlled trial. J Rehabil Med. 2007;39(1):81–7.
18. Eriksen W, Bruusgaard D, Knardahl S. Work factors as predictors of sickness absence attributed to airway infections; a three month prospective study of nurses' aides. Occup Environ Med. 2004;61(1):45–51.
19. Jansen JP, Morgenstern H, Burdorf A. Dose–response relations between occupational exposures to physical and psychosocial factors and the risk of low back pain. Occup Environ Med. 2004;61(12):972–9.
20. Harling M, Schablon A, Nienhaus A. Validation of the German version of the Nurse- Work Instability Scale: baseline survey findings of a prospective study of a cohort of geriatric care workers. J Occup Med Toxicol. 2013;8:33.
21. Peter Koch P, Aki Pietsch A, Melanie Harling M, Susanne Behl-Schön S, Albert Nienhaus A. Evaluation of the Back College for nursing staff. J Occup Med Toxicol. 2014;9:32.
22. Harling M, Schablon A, Peters C, Nienhaus A. Predictive values and other quality criteria of the German version of the Nurse-Work Instability Scale (Nurse-WIS) - follow-up survey findings of a prospective study of a cohort of geriatric care workers. J Occup Med Toxicol. 2014;9:30.
23. Bardak AN, Erhan B, Gündüz B. Low back pain among caregivers of spinal cord injured patients. J Rehabil Med. 2012;44(10):858–61.
24. Mitchell T, O'Sullivan PB, Smith A, Burnett AF, Straker L, Thornton J, et al. Biopsychosocial factors are associated with low back pain in female nursing students: a cross-sectional study. Int J Nurs Stud. 2009;46(5):678–88.
25. Feng C-K, Chen M-L, Mao I-F. Prevalence of and risk factors for different measures of low back pain among female nursing aides in Taiwanese nursing homes. BMC Musculoskelet Disord. 2007;8:52.

26. Bos E, Krol B, van der Star L, Groothoff J. Risk factors and musculoskeletal complaints in non-specialized nurses, IC nurses, operation room nurses, and X-ray technologists. Int Arch Occup Environ Health. 2007;80(3):198–206.
27. Alexopoulos EC, Burdorf A, Kalokerinou A. A comparative analysis on musculoskeletal disorders between Greek and Dutch nursing personnel. Int Arch Occup Environ Health. 2006;79(1):82–8.

7

Wellbeing and occupational risk perception among health care workers: a multicenter study in Morocco and France

Doina Ileana Giurgiu[1,2], Christine Jeoffrion[3], Christine Roland-Lévy[4], Benjamin Grasset[1,3], Brigitte Keriven Dessomme[5], Leila Moret[5], Yves Roquelaure[6], Alain Caubet[7], Christian Verger[7], Chakib El Houssine Laraqui[8], Pierre Lombrail[9], Christian Geraut[1] and Dominique Tripodi[1,3*]

Abstract

Background: The study analyzes health care workers' (HCWs) occupational risk perception and compares exposure to occupational risk factors in Moroccan and French hospitals.

Method: Across nine public hospitals from three Moroccan regions (north, center and south), a 49 item French questionnaire, based on the Job Content Questionnaire, and 4 occupational risks subscales, was distributed to 4746 HCWs. Internal consistency of the study was determined for each subscale. Confirmatory factor analysis was conducted on the Moroccan questionnaire. Psychosocial job demand, job decision latitude and social support scores analysis was used to isolate high strain jobs. Occupational risks and high strain perception correlation were analyzed by univariate and multivariate logistic regression. A comparative analysis between Moroccan and French (Nantes Hospitals) investigations data was performed.

Results: In Morocco, 2863 HCWs (60 %) answered the questionnaire (54 % women; mean age 40 years; mean work seniority 11 years; 24 % physicians; 45 % nurses). 44 % Moroccan HCWs are at high strain. Casablanca region (1.75 OR; CI: 1.34–2.28), north Morocco (1.66 OR; CI: 1.27–2.17), midwives (2.35 OR; 95 % CI 1.51–3.68), nursing aides (1.80 OR; 95 % CI: 1.09–2.95), full-time employment (1.34 OR; 95 % CI 1.06–1.68); hypnotics, sedatives use (1.48 OR; 95 % CI 1.19–1.83), analgesics use (1.40 OR; 95 % CI 1.18–1.65) were statistically associated to high strain. 44% Moroccan HCWs are at high strain versus 37 % French (Nantes) HCWs ($p < 0.001$).

Conclusion: Moroccan HCWs have high strain activity. Moroccan HCWs and more Moroccan physicians are at high strain than Nantes HCWs. Moroccan and French's results showed that full time workers, midwives, workers using hypnotics, and analgesics are at high strain. Our findings underscore out the importance of implementing a risk prevention plan and even a hospital reform. Further research, with an enlarged study pool will provide more information on psychosocial risks (PSR) and HCWs' health.

Keywords: Occupational stress, Risk exposure, High strain, Public hospital, Medication use

* Correspondence: dominique.tripodi@chu-nantes.fr
[1]Department of Occupational Medicine and Environment Health, HCWs Research Laboratory, 5 rue du doyen Boquien, Nantes University Hospital, Nantes 44 093, France
[3]Psychology Laboratory of Pays de la Loire (LPPL - UPRES EA 4638), Department of Psychology, University of Nantes, BP 81 227 44312 Nantes cedex 3, France
Full list of author information is available at the end of the article

Background

The workplace is now regarded as a key player in the origin of various illnesses and as a determinant of the individual's well-being, along with the individual's lifestyle. In recent years occupational health, particularly occupational mental health, has been the subject of particular attention. Health at work has become a major concern in our society and a priority in public health [1]. Among numerous risks found in the workplace, one group, covering various risks, has lately emerged as a major public health concern and a challenge to the occupational health research field: the psychosocial risks (PSR). PSR are not just another type of risk factors, but one to be found at the center of the complex architecture of work conditions.

The French Ministry of Work and Employment (2013) describes the concept of PSR as "risks to health, mental as well as physical, created at least by work through social and psychological mechanisms". PSR include stress, internal violence and external violence (INRS[1]). Internal violence involves physical or verbal abuse, bullying, intimidation, and conflicts with colleagues or managers; it includes situations of moral and sexual harassment. People in the workplace produce PSR towards others. External violence is carried out towards employees, in the working context, by people from outside the organization it-self (users, families, providers and suppliers, customers, consumers, etc.). The most exposed workstations are those in contact with the public, specifically when dealing with people in precarious situations or having psychological problems.

It seems necessary to distinguish the concept of "risk", i.e. the probability of being confronted to risk, thus creating "risk factors", from "disorder", which is a consequence of exposure to risk. A large number of studies, in the medical sector and particularly in the hospital context [2–6], have shown the importance of PSR in terms of consequences on both physical and mental health. These studies show that the influence of negative organizational climate on nurses' health [7], along with interactions between physical and PSR factors which can generate musculoskeletal disorders [8]. The impact of occupational safety climate in hospitals confirms the link between PSR and workers' health [9]. In Europe, according to recent work conditions surveys, the influence of psychosocial risk factors in the workplace ranked second in the recent major developments hierarchy [10]. The European Agency for Safety and Health at Work (EU-OSHA), in its report on emerging risks [11] indicated that there is a strong correlation between eight variables (size of establishment; whether the establishment is a part of a larger entity; sector (public or private); gender composition of establishment's workforce; age; composition of establishment's workforce; proportion of foreigners in establishment's workforce; sector of activity; country) considered for inclusion in the Occupational Safety Health composite score. An imbalance between the number of industrial accidents and the number of occupational illnesses has also been noted: even if the first is decreasing, the latter is increasing [12]. In France, indicators defined by experts enable us to demonstrate that the workplace PSR factors often contribute to the occurrence of health problems, such as cardiovascular diseases, mental health disorders or musculoskeletal disorders [13].

As the workforce in the European Union (EU) is ageing and the work intensity is constantly increasing, questions on steps to be taken to keep the workforce active have arisen along with the need for a well-designed policy [14]. The over 40 million people in the EU suffering from consequences of work-related stress, which translates into over 20 billion € of health and absenteeism costs [15], contributes to underlining the economic and social importance of addressing the issue of work-related PSR.

The guidelines of the European Commission (EC) on work-related stress itemized the steps to be taken, of which the first was identifying the risk, with its sources and consequences, by the means of monitoring "job content, working conditions, terms of employment, social relations at work, health, well-being and productivity" [16]. One of the important methods for detecting work-related stress, i/e. PSR, is to use a risk-perception evaluation; the individual's subjective experience will be the generator of symptoms and diseases, going from transient increase in heart rate and blood pressure to developing cardiovascular diseases, and from brief anxiety or depression to serious mental health problems. The EC, in its *Improving quality and productivity at work. Community strategy 2007–2012 on health and safety at work*, has identified a significant proportion of employees who acknowledged the impact work has on their health: "35% of workers on average feel that their job puts their health at risk" [17].

Psycho-social strain is not limited to European workplaces. However, intercontinental comparisons of stress in the workplace are rare. Among these few studies, this study compares Morocco and France, which is quite interesting as labour laws in Morocco are close to French laws. Furthermore, in hospitals, the work organization is similar in both countries. Therefore, in this paper, we analyse the Moroccan situation and compare it to the French one. Currently, international comparative studies on occupational risks in the public hospitals are scarce and only few researchers concentrated on psychosocial stress in Moroccan HCWs [18–22].

Even though Karasek's JCQ was translated, tested and used in many different countries [23–30], none focused on Moroccan HCWs' PSR perception. Studies in health care concentrate mainly on nurses, probably because it is a rather homogenous group that is quite easy to access, contrary to more sensitive groups such as physicians, who are a complex target. In fact, some studies even excluded physicians because of the difficulty in obtaining a significant number of responses [27]. As Robert Karasek has already stated in his 1998 study on psychosocial job assessment through JCQ [28], one of the problems with demanding jobs holders is their reluctance to participate in research projects.

The aim of the present study is twofold: (i) to assess risk perception among Moroccan HCWs, including physicians, using a validated questionnaire; and (ii) to make an analysis of exposure to occupational risk factors variance in Moroccan public hospitals. Special attention was given to the different aspects which influence the occurrence of "high strain" situations: mainly ergonomics and overall working conditions. The study aimed at making a comparative evaluation of perceived risks in the healthcare sector of Morocco and France, by analyzing comparable structures. The main goal was to find out if, in comparable structures from different cultures, with similar occupational categories, stress was perceived in the same manner or not. The concluding goal was to develop a model for high strain perception to be of use for crafting and implementing a specific prevention plan.

Methods

The study was a cross-sectional multicenter investigation, conducted in French and Moroccan public hospitals, in which labor laws, as well as the work organization, are very similar.

Moroccan public hospitals were selected from the three Moroccan regions: north, center and south. On Morocco, the north region hospitals were those of Kenitra, Oujda and Larache; the southern region hospitals were those of Agadir and Marrakech. The center region or the Casablanca region covered Baouafi, Sekkat, Settat and Khouribga's hospitals. The Moroccan Public Health Ministry's authorization was obtained before beginning the investigation.

The same investigation was conducted in three French public hospitals, covering all departments through the same self-administered questionnaire.

The study population is composed of all Health Care Workers (HCWs). The activity sectors were Anesthesia and Intensive Care, Biology, Oncology, Digestive, Emergency, Geriatric Care, Medicine, Mother and Child Hospital, Nephrology, Urology and Transplant, Neuroscience, Dentistry, Orthopedics, Physiotherapy and Occupational therapy, Psychiatry, Public Health and Occupational Medicine, Head and Neck, Imaging, Research, Teaching, and the Chest department.

A steering committee, involving the university hospital management, engineers and public health and occupational medicine staff created a self-administrated questionnaire targeting occupational hazards and the main psychological factors encountered. The workplace health and safety committee (WPHSC), in agreement with the French labor law, approved the study protocol.

The questionnaire includes 49 questions grouped in four subscales. The first 29 items on work and psychosocial relations were extracted from Karasek's Job Content Questionnaire (JCQ) [23] and were validated in France by Niedhammer [26]. The next items stemmed from the French study, with authorization of use provided by the authors [24, 25]: eight items targeted workplace ergonomics; three items addressed workplace environment risk. The last 8 items focused on passive smoking, alcoholism and medication use (hypnotics, sedatives and analgesics) and were taken from the French National Institute of Prevention and Health Education's "Adults Health Barometer". The first cluster corresponded to the main variable, which is the psychosocial risk factor. The two other clusters were cofactors for the analysis of risks related to ergonomic, biomechanical, organizational, environmental, toxic and addictive factors (French version of CAGE questionnaire for alcoholism screening).

The questionnaire was distributed and collected upon completion by Moroccan medical students who first informed the personnel of its purpose, items and anonymity. All 4 746 employees from the nine public hospitals were considered eligible.

Data capture was made by students, by means of an Excel mask designed by the Medical Evaluation and Therapeutic Education Office of the Medical Information and Public Health Evaluation Department of Nantes University Hospital. Data was analyzed with SAS/STAT 8.2 and SPSS 13.0. Questionnaires with missing answers were excluded from the analysis. Descriptive analysis of data was made: percentage of answers for qualitative variables, mean and Standard Deviation for quantitative variables. Job Decision Latitude (JDL), Psychological Job Demand (PJD) and Social Support (SoSu) scores were calculated according to Karasek et al. [23] and Niedhammer et al. [26]. Threshold values for high PJD, low JDL and low SoSu were respectively set to 24, 72 and 22 [26]. High strain occupations had PJD score over 24, JDL score under 72 and SoSu score under 22.

Categorical variables correlations (e.g., between medication use and alcohol consumption) were analyzed by chi-squared tests. Quantitative correlations were analyzed by Student's *t*-tests. Other qualitative variables correlations (e.g., between scores and age) were estimated by Pearson's correlation coefficient. Factors influencing the scores were determined by one-way ANOVA and by

MANOVA for occupational categories adjustment. Step-by-step logistic regression and multivariate analysis was used for identifying factors connected to high PJD associated with low JDL. A comparative analysis of Moroccan and French (Nantes Hospitals) investigative data was performed. The studies in Morocco and France were carried out a few months apart. Moroccan hospitals have the same ward structure and occupational categories as French hospitals. The France data was extracted from the 2012 published study [25] with permission from authors. Confirmatory factor analysis was conducted on the Moroccan questionnaire.

Results

Descriptive data

In Morocco, 2,863 HCWs (60 % of the total hospital staff) answered the questionnaire, of whom 54 % were women. The mean age of the sample was 40.4 years [SD ± 10.2]. The mean work seniority was 11.3 years [SD ± 9.9]. 97 % of HCWs had a permanent employment contract and 79 % worked full-time. One should note thatin Morocco many HCWs have a second job because of the low salary they receive. The participation rate varied among the different hospitals, with leading scores from Larache (North Morocco) and Sekkat (Casablanca) hospitals (94 % and 91 %) and the lowest score (38 %) from Marrakech hospital (South Morocco). The participation rate was higher in the administration departments (67 %) and lower in surgery and technical-medical departments (57 %). The technical-medical personnel had the highest participation rate (74 %), followed by the janitors and the administrative personnel (73 %, 70 %), with the technical staff (27 %), the psychologists (33 %) and the nursing assistants (37 %) having least participated in the study.

Questionnaire' validity

Cronbach alpha coefficients for the French and Moroccan models are presented in Table 1.

Internal consistency of the study was determined for each subscale; in the Moroccan study, Cronbach's alpha coefficients were 0.596 for JDL, 0.383 PJD, 0.764 for SoSu, 0.737 for workplace ergonomics, 0.450 for environmental risks and 0.516 for medication use. Cronbach's alpha for PJD was clearly low, and after confirmatory factorial analysis, excluding two inversed question of JCQ, it was adjusted at 0.490. This low score was probably due to a poor understanding of the French nuances. PJD and SoSu scores were not correlated ($r = -0.025$, NS). JDL and PJD scores were weakly correlated ($r = 0.110$, $p < .01$), as well as JDL and SoSu scores ($r = 0.248$; $p < 0.01$).

Psychosocial risks

JDL, PJD and SoSu scores were diverse among occupational categories ($p < 0.001$) (Table 2).

Moroccan results: the respondents with the highest risk (High strain: occupational categories with the riskier combination of low job decision latitude, high psychological demand and low social support) were technical staff and care management personnel, but physicians, nurses and specialized nurses also had a high risk (Table 3). No occupational category placed itself in the active job quadrant—high demand and high control (Fig. 1).

JDL, PJD and SoSu were dependent of gender (adjusted OR = 1.26, Table 4)... Temporary employees had higher social support ($p < 0.001$). Full-time employees scored lower in JDL and SoSu ($p < 0.001$), but higher in PJD ($p < 0.001$). 20 % of the respondents reported using hypnotics or sedatives on a fairly regular basis (more than once during the week preceding the investigation), with an equal proportion of men and women. These respondents were older (43.2 years [SD ± 9.9] versus 40.3 years [SD ± 10.0], $p < 0.001$). 41 % of the respondents reported taking analgesics fairly regularly (more than once during the week preceding the investigation). Among them, more were women (43 % women versus 39 % men, $p < 0.05$) and they were older (41.9 [SD ± 10.1 years] versus 40.3 [SD ± 9.9 years], $p < 0.001$). Use of hypnotics or sedatives was significantly correlated to low JDL ($p < 0.001$). It was also correlated to a high PJD ($p < 0.05$) and to a lower SoSu ($p < 0.01$). Use of analgesic could be explained by high prevalence of musculoskeletal disorders. Use of hypnotics could be explained first by a high level of strain and second by sleeping disorders. Alcohol intake investigation did not show significant results, as the survey was incidentally carried out in the month of Ramadan, when, in accordance with a religious principle, the use of alcohol is prohibited, which

Table 1 Internal consistency of the French and Moroccan questionnaire

Cronbach's alpha coefficients	French questionnaire submitted to French HCWs	French questionnaire submitted to Moroccan HCWs
Job Decision Latitude scale	0.771	0.596
Psychological Demand scale	0.713	0.3832[a]
Social Support scale	0.814	0.764

[a]Cronbach's alpha for PJD was clearly low; and after confirmatory factorial analysis, excluding the two inversed questions of JCQ, it was adjusted at 0.490

Table 2 Moroccan-French decision latitude and psychological demand scales

Psycological demand scale France (Nantes)				Psychological demand scale Morocco			
Occupational category	Mean*	N	SD	Occupational category	Mean*	N	SD
Psychologist	21,5	17	2,8	Psychologist	23.0	2	0
Janitor	22,3	59	3,9	Rehabilitation personnel	23.1	39	3.2
Technical-medical personnel	22,7	116	3,0	Nursing assistant	23.3	39	2.7
Technical staff	23,4	92	3,2	Administrative	23.6	299	3.4
Other	23,5	30	3,9	Social/Educational staff	24.0	16	3.5
Social/Educational staff	23,8	26	3,7	Other	24.1	53	2.7
Nursing-assistant	24,4	237	3,4	Technical staff	24.2	27	2.8
Rehabilitation personnel	24,7	32	3,6	Specialist nurse	24.2	463	3.3
Administrative	24,7	222	3,7	Technical-medical personnel	24.4	88	3.4
Midewife	24,8	20	2,1	Janitor	24.6	60	2.5
Nurse	24,8	103	3,2	Nurse	24.7	717	3.2
Physician	25,3	204	3,4	Physician	25.0	630	3.3
Non specialist nurse	25,6	355	3,5	Care management	25.2	26	2.8
Care Management	25,9	127	3,4	Midwife	25.8	148	3.1
Total	24,6	1640	3,6	Total	24.6	2607	3.3

Decision Latitude scale France (Nantes)				Decision Latitude scale Morocco			
Occupational category	Mean	N	SD	Occupational category	Mean	N	SD
Janitor	61,4	59	11,4	Technical staff	53.9	25	10.4
Nurse-assistant	63,6	235	8,8	Other	62.1	58	9.3
Technical-medical personnel	66,4	114	9,2	Administrative	62.9	297	9.9
Administrative	67,9	223	11,2	Social/Educational staff	62.9	13	10.4
Non specialist nurse	68,6	359	8,7	Janitor	64.3	60	13.8
Nurse	69,1	109	8,3	Nursing assistant	64.4	41	6.8
Technical staff	70,3	91	11,1	Technical-medical personnel	65.1	88	10.6
Psychologist	72,7	17	19,5	Care management	65.4	27	7.8
Other	73,1	30	11,6	Midwife	65.6	142	9.9
Social/Educational staff	74,1	27	7,5	Nurse	66.2	729	9.4
Midewife	74,3	20	9,0	Specialist nurse	66.9	461	8.8
Rehabilitation personnel	75,2	36	5,9	Physician	69.5	630	9.0
Care management	76,3	128	8,0	Rehabilitation personnel	74.5	38	9.9
Physician	77,1	203	8,4	Psychologist	83.0	2	9.9
Total	69,6*	1651	10,4	Total	66.5*	2611	9.8

SD Standard Deviation
*$p < 0.001$

implies that even if some participants were taking alcohol, they would not mention it. After adjustment and multivariate analysis, high strain perception was strongly correlated with north and center morocco hospitals, sex (males are more at risk), employment contract and type of contract (full time HCWs are more at risk), occupational category (midwifes), workplace environment (bad accessibility, noise, brightness at workstation), the use of hypnotics and sedatives (see Table 4). Moroccan—-French hospitals comparison (Fig. 1, Fig. 2, Table 3, Table 5). Comparative analysis of Moroccan and French (Nantes) investigations showed that 76 % of the Moroccan HCWs and 62 % of the Nantes University Hospital HCWs experienced low JDL situations ($p < 0.001$). High strain situations (low JDL and high PJD) were recorded for 44 % of Moroccan HCWs, versus 37 % of Nantes

Table 3 Comparative analysis of Moroccan-French high strain and iso strain

	Moroccan HCWs $N = 2863$	Nantes HCWs $N = 1612$	*p*
High PJD	62 %	66 %	< 0.01
Low JDL	76 %	62 %	< 0.001
High Strain (high PJD, low JDL)	44 %	37 %	< 0.001
Iso Strain (high PJD, low JDL, low SoSu)	25 %[a]	19 %[b]	< 0.001
	Decision Latitude scale comparison		
Region	Mean	*N*	SD
North Morroco	64,8	821	9,7
Center Morocco	65,4	862	9,4
South Morocco	68,8	947	9,7
France (Nantes)	69,5	1661	10,4
Total	67,6	4291	10,2
	Psychological demand scale comparison		
Region	Mean	*N*	SD
South Morocco	24,42	933	3,38
North Morocco	24,59	816	3,59
Center Morocco	24,62	879	2,80
France (Nantes)	25,27	1640	4,01
Total	24,82	4268	3,59
	Nantes $n = 1612$	Morocco $n = 2863$	*p*
Decision latitude scale	69,5 +/- 10,5	66,4 +/- 9,8	*
Psychological demand scale	25,2 +/- 4,0	24,5 +/- 3,3	*

SD Standard Deviation
*$p < 0.001$
[a]technical staff, care management
[b]nurse assistant, technical-medical personnel, non specialist nurse

University Hospital HCWs ($p < 0.001$). Adding social isolation, the high strain quadrant grouped another 25 % of Moroccan HCWs, opposed to the 19 % of Nantes HCWs ($p < 0.001$). In order to analyze high strain in all HCWs, the HCWs Moroccan and French groups were merged. The risk factors which were strongly associated with a problematic context (high PJD and low JDL), in univariate and multivariate analysis of the merged Moroccan and Nantes groups, were the Moroccan group, with a higher strain in Northern Morocco and the

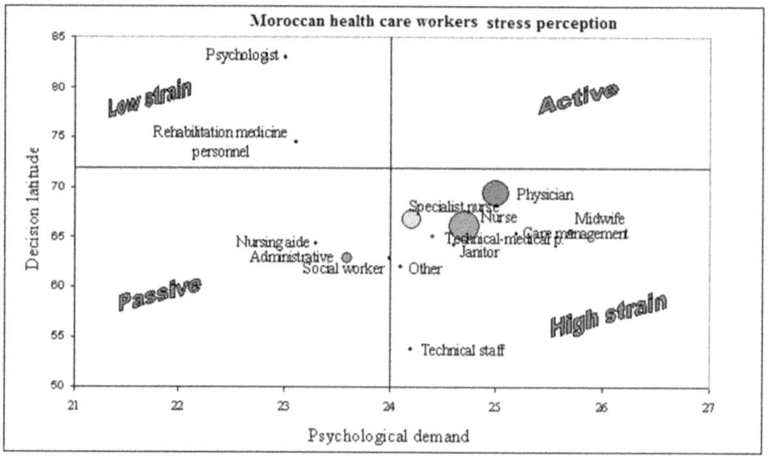

Fig. 1 Moroccan Health care workers stress perception

Table 4 High Strain and occupational risk factors in Moroccan HCWs, univariate and multivariate analysis

Problematic context =	high strain	*n*	%	Crude OR	Crude CI	Adjusted OR	CI
Group *n* = 2472	Casablanca region (control)	387	50	1		1	
	North Morocco	399	51	0.62	0.50–0.75	1.03	0.82–1.31
	South Morocco	353	38	1.05	0.86–1.29	0.73	0.56–0.96
Gender	Female	620	48	1		1	
n =2453	Male	512	45	0.89	0.76–1.05	1.26	1.04–1.53
Employment Contract	Permanent	1096	46	1		-	-
n =2462	Temporary	37	48	1.09	0.67–1.75		
Employment type	Full-time	923	49	1.68	1.37–2.05	1.65	1.24–2.19
n =2448	Part-time	201	36	1		1	
Occupational category *n* =2452	Administrative	123	45	1		1	
	Care management	16	62	1.94	0.80–4.79	2.10	0.85–5.23
	Specialist nurse	181	42	0.87	0.63–1.20	0.79	0.56–1.12
	Nurse	335	49	1.15	0.86–1.53	1.07	0.77–1.48
	Nursing assistant	16	46	1.02	0.48–2.18	0.96	0.42–2.21
	Janitor	27	45	0.99	0.54–1.80	0.95	0.51–1.78
	Midwife	94	69	2.71	1.72–4.29	2.33	1.41–3.85
	Rehabilitation medicine personnel	7	18	0.27	0.11–0.68	0.24	0.09–0.62
	Social worker	6	50	1.21	0.34–4.37	1.34	0.36–5.08
	Physician	244	41	0.84	0.62–1.13	0.65	0.47–0.91
	Technical-medical personnel	45	54	1.43	0.85–2.42	1.33	0.75–2.34
	Technical staff	12	50	1.21	0.49–3.00	0.44	0.15–1.31
	Other	21	45	0.98	0.50–1.90	1.12	0.52–2.42
Accessibility in the workplace *n* = 2504	Satisfactory	750	42	1		1	
	Unsatisfactory	363	52	1.50	1.26–1.78	1.24	1.01–1.53
Comfortable work posture *n* = 2423	Satisfactory	379	41	1		-	-
	Unsatisfactory	698	47	1.30	1.10–1.53		
Work plan height *n* = 2266	Satisfactory	417	41	1		-	-
	Unsatisfactory	587	47	1.31	1.11–1.55	-	-
Manual handling *n* = 2136	Easy	489	43	1		-	-
	Difficult	495	49	1.27	1.07–1.51	-	-
Noise level *n* = 2520	Correct	563	39	1		1	
	Incorrect	556	51	1.65	1.40–1.93	1.31	1.08–1.60
Lighting or brightness level *n* = 2537	Correct	501	38	1		1	
	Incorrect	624	52	1.76	1.50–2.06	1.45	1.19–1.76
Ambient temperature level *n* = 2547	Acceptable	409	40	1		-	-
	Unacceptable	721	48	1.38	1.17–1.62		
Exposure to hazardous chemicals *n* = 2324	Satisfactory	279	47	1		-	-
	Unsatisfactory	792	46	0.96	0.79–1.16		
Exposure to radiation *n* = 2330	Satisfactory	185	43	1		-	-
	Unsatisfactory	881	47	1.17	0.94–1.45		
Safety instructions *n* = 2383	Present or available	287	40	1		-	-
	Absent or unavailable	777	47	1.29	1.08–1.54	-	-
Use of hypnotics or sedatives *n* =2384	Yes	250	53	1.50	1.22–1.85	1.41	1.11–1.79
	No	811	43	1		1	
Use of analgesics *n* =2413	Yes	499	50	1.36	1.15–1.61	1.37	1.13–1.66
	No	587	42	1		1	

CI Confidence Interval
OR Odds Ratio

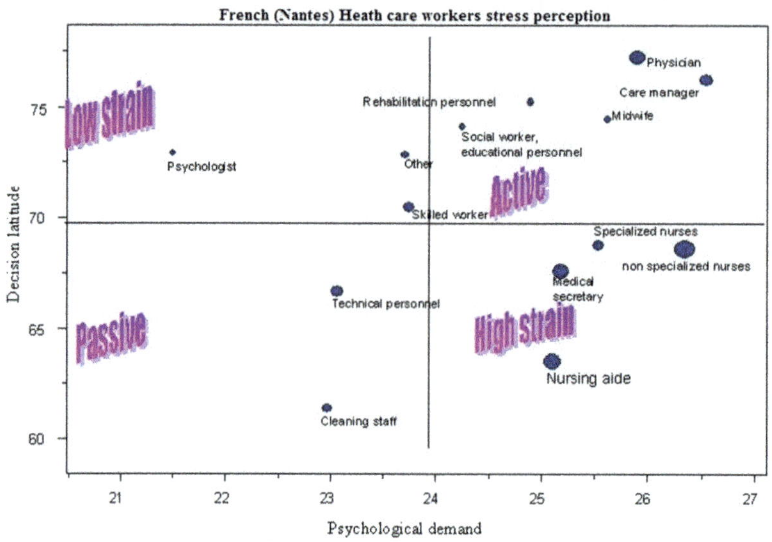

Fig. 2 French (Nantes) Health care stress perception

Table 5 High Strain in Moroccan and Nantes HCWs, multivariate analysis

Problematic context = High strain		*n*	%	Adjusted OR	CI
Group	Nantes	606	39	1	
n = 4011	North Morocco	399	51	1.66	1.27–2.17
	South Morocco	353	38	1.07	0.83–1.38
	Casablanca region	387	50	1.75	1.34–2.28
Employment type	Full-time	1295	46	1.34	1.06–1.68
n = 3717	Part-time	331	37	1	
Occupational category	Administrative	208	43	1	
n = 3984	Care management	48	33	0.64	0.35–1.16
	Specialist nurse	232	44	0.81	0.56–1.09
	Nurse	513	50	1.03	0.78–1.35
	Nursing assistant	129	52	1.80	1.09–2.95
	Janitor	48	43	0.87	0.52–1.45
	Midwife	104	67	2.35	1.51–3.68
	Rehabilitation medicine personnel	10	15	0.26	0.12–0.55
	Social worker	13	35	0.77	0.28–2.14
	Physician	287	36	0.70	0.53–0.94
	Technical staff	32	29	0.52	0.28–0.97
	Other	27	36	0.91	0.47–1.75
Seniority *n* = 3095		–	–	1.02	1.01–1.04
Use of hypnotics	Yes	315	53	1.48	1.19–1.83
n = 3799	No	1342	42	1	
Use of analgesics	Yes	691	49	1.40	1.18–1.65
n = 3835	No	991	41	1	

CI Confidence Interval *OR* Odds Ratio

Casablanca region, especially among midwives and nursing aides, more with full-time employment with a greater seniority in workplace, which includes those who use hypnotics and analgesics (see Table 5).

Discussion

The goal of the present study was to assess risk perception among Moroccan HCWs with a validated questionnaire, in order to make an analysis of exposure in relation to occupational risk factors variance in Moroccan public hospitals, and to compare the results with French HCWs (Nantes). The Labor Law in Marocco and the work organization on public hospitals are very similar to French ones which allowed meaningful comparisons of data over time.

The first strength of this investigation is the size and diversity of the HCWs' group, with a 60 % participation rate in the health care sector and a 67 % response rate by physicians constituting trustworthy data for analysis. The second originality of this paper is that it compares two cultures, French and Moroccan participants, knowing that we did not find any study of the kind comparing participants from Morocco.

The data show that significantly more Moroccan HCWs are exposed to high strain than Nantes Hospital HCWs. North Morocco and Casablanca region HCWs are subjected to higher strain than both South Morocco and French HCWs. Whereas the French study found many active jobs: physician, care management, midwife, the Moroccan study brought to attention a crowded high-strain quadrant in the JDL-PJD diagram (Fig. 1), which included all of the above occupations, alongside nurses and even janitors, which were passive category in the French survey. On the contrary, none of the Moroccan HCW jobs qualified as active. There might be a cultural mark involved, but the main reasons were economic and organizational: Moroccan physician and nurse staff appeared to be clearly insufficient in number; the doctors' activity was always intense and they complained of suffering from excessive time pressure and the technical equipment was often inadequate, outdated or faulty. Moreover, the staff was poorly paid and had a low degree of job independence, which led to the fact that many HCWs had to have a second job because of low pay.

Among the main perceived occupational risks, HCWs also indicated aggression, additional workload, musculoskeletal disorders and stress. Though physicians and nurses were considered as holding and active jobs [23], there are many investigations with opposite results. Columbian nurses had high demands but also high control [24]. The 2004 French report [31] on public hospitals HCWs showed an high level of job autonomy for physicians, but a much lower one for nurses and nursing assistants. The 2011 Italian study on risk factors in healthcare professionals [32] showed low JDL and SoSu scores for ancillary workers, but no significant variation in PJD, which is consistent with our findings. But differences in job demands are not unusual between countries and cultures. Pisanti et al. [33] brought evidence of higher pressure among Italian nurses, as opposed to Dutch nurses, which is also consistent with the differences between PJD scores for our French and Moroccan nurses. But there are many elements that can influence job perception and thus job satisfaction: the difficult climate of today's economic crisis leaves its mark on job security, even if all three scores of PJD, JDL and SoSu are high enough to place the nurses in the active jobs category [29].

High strain among nurses is also not uncommon and the reasons outlined by researchers mainly reside in gender disparity: women report lower levels of decision latitude [23]. Nevertheless, no gender influence on high-strain scores was found here. However there are grounds for high strain in women: cultural elements, tradition, or increased workload (based on unclear competencies) forced on nurses [34]. Moroccan women have a specific social status: Moroccan traditional family structure gives them the household responsibilities, which may in turn increase their general stress level [35]. Social status and high or low level of education can also influence the understanding of any questionnaire content and purpose, and may affect answer, bringing in bias [36].

As already mentioned, this is the first cross-sectional multicenter study to assess PSR perception and to estimate occupational stress in Moroccan non-university public hospitals. It showed a good overall participation rate and a very strong willingness of hospital HCWs to participate in the survey (94 % participation rate in Sekkat Casablanca and 91 % participation rate in Larache); we believe this speaks in itself about both the awareness and the need for changes in working conditions. Besides evaluating, another study purpose was to build ground base for organizational and work environment changes, to decrease occupational stress and to increase job control and social support. It has already been shown that, among many consequences, high JDL and SoSu enhanced safety participation [37]. This may not be the case yet for our study group, which has unsatisfying levels of JDL for the majority of HCWs, but constitutes another trigger for policy design. If an intervention plan was to be implemented in all Moroccan public hospitals, once started, an evaluative re-analysis of PSR would be not only necessary but highly useful [38].

Our study showed no positive correlation between age and high strain (0.97 adjusted OR, CI: 0.96–0.99), similar to results from larger and more heterogeneous groups [23], though JDL and SoSu perception decreased with age, which is similar to the Nantes study results [19]. But, we must consider the risk of cardiovascular disease (CVD) that comes with age, one which is already linked to job strain [39]. In a meta-analysis of 14 prospective cohort studies, Kivimäki et al. (2006) suggested an average 50 % excess risk of coronary heart disease when occupational stress was present [40]. A connection between occupational stress and inflammation appears to exist, the latter triggering CVDs [41].

Since we found no explanation for temporary HCWs having higher SoSu and for senior workers having lower SoSu, there is need for further investigation here. Full-time employees experienced more stress than part-time employees, which was consistent with findings in the Nantes' study. There was certainly more pressure in full-time contract and the perceived responsibility increased for these. Longer working time enhanced a greater workload and more stress, as its imprints on scores showed: lower JDL (65.5 [SD ± 9.6]), lower SS (21.6 [SD ± 3.9]) and higher PJD 24.7 [SD ± 3.3].

Moroccan HCWs took significantly more hypnotics and sedatives (20 %) and more analgesics (40 %) than Nantes HCWs (9 % and 25 %); the use of medication was significantly associated to high strain ($p < .001$). Medication use in Moroccan HCWs proved to be much higher than other reports from hospital environments. Virtanen et al. conducted a study in 21 Finnish hospitals and found lower usage rate: 5 % for anxiolytic and hypnotic medication and 16 % for pain-killers [42]. Use of sedatives and hypnotics is certainly linked to alternative shifts, night work, stress, workload and fatigue. Analgesics use was associated to musculoskeletal disorders, even if the declared average weight lifted by Moroccan HCWs [51.1kg SD ± 109.1 kg] was much lower than the average weight lifted by Nantes HCWs [130.7 kg SD ± 255.9 kg]. However we can question the use of such drugs which presupposes often the presence of psychological and/or psychiatric disorders in these subjects and we regret not having evaluated these people with some specific tests for the psychiatric screening. Further studies should have recourse to such tests. Alcohol intake in Moroccan HCWs could not be compared to that of Nantes HCWs, because of the alcohol prohibition during the Ramadan month, which we had not taken into account when designing the investigation time schedule, therefore leading to a limitation.

Though PJD was lower in Moroccan HCWs, it still held a high score, and when associated to low JDL it concentrated a higher percentage of high strain HCWs (44 %) than the ones reported in other studies: 16.5 % in Taiwanese HCWs [28], 25 % in European workers [43]. This raises high concern and it calls for an immediate intervention. As for the different occupational categories, it must be noted that Moroccan physicians were at a higher level of strain than physicians from any other country. In our study they were not considered an active occupation. Work overload, insufficient staffing, poor doctor-patient relationship, low hospital budget are all triggers of occupation status corrosion. All studies on perceived stress focusing on or including doctors have placed them in the high demand-high control job category. This indicates a higher risk degree in Moroccan doctors for developing CVDs and mental disorders. Higher depression rates than in general population have been reported in physicians with high work demands [44]. On the other hand, Moroccan rehabilitation medicine personnel had passive jobs, similar to other reports [44, 45], but unlike its Nantes counterpart, which found itself in the active quadrant of Karasek's JCQ model. This proved a much lower degree of independence.

Our study has encountered a number of limitations. The weak points of self-reporting must first be restated. There is no solution to avoid or limit individual variation in PSR perception. In the Moroccan study, Cronbach's alpha for PJD was clearly low, and after factorial analysis, excluding two inversed question of JCQ, it was adjusted at 0.490. This low score was probably due to a poor comprehension of French language. The target is personal, subjective sensation and understanding and not objective quantification. But there is sufficient evidence that perception is at the origin of changes in well-being and of ill health, and their prevention is occupational medicine's ultimate goal. Participants in the study have not been randomly selected. Reasons for unresponsiveness were not requested. Results may have been influenced by exclusion of participants due to missing item answers. Karasek's demand-control model leaves out the effort-reward balance and the patient-caregiver relationship, and there is no data on absenteeism, presence, patient admission rates, factors to be taken into account in future investigation. The study did not take into account the patients/staff ratio and did not investigate differences in staff norming between the analyzed healthcare structures in Morocco and France. The questionnaire version used in Morocco wasn't perfectly identical to that used in the Nantes study, since some workstation ergonomics items weren't identical and therefore could not be mentioned. However, the study provides an accurate picture of PSR in Moroccan public hospitals. It brings forward a map of stressful occupations and it points out priorities for action.

Conclusions

This paper is innovative by comparing hospital staff in two different countries which were not compared before. More Moroccan HCWs in general and more Moroccan physicians are at high strain than Nantes' HCWs and physicians. Use of hypnotics and analgesics is at high level in Moroccan HCWs. Full time workers, midwives and workers using hypnotics, sedatives and analgesics are under high strain. Our results provide elements for improving the working conditions and well-being of health care workers in Morocco. They stress out the importance of implementing a risk prevention plan and even a hospital reform. Further research, with an enlarged study pool and a more exhaustive analysis, will bring more information on PSR and HCWs' health.

Competing interests
The authors declare that they have no competing interests.

Authors' contributions
DIG contributed to methods, to data analysis, interpretation and discussion, wrote and revised the manuscript. DT designed the questionnaire and methods, contributed to discussion and manuscript revision, mentored DIG in research internship in the Department of Occupational Medicine and Occupational Hazards, University Hospital of Nantes and mentored the Moroccan medicine students. BG contributed to data analysis and interpretation. CJ contributed to data interpretation and commented on drafts of the manuscript. BKD advised on and contributed to data analysis and interpretation; LM, YR, AC, CV and CG commented on drafts of the manuscript. CEHL mentored the Moroccan medicine students and commented on drafts of the manuscript, CRL commented draft and reviewed the paper as a native speaker. All authors read and approved the final manuscript.

Acknowledgements
The authors acknowledge the participation and help of the Moroccan medicine students. DIG's contribution to the study is part of research carried out within the framework of POSDRU/CPP107/DMI1.5/S/76851 project, co-financed by the European Social Fund through the Sectorial Operational Programme Human Resources Development 2007–2013.

Author details
[1]Department of Occupational Medicine and Environment Health, HCWs Research Laboratory, 5 rue du doyen Boquien, Nantes University Hospital, Nantes 44 093, France. [2]"Lucian Blaga" University of Sibiu, 10 Victoriei Boulevard, Sibiu 550024, Romania. [3]Psychology Laboratory of Pays de la Loire (LPPL - UPRES EA 4638), Department of Psychology, University of Nantes, BP 81 227 44312 Nantes cedex 3, France. [4]Cognition, Health, Socialization, EA6291 University of Reims Champagne-Ardenne, 57, rue Pierre-Taittinger, Reims 51 096, France. [5]Department of Public Health, Nantes University Hospital, 35 rue Saint Jacques, Nantes 44 000, France. [6]Laboratory of Ergonomics Epidemiology Health and Work, LEEST-UA InVS - IFR 132- UPRES EA 4336, University of Angers, Faculty of Medicine, University Hospital, 4 rue Larrey, 49933 Angers Cedex, France. [7]Occupational Medicine Department, 6 rue Henri Le Guilloux, University Hospital of Rennes, Rennes 35 000, France. [8]Graduate School of Health Engineering and Project Management, 24 rue Lafontaine, Quartier Racine, Casablanca 20 100, Morocco. [9]Public Health Department, SMBH, Paris 13 University, 74 avenue Marcel Cachin, Bobigny 93017, France.

References

1. Roland-Lévy C, Lemoine J, Jeoffrion C. Health and Well-being at Work: The Hospital Context. Eur Rev Appl Psychol. 2014;64(2):53–62.
2. Eriksen W, Bruusgaard D, Knardahl S. Work factors as predictors of intense or disabling low back pain; a prospective study of nurses' aides. Occup Environ Med. 2004;61(5):398–404.
3. Eriksen W, Bruusgaard D, Knardahl S. Work factors as predictors of sickness absence attributed to airway infections; A three-month prospective study of nurses' aides. Occup Environ Med. 2004;61(1):45–51.
4. Jhun HJ, Cho SI, Park JT. Changes in job stress, musculoskeletal symptoms, and complaints of unfavorable working conditions among nurses after the adoption of a computerized order communication system. Int Arch Occup Environ Health. 2004;77(5):363–7.
5. Violante FS, Fiori M, Fiorentini C, Risi A, Garagnani G, Bonfiglioli R, Mattioli, S. Associations of psychosocial and individual factors with three different categories of back disorder among nursing staff. J Occup Health. 2004;46(2):100–8.
6. Yip Y. A Study of work Stress, patient handing activities and the risk of Low back pain among nurses in Hong Kong. J Adv Nurs. 2001;36(6):794–803.
7. Gershon RRM, Stone PW, Zeltser M, Faucett J, Macdavitt K, Chou SS. Organizational Climate and Nurse Health Outcomes in the United States: A Systematic Review. Ind Health. 2007;45:622–36.
8. Devereux JJ, Vlachonikolis IG, Buckle PW. Epidemiological study to investigate potential interaction between physical and psychosocial factors at work that may increase the risk of symptoms of musculoskeletal disorder of the neck and upper limb. Occup Environ Med. 2002;59:269–77.
9. Smith DR, Muto T, Sairenchi T, Ishikawa Y, Sayama S, Yoshida A, Townley-Jones M. Hospital safety climate, psychosocial risk factors and needlestick injuries in Japan. Ind Health. 2010;48(1):85–95.
10. European Foundation for the Improvement of Living and Working Conditions: Rise in psychosocial risk factors at the workplace [http://www.eurofound.europa.eu/ewco/surveyreports/FR0909019D/FR0909019D.pdf]. Accessed 20 Apr 2016.
11. Van Stolk C, Staetsky L, Hassan E, Chong WK. European Agency for Safety and Health at Work (EU-OSHA): Management of PSR at work: An analysis of the findings of the European Survey of Enterprises on New and Emerging Risks (ESENER). European Risk Observatory (Report). Luxembourg: Publications Office of the European Union; 2012.
12. European Foundation for the Improvement of Living and Working Conditions: A review of working conditions in France. [http://www.eurofound.europa.eu/ewco/surveys/FR0603SR01/FR0603SR01.pdf].
13. Collège d'expertise sur le suivi statistique des risques psychosociaux au travail: Indicateurs provisoires de facteurs de risques psychosociaux au travail [http://www.collegerisquespsychosociauxtravail.fr/site/medias/Indicateurs-provisoires.pdf]
14. Parent-Thirion A, Vermeylen G, Van Houten G, Lyly-Yrjänäinen M, Biletta I, Cabrita J, Niedhammer I. European Foundation for the Improvement of Living and Working Conditions. Fifth European Working Conditions Survey: Overview Report. Luxembourg: Publications Office of the European Union. 2012–151 p. doi:10.2806/34660.
15. Leka S, Cox T. PRIMA-EF Guidance on the European Framework for Psychosocial Risk Management: A Resource for Employers and Worker Representatives. Geneva: World Health Organization; 2008.
16. European Commission. Guidance on work-related stress – Spice of life or kiss of death? Luxembourg: Office for Official Publications of the European Communities; 2002.
17. European Commission: Communication from the Commission to the European Parliament, the Council, the European Economic and Social Committee and the Committee of the Regions. Improving quality and productivity at work: Community strategy 2007-2012 on health and safety at work. February 2007. [http://eur-lex.europa.eu/LexUriServ/LexUriServ.do?uri=COM:2007:0062:FIN:EN:PDF]. Accessed 20 Apr 2016.
18. Goedhart G, Snijders AC, Hesselink AE, van Poppel MN, Bonsel GJ, Vrijkotte TG. Maternal depressive symptoms in relation to perinatal mortality and morbidity: results from a large multi-ethnic cohort study. Psychosom Med. 2010;72(8):769–76.
19. Crone MR, Bekkema N, Wiefferink CH, Reijneveld SA. Professional identification of psychosocial problems among children from ethnic minority groups: room for improvement. J Pediatr. 2010;156(2):277–84.
20. Eichelsheim VI, Buist KL, Deković M, Wissink IB, Frijns T, van Lier PA, Koot HM, Meeus WH. Associations among the parent-adolescent relationship, aggression and delinquency in different ethnic groups: a replication across two Dutch samples. Soc Psychiatry Psychiatr Epidemiol. 2010;45(3):293–300.
21. Abourazzak FE, Allali F, Rostom S, Hmamouchi I, Ichchou L, El Mansouri L, Bennani L, Khazzani H, Abouqal R, Hajjaj-Hassouni N. Factors influencing quality of life in Moroccan postmenopausal women with osteoporotic vertebral fracture assessed by ECOS 16 questionnaire. Health Qual Life Outcomes. 2009;7:23.

22. Laraqui O, Laraqui S, Tripodi D, Caubet A, Verger C, Laraqui CH. Evaluation du stress chez le personnel de santé au Maroc : à propos d'une étude Multicentrique. Stress assessment among health care workers in Morocco. Arch Mal Prof Env. 2008;69:672–82.
23. Karasek RA, Brisson C, Kawakami N, Houtman I, Bongers P, Amick B. The Job Content Questionnaire (JCQ): an instrument for internationally comparative assessments of psychosocial job characteristics. J Occup Health Psychol. 1998;3:322–55.
24. Tripodi D, Keriven-Dessomme B, Lombrail P, Bourut Lacouture M, Chabot AS, Houdebine MT, Gordeeff C, Durand Perdiel MH, Moret L, Dupas D, Cantineau A, Geraut C. Evaluation des risques professionnels perçus chez le personnel du centre hospitalo-universitaire de Nantes. Arch Mal Prof Env. 2007;68:457–73.
25. Tripodi D, Roedlich C, Laheux MA, Longuenesse C, Roquelaure Y, Lombrail P, Geraut C. Stress perception among employees in a French University Hospital. Occup Med (Lond). 2012;62(3):216–9.
26. Niedhammer I. Psychometric properties of the French version of the Karasek Job Content Questionnaire: a study of the scales of decision latitude, psychological demands, social support, and physical demands in the GAZEL cohort. Int Arch Occup Environ Health. 2002;75(3):129–44.
27. Araújo TM, Karasek R: Validity and reliability of the job content questionnaire in formal and informal jobs in Brazil. SJWEH 2008, (Suppl 6): 52–59. [www.sjweh.fi/download.php?abstract_id=1251]. Accessed 20 Apr 2016.
28. Chien TW, Lai WP, Wang HY, Hsu SY, Castillo RV, Guo HR, Chen SC, Su SB. Applying the revised Chinese Job Content Questionnaire to assess psychosocial work conditions among Taiwan's hospital workers. BMC Public Health. 2011;11:478.
29. Eum KD, Li J, Jhun HJ, Park JT, Tak SW, Karasek R, Cho SI. Psychometric properties of the Korean version of the job content questionnaire: data from health care workers. Int Arch Occup Environ Health. 2007;80(6):497–504.
30. Gomez Ortiz V. Evaluación de estresores psicosociales en el trabajo: propiedades psicométricas del Cuestionario del contenido del trabajo (JCQ) con trabajadores colombianos. Rev Latinoam Psicol. 2011;43(2):329–42.
31. Le Lan R., Baubeau D: Les conditions de travail perçues par les professionnels de santé. Études et résultats, DREES No 335, 2004. [http://www.drees.sante.gouv.fr/IMG/pdf/er335.pdf]. Accessed 20 Apr 2016.
32. Albini E, Zoni S, Parrinello G, Benedetti L, Lucchini R. An integrated model for the assessment of stress-related risk factors in health care professionals. Ind Health. 2011;49(1):15–23.
33. Pisanti R, van der Doef M, Maes S, Lazzari D, Bertini M. Job characteristics, organizational conditions, and distress/well-being among Italian and Dutch nurses: a cross-national comparison. Int J Nurs Stud. 2011;48(7):829–37.
34. Bojtor A. The importance of social and cultural factors to nursing status. Int J Nurs Pract. 2003;9(5):328–35.
35. Chahraoui K, Bioy C, Gilles F, Laurent A, Valache B, Quenot JP. Vécu psychologique des soignants en réanimation : une étude exploratrice et qualitative. Ann Fr Anesth Reanim. 2001;30:342–8.
36. Hökerberg YH, Aguiar OB, Reichenheim M, Faerstein E, Valente JG, Fonseca Mde J, Passos SR. Dimensional structure of the demand control support questionnaire: a Brazilian context. Int Arch Occup Environ Health. 2010;83(4): 407–16.
37. Turner N, Stride CB, Carter AJ, McCaughey D, Carroll AE. Job Demands-Control-Support model and employee safety performance. Accid Anal Prev. 2012;45:811–7.
38. Bourbonnais R, Brisson C, Vézina M. Long-term effects of an intervention on psychosocial work factors among healthcare professionals in a hospital setting. Occup Environ Med. 2011;68(7):479–86.
39. Belkic KL, Landsbergis PA, Schnall PL, Baker D. Is job strain a major source of cardiovascular disease risk? Scand J Work Environ Health. 2004;30(2):85–128.
40. Kivimäki M, Virtanen M, Elovainio M, Kouvonen A, Väänänen A, Vahtera J. Work stress in the etiology of coronary heart disease–a meta-analysis. Scand J Work Environ Health. 2006;32(6):431–42.
41. Poantă L, Crăciun A, Dumitraşcu DL. Professional stress and inflammatory markers in physicians. Rom J Intern Med. 2010;48(1):57–63.
42. Virtanen M, Vahtera J, Batty GD, Tuisku K, Oksanen T, Elovainio M, Ahola K, Pentti J, Salo P, Vartti AM, Kivimäki M. Health risk behaviors and morbidity among hospital staff-comparison across hospital ward medical specialties in a study of 21 Finnish hospitals. Scand J Work Environ Health. 2012;38(3):228–37.
43. Niedhammer I, Sultan-Taïeb H, Chastang JF, Vermeylen G, Parent-Thirion A. Exposure to psychosocial work factors in 31 European countries. Occup Med (Lond). 2012;62(3):196–202.
44. Wang LJ, Chen CK, Hsu SC, Lee SY, Wang CS, Yeh WY. Active job, healthy job? Occupational stress and depression among hospital physicians in Taiwan. Ind Health. 2011;49(2):173–84.
45. Campo MA, Weiser S, Koenig KL. Job strain in physical therapists. Phys Ther. 2009;89(9):946–56.

8

Health behaviour, health status and occupational prospects of apprentice nurses and kindergarten teachers in Germany

Tanja Wirth[1*], Agnessa Kozak[2], Grita Schedlbauer[1] and Albert Nienhaus[1,2]

Abstract

Background: Apprentices in human service professions are exposed to emotional and physical stresses in their workplaces. Moreover, they are in the vulnerable phase of becoming an adult. Their lifestyle and health therefore seem to be particularly unstable. This study aims to evaluate and compare the health behaviour, health status and occupational prospects of apprentices in nursing and early childhood education and to identify factors associated with their physical and mental health.

Methods: A cross-sectional study based on self-administered questionnaires was carried out at eight vocational schools in Hamburg, Germany. Four hundred two apprentice geriatric nurses, hospital nurses and kindergarten teachers/assistants participated (response rate: 99 %). Apprentices were compared in terms of their physical activity, dietary patterns, cigarette and alcohol consumption, body mass index, self-rated health, previous diseases, job satisfaction and occupational prospects. Factors associated with the participants' musculoskeletal or mental disorders were identified using logistic regression.

Results: Around 33 % of apprentice geriatric nurses and kindergarten teachers/assistants were overweight or obese. Fifty-five percent of geriatric nurses were smokers. Job satisfaction was lowest among hospital nurses. More than one third of the apprentices suffered from musculoskeletal or mental disorders. The ages of 23–26 years and mental disorder were associated with musculoskeletal disorders (OR 3.1, 95 % CI 1.4–6.7; OR 1.8, 95 % CI 1.1–3.1). Being an apprentice in early childhood education was associated with an increased chance of mental disorder (OR 2.9, 95 % CI 1.4–6.0). Additionally, musculoskeletal disorders, self-efficacy and irritation were associated with mental disorder.

Conclusions: Differences between the occupational groups indicate the need for specific work-related health promotion for apprentices at an early stage in their careers. Future projects should focus on the implementation and evaluation of these measures.

Keywords: Health behaviour, Health status, Job satisfaction, Mental disorder, Musculoskeletal disorders, Observational study, Student nurses

* Correspondence: t.wirth@cvcare.de
[1]Institution for Statutory Accident Insurance and Prevention in the Health and Welfare Services, Department for the Principle of Prevention and Rehabilitation, Pappelallee 33/35/37, 22089 Hamburg, Germany
Full list of author information is available at the end of the article

Background

Hospital and geriatric nurses as well as kindergarten teachers belong to the human service professions, which are becoming increasingly important in our society. Due to an ageing population in the course of demographic change, there is a growing demand for professional nursing care, which will be difficult to cover. Projections estimate that there will be a lack of up to half a million full-time employees in outpatient and inpatient care in Germany by the year 2030 [1]. Similarly, early childhood education has been expanded in Germany in recent years, also leading to a need for more employees in this occupational field. However, nursing professions in particular are not very attractive to graduates. One reason is that these professions are associated with high emotional and physical stress [2]. Besides increasing time pressure at work, dealing with suffering and dying patients is a major challenge in nursing. Kindergarten teachers are exposed to a continuously high level of noise and usually work in bent and twisted postures. Consequently, these professions show high rates of occupational disabilities and dropouts [3, 4], also among young employees [2]. Promoting health early in their careers could be one strategy to prevent high turnover in these professions.

Germany has a practically oriented apprenticeship system. In addition to school education, apprentices spend a large part of their vocational training in the workplace. Thus, apprentices in human service professions are exposed to both performance stress at school and a high degree of stress in their occupations. Moreover, most apprentices are still in the process of becoming an adult, a vulnerable phase in human life, during which one is susceptible to adjusting to an unhealthy lifestyle [5].

Results from the German Health Interview and Examination Survey (DEGS1) indicate that smoking and at-risk drinking are common among a representative sample of young adults aged 18 to 29 years. Forty percent of women in this youngest age group smoked; 36 % consumed alcohol at hazardous levels [6, 7]. According to the DEGS1, 30 % of young women in Germany are overweight [8].

Studies of students in general nursing support the concerns that they also do not follow a healthy lifestyle. A systematic review showed that the smoking rates among nursing students vary considerably depending on the country of study; from 3 % in Iran, to around 30 % in Great Britain, to over 60 % reported in one Australian survey [9]. With regard to Germany, studies consistently reported high smoking rates of over 40 % [10–15]. In a Scottish survey, 74 % of student nurses and midwives practiced harmful alcohol consumption [16]. Around one third of nursing students in Germany consumed alcohol at harmful levels [10]. The highest proportion (45 %) of overweight and obesity among nursing students was found in the US [17]. Rates reported by German studies of apprentices in the nursing field ranged from 20 to 32 % [12, 13]. A German survey reported that 58 % of apprentices at nursing schools consumed fast food at least once a week [14]. Symptoms of musculoskeletal disorders (MSD) and mental disorders such as depression or burnout have also been observed among nursing students [18, 19].

In Germany, separate vocational training is offered for the two disciplines of geriatric and hospital nursing. Most studies do not distinguish between these two professions; to the best of our knowledge, differentiated analyses among students with respect to health behaviour and health status are missing. Studies examining the health status and behaviour of young apprentices in early childhood education are also lacking. However, analyses of older employees in childcare showed that kindergarten teachers were less likely to be smokers compared to the general German population. In the same study, the prevalence rates for overweight and obesity were 41 and 18 % respectively [20]. Similarly, a study from Georgia reported that 50 % of female childcare providers were overweight or obese [21]. Most early childhood workers in a study from New Zealand believed that they have good nutrition and perceived their health as good or excellent. However, they reported an increase in physical symptoms, such as back pain, muscle strain and fatigue, since they started working in this setting [3].

Dual vocational training at schools and in workplaces provides a unique opportunity for the implementation of health promotion programmes that may increase the awareness of a healthy lifestyle and reduce the effects of occupational stresses. To identify needs for specific measures at vocational schools and workplaces, the health behaviour and status of apprentices must be determined. We have chosen the professions of geriatric nurses, hospital nurses and kindergarten teachers/assistants, as they work in settings with high emotional and physical demands; the constant and intense interactions with patients/clients require a high level of dedication and empathy. In addition, apprentices in these professions serve as role models for patients/clients with respect to their health behaviour. All three occupations also have in common the fact that they are mostly practiced by women and share the same required level of education (general certificate of secondary education).

The objectives of this study were (i) to describe the health status, health behaviour and prospects of apprentice geriatric nurses, hospital nurses and kindergarten teachers/assistants, (ii) to examine differences between these three groups and (iii) to identify factors associated with MSD and mental disorders of apprentices.

Methods

Study design, participants and procedures

A cross-sectional survey was carried out in Hamburg, Germany. Apprentice geriatric nurses, hospital nurses and kindergarten teachers/assistants were eligible for inclusion in the study. Apprentices in all years of vocational training, of both sexes and all ages were included at this stage. We calculated an estimate of the required sample size based on the prevalence of overweight, as defined by the body mass index (BMI). Overweight is an indicator for health behaviour and a factor influencing the health status. A mean prevalence of 30 % of overweight was assumed among apprentices [12, 13]. For a 95 % chance of our sample estimate being within five percentage points of this assumed prevalence (30 ± 5 %), a sample size of $n = 322$ was needed. We oversampled by 20 % in order to account for non-response and missing data. We therefore aimed to recruit approximately 403 apprentices.

Sixteen out of 20 vocational schools in Hamburg identified for the target professions were contacted at random. Eight of them gave their consent to participate in the study. The schools were responsible for selecting classes by convenience in which questionnaires could be distributed to apprentices during lessons. Apprentices were informed by a project member of the aim and content of the study, of measures to ensure confidentiality and of the voluntary nature of participation. By completing the questionnaires, participants provided their informed consent to take part in the study. Ethical approval was obtained from the Hamburg Medical Council Ethics Committee (# PV4649).

Data collection took place from January to March 2014. In total, 402 apprentices participated in the study (response rate: 98.8 %). The recruitment process is shown in Fig. 1. The age of participants varied greatly from 16 to 52 years. The health behaviour of younger apprentices differs considerably from that of older ones. For example, apprentices under the age of 30 years showed hazardous alcohol consumption ($\chi^2 = 9.9$ [df = 1], $p < 0.01$) and unfavourable dietary patterns ($\chi^2 = 11.4$ [df = 2], $p < 0.01$) significantly more often than their older counterparts. The study sample was therefore reduced to participants aged 16 to 30 years ($n = 354$). We set the cut-off at the age of 30 years to ascertain its comparability with the age group of 18 to 29-year-olds applied in the DEGS1 survey [6–8].

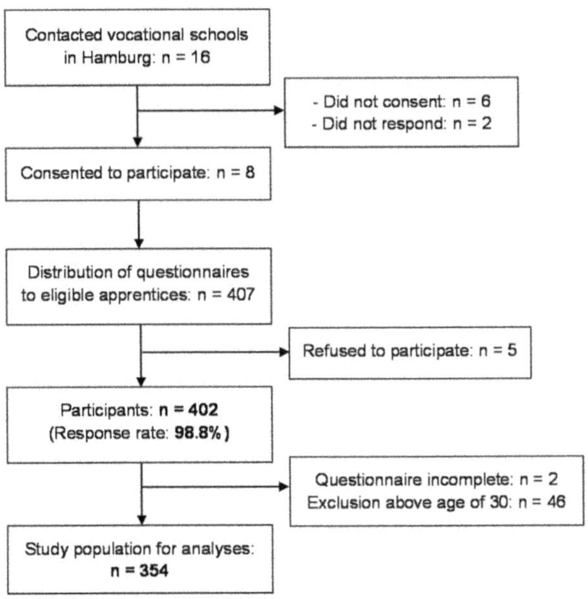

Fig. 1 Flow diagram of the recruitment process

Measures

A self-administered questionnaire was compiled from validated scales and single items which were applied in previous studies. An overview of the scales and items used in the analyses is given in Table 1. The internal consistencies of the self-efficacy, irritation and job satisfaction scale were good (Cronbach's $\alpha = 0.81$ to 0.88) and comparable to validation studies [22–24]. The applicability and comprehensibility of the instrument was verified in a pre-test with one class of apprentice geriatric nurses ($n = 15$). This class was not included in the final study sample.

Information on the socio-demographic characteristics of participants included age, sex, height, weight, migration background, socioeconomic status (SES) and year of education. Apprentices were classified according to their BMI (kg/m^2) as underweight (<18.5), normal weight (18.5 to 24.9), overweight (25 to 30) or obese (≥30). Migration background was assumed if apprentices themselves had immigrated to Germany and at least one of their parents was not born in Germany or was not of German nationality, or if both parents had immigrated or were not of German nationality [25]. The SES was determined from the highest educational level of apprentices and the current parental occupation. The following scores were administered to educational levels: 1 = comprehensive school qualification, 2 = general certificate of secondary education, 3 = technical college entrance qualification, 4 = university entrance qualification and 5 = technical college entrance qualification or university entrance qualification plus university degree. Parents' occupations were coded according to the International Standard Classification of Occupations (ISCO-88) [26]. By using the International Socio-Economic Index of Occupational Status (ISEI), values from 16 to 90 were assigned to these codes [27]. Scoring categories were defined by quintiles. Scores for educational level were added to scores for the parental occupation with the higher ISEI value. The SES was classified as low (2 to 4), middle (5 to 7) or high (8 to 10) [28].

The health behaviour of apprentices was assessed by physical activity, dietary patterns, smoking habits and

Table 1 Variables of the study instrument used in the analyses

Variables	Name and source of the original scales and items	α	Items (n)
Socio-demographic factors[a]			18
Health behaviour			
Physical activity	Health Questionnaire age 18–64 years [29]	–	1
Dietary habits	Food Frequency Questionnaire [30]	–	15
Smoking	Health Questionnaire age 18–64 years [7]	–	2
Alcohol consumption	AUDIT-C [31, 32]	–	3
Health status			
General health status	Survey in vocational schools in Bielefeld [36]	–	1
Diseases and complaints	Work Ability Index – Questionnaire [33]	–	6
Self-efficacy	Self-efficacy scale [24]	0.85	10
Irritation	Irritation scale [22]	0.88	8
Occupational situation and prospects			
Job satisfaction	COPSOQ: German standard version [23, 34]	0.81	7
Job strain and prospects	Additional questions (e.g., taking into account the current work situation, do you want to stay in this profession for the next five years?)	–	3

[a]Included age, sex, height, weight, migration background, socioeconomic status and year of education
α = Cronbach's alpha, *AUDIT-C* Alcohol Use Disorder Identification Test, *COPSOQ* Copenhagen Psychosocial Questionnaire

alcohol consumption. Regular physical activity was defined as a planned, structured and ongoing activity for increasing physical fitness. For the analysis, activity levels were classified as "no physical activity", "up to 2 h/week" and "regularly, at least 2 h/week" [29]. A food frequency scale, ranging from never to daily, was applied to examine the consumption of fifteen food items. Each item had an individual scoring system from 0 = deviant to 2 = optimal. Scores were added together and classified according to the tertiles of the index [30]. A distinction was made between daily, occasional, former and never smokers. Apprentices smoking ≥20 cigarettes/day were classified as heavy smokers [7]. The Alcohol Use Disorder Identification Test (AUDIT-C) was performed to detect hazardous drinking behaviour. The cut-offs were >3 for women and >4 for men [31, 32].

The health status was rated on a five-point scale ranging from "excellent" to "poor". Questions regarding diseases they had experienced during the previous twelve months were adapted from the Work Ability Index. Response categories were predefined as "no", "yes, own opinion" or "yes, physician's diagnosis" [33]. Two scales evaluated mental health. The General Self-Efficacy Scale identifies resources for coping with life's challenges. It consists of ten items on a four-point Likert scale, with higher scores indicating better self-efficacy [24]. The Irritation scale measures emotional and cognitive psychological strain in occupational contexts. A higher score on a seven-point Likert scale reflects greater irritation [22].

Job satisfaction, motivation to stay in the profession, as well as occupational stresses and wishes were considered as prospects. Job satisfaction was measured by seven items on a four-point Likert scale. Response categories were transformed to 0 = very dissatisfied, 33 = dissatisfied, 66 = satisfied and 100 = very satisfied [23, 34]. Intentions to stay in the profession for the next five years were predefined as "yes", "no" or "don't know". Two open questions asked about occupational stresses and wishes for the work situation. Out of the free texts, entries categories were formed, which were analysed quantitatively.

Statistical analyses

Frequency distributions and percentages as well as means with corresponding standard deviations (SD) were calculated. Differences between the three professional groups were analysed using the chi-square test for categorical variables. Fisher's exact test was performed if the expected cell frequencies were less than five. Mean differences were evaluated using one-way ANOVA and Scheffé post-hoc tests. If assumptions of normal distribution and homogeneity of variance were not met, non-parametric tests were used. Associations between health-related factors and binary outcome variables (MSD and mental disorder) were examined by logistic regression. Firstly, all variables with a significance value of $p < 0.05$ from univariate analyses were included in a hierarchical model. Secondly, variables with p-value <0.25 were added [35]. If the model did not improve significantly through the second step, a final model with all the variables from the first step was calculated using the "enter" method. Odds ratios with corresponding 95 % confidence intervals and explained variances (Nagelkerke's Pseudo R^2) were calculated from logistic regression analyses. Statistical significance was set at $p < 0.05$. All statistical analyses were performed using SPSS version 20.

Results

The socio-demographic characteristics of the study participants are presented in Table 2. More than 75 % of apprentices were female. Geriatric nurses were slightly older (23.2 SD 3.3 years) than hospital nurses (21.9 SD 2.4 years) and kindergarten teachers/assistants (21.7 SD 3.5 years, $p < 0.01$). Twenty-seven percent of apprentices were overweight or obese. Among geriatric nurses and kindergarten teachers/assistants, this applied to nearly one third. The SES differed significantly between the groups ($p < 0.001$).

More hospital nurses regularly took part in physical activities (37 %, ≥2 h/week) compared to kindergarten teachers/assistants (31 %) and geriatric nurses (25 %, $p = 0.16$). The dietary patterns of geriatric nurses and kindergarten teachers/assistants tended to be unfavourable (41 and 46 %) more often than those of hospital nurses (28 %, $p < 0.05$). The proportion of daily and occasional smokers was highest among geriatric nurses (55 %, $p < 0.01$). Twenty-one percent were classified as heavy smokers (≥20 cigarettes per day), whereas only 12 % of hospital nurses and 4 % of kindergarten teachers/assistants were classified as such. Hazardous drinking behaviour was equally common ($p = 0.69$) (Table 3).

Around half of the apprentices in each occupational group rated their health as good. Between 31 and 49 % of apprentices reported a mental disorder ($p < 0.05$), either in their own opinion or according to a physician's diagnosis. MSD were the second most prevalent complaint, with proportions exceeding 30 % (Table 3). The body regions most frequently affected were the back, knees or knee joints. Kindergarten teachers/assistants had the lowest self-efficacy and highest irritation. Differences between the groups did not reach statistical significance (Table 3). Irritation was significantly higher among apprentices in their third (24.0 SD

Table 2 Characteristics of the study population

Items	Geriatric nursing ($n = 130$) n (%)	General healthcare and nursing ($n = 142$) n (%)	Early childhood education ($n = 82$) n (%)	*p*-value
Age groups (years)				<0.001
16–19	20 (15.4)	24 (16.9)	24 (29.3)	
20–22	38 (29.2)	62 (43.7)	29 (35.4)	
23–26	46 (35.4)	49 (34.5)	20 (24.4)	
27–30	26 (20.0)	7 (4.9)	9 (11.0)	
Sex				0.07
Female	98 (75.4)	122 (85.9)	63 (76.8)	
Male	32 (24.6)	20 (14.1)	19 (23.2)	
Body mass index				0.15
< 18.5	4 (3.1)	9 (6.3)	7 (8.5)	
18.5–24.9	78 (60.0)	95 (66.9)	45 (54.9)	
25–30	26 (20.0)	26 (18.3)	18 (22.0)	
≥ 30	14 (10.8)	5 (3.5)	6 (7.3)	
Migration background				0.13
No	90 (69.2)	110 (77.5)	57 (69.5)	
Yes	38 (29.2)	28 (19.7)	25 (30.5)	
Socioeconomic status[a]				<0.001
Low	64 (49.2)	25 (17.6)	37 (45.1)	
Middle	52 (40.0)	79 (55.6)	36 (43.9)	
High	4 (3.1)	30 (21.1)	3 (3.7)	
Year of education				<0.001
1st	32 (24.6)	59 (41.5)	29 (35.4)	
2nd	66 (50.8)	35 (24.6)	53 (64.6)	
3rd	32 (24.6)	48 (33.8)	/	

[a]Derived from educational level of apprentices and parental occupation
Missing values: Body mass index $n = 21$ (5.9 %); Migration background $n = 6$ (1.7 %); Socioeconomic status $n = 24$ (6.8 %)

Table 3 Group comparisons of health behaviour, health status and occupational prospects

	Geriatric nursing ($n = 130$)	General healthcare and nursing ($n = 142$)	Early childhood education ($n = 82$)		
Items	n (%)	n (%)	n (%)	Chi² (df)	*p*-value
Health behaviour					
Physical activity				6.5 (4)	0.16
No physical activity	33 (25.4)	22 (15.5)	18 (22.0)		
< 2 h/week	62 (47.7)	66 (46.5)	39 (47.6)		
≥ 2 h/week	32 (24.6)	52 (36.6)	25 (30.5)		
Dietary patterns				9.9 (4)	<0.05
Unfavourable	53 (40.8)	39 (27.5)	38 (46.3)		
Normal	36 (27.7)	49 (34.5)	22 (26.8)		
Favourable	26 (20.0)	42 (29.6)	18 (22.0)		
Smoking habits				17.6 (6)	<0.01
Daily	58 (44.6)	43 (30.3)	29 (35.4)		
Occasionally	14 (10.8)	7 (4.9)	7 (8.5)		
Former	17 (13.1)	15 (10.6)	5 (6.1)		
Never	41 (31.5)	77 (54.2)	41 (50.0)		
Hazardous alcohol consumption				0.7 (2)	0.69
Yes	53 (40.8)	60 (42.3)	38 (46.3)		
No	72 (55.4)	80 (56.3)	41 (50.0)		
Health status					
Self-rated health status				9.2 (4)	0.06
Excellent/very good	52 (40.0)	55 (38.7)	25 (30.5)		
Good	65 (50.0)	74 (52.1)	40 (48.8)		
Not so good/poor	11 (8.5)	13 (9.2)	17 (20.7)		
Diseases and complaints					
Mental disorder	50 (38.5)	44 (31.0)	40 (48.8)	7.9 (2)	<0.05
MSD	45 (34.6)	52 (36.6)	26 (31.7)	0.5 (2)	0.79
Neurological or sensory disease	47 (36.2)	39 (27.5)	25 (30.5)	2.3 (2)	0.32
Respiratory disease	34 (26.2)	48 (33.8)	23 (28.0)	1.9 (2)	0.38
Skin disease	33 (25.4)	47 (33.1)	23 (28.0)	2.0 (2)	0.37
Injury due to an accident	37 (28.5)	28 (19.7)	25 (30.5)	4.0 (2)	0.13
	Mean (SD)	Mean (SD)	Mean (SD)	F (df1/df2)	*p*-value
Self-efficacy (10–40)	29.3 (4.5)	29.2 (4.2)	28.1 (4.9)	1.9 (2/338)	0.15
Irritation (8–56)	23.4 (11.1)	21.9 (9.9)	24.7 (10.2)	1.8 (2/343)	0.17
Occupational prospects					
Job satisfaction (0–100)	62.1 (15.9)	57.4 (15.2)	68.2 (16.7)	12.3 (2/350)	<0.001

Missing values: Physical activity $n = 5$ (1.4 %); Dietary patterns = 31 (8.8 %); Hazardous alcohol consumption $n = 10$ (2.8 %); Self-rated health status $n = 2$ (0.6 %)
SD standard deviation, *df* degrees of freedom, *MSD* musculoskeletal disorders

11.6) and second years (24.2 SD 10.5) of education than for those in their first year (21.1 SD 9.4, $p < 0.05$).

Kindergarten teachers/assistants were significantly more satisfied with their job than geriatric and hospital nurses ($p < 0.001$) (Table 3). Moreover, job satisfaction was highest among apprentices in the first year (68.6 SD 13.8), compared to the second (60.6 SD 15.6) and third years of education (53.1 SD 16.9, $p < 0.001$). With respect to occupational stresses, geriatric nurses most frequently reported time pressure and stress (39 %), physical and mental exertion (30 %) as well as a lack of staff (26 %). Besides these aspects, a high proportion of hospital nurses perceived the team situation and interaction with colleagues as burdensome (26 %). Kindergarten teachers/assistants listed physical and mental exertion (35 %) as well as working hours (26 %) most often. The majority of them intended to stay in their profession for the next five years (62 %). This also applied to nearly half of geriatric nurses, but only to 36 % of hospital nurses. Motivation to stay in the profession was significantly lower in the third year of education (35 %) than in the second (47 %) and first years (57 %, $p < 0.001$). More than half of apprentices in all occupational groups demanded higher wages and better public standing for their profession. There was a strong wish for more staff among geriatric and hospital nurses (44 and 53 %). Kindergarten teachers/assistants requested an improvement in working atmosphere and teamwork (25 %).

The variables age, SES, mental disorder, irritation and job satisfaction were significantly related to MSD in univariate analyses and therefore included in a logistic regression model. The ages of 23–26 years (OR 3.1, 95 % CI 1.4–6.7) and mental disorder (OR 1.8, 95 % CI 1.1–3.1) were associated with MSD; the model explained 18 % of the variance in the outcome variable (Table 4).

A logistic regression model for the outcome of mental disorder was formed with the variables apprenticeship trade, SES, MSD, self-efficacy, irritation and job satisfaction. Being an apprentice in early childhood education was associated with an increased chance of mental disorder (OR 2.9, 95 % CI 1.4–6.0). Additionally, MSD, self-efficacy and irritation were significantly associated with mental disorder; the model explained 25 % of the variance in the outcome variable (Table 4).

Discussion

This study was the first to provide a comparison of the health of apprentices in nursing professions and early childhood education. Results show that the health behaviour of geriatric nurses and kindergarten teachers/assistants is particularly worrying. Overall, more than one third of participants reported MSD or mental disorder.

In the present study, only 25 % of geriatric nurses were engaged in sports (≥2 h/week). This proportion was considerably lower than among young adults aged 18 to 29 years (37 %) in a recent German survey (DEGS1) [29]. We applied a food frequency index to evaluate the dietary patterns of apprentices, which extends beyond a simple enumeration of consumption frequencies. According to this index, around 46 % of kindergarten teachers/assistants had unfavourable dietary patterns, although teaching a healthy diet is part of their curriculum in Germany. The prevalence of overweight and obesity ranged from 22 % for hospital nurses to 31 % for geriatric nurses. These rates were similar to those of the corresponding age group in the general female population in Germany (30 %) [8]. However, apprentices engaged mainly in technical and commercial occupations showed a lower prevalence of overweight and obesity (19 %) [36].

We detected high smoking rates among geriatric nurses (55 %) and kindergarten teachers/assistants (44 %) which exceeded the smoking rate of 40 % found among young female adults in the general population [7]. However, our findings are in line with the results of studies of nursing students in Germany (smoking rates over 40 %) [10–12, 14, 15]. When compared to international studies, our smoking rates were considerably higher [9]. The proportions of apprentices classified as hazardous drinkers ranged from 41 to 46 % in our study. These were slightly higher than in women from the general population aged 18 to 29 years (36 %) [6].

A considerable proportion of apprentices in our study had suffered from MSD during the previous twelve months (32 to 37 %). Also, high prevalence rates (25 to 53 %) were detected by other investigations of nursing students and professionals in early childhood education [3, 14, 18]. We found that apprentices aged 23 to 26 years were more likely to suffer from MSD than younger apprentices (16 to 19 years). However, the ages of 27 to 30 years was not associated with an increased chance of MSD, meaning that we could not prove a consistent age effect. Other investigations confirm an age trend [37, 38]. It cannot be ruled out that our findings result from the narrow categorisation of age groups chosen for the analysis.

In the present analysis, low SES was associated with a low prevalence of MSD. Previous studies have found inconsistent results. A review reported that low SES was associated with a higher prevalence of musculoskeletal pain [39]. One reason for the inconsistencies could be differences in the methods used to measure the SES. Additionally, we observed a significant correlation between age and SES. Therefore, age could have influenced the association between SES and MSD in our study.

An overview of systematic reviews found strong evidence that poor job satisfaction is a risk factor for the development of low back pain in adults aged 18 years and older [40]. In our study, no association between job satisfaction and MSD was found. Job satisfaction has probably not yet had any substantial influence on the physical health of apprentices, as they have just entered the profession.

Mental disorders measured in our study included several symptoms such as depression, anxiety and chronic insomnia. With frequencies between 8 and 18 % of mental disorders confirmed by a physician's diagnosis, we observed higher twelve-month prevalence rates than the survey of the general German population (4 % in adults aged 18 to 29 years). This prevalence included only diagnosed depressions and no other symptoms which could explain the difference in prevalence rates [41]. Nevertheless, our results of mental disorders could indicate that apprentices suffer from high occupational stress in their workplaces and performance stress due to their involvement in exams at vocational schools, since we

Table 4 Variables associated with musculoskeletal and mental disorders

Musculoskeletal disorders (MSD)			
Independent variables	MSD n (%)	Crude OR (95 % CI)	Adjusted OR[a] (95 % CI)
Age (years)			
16–19	17 (25.0)	1	1
20–22	38 (29.7)	1.3 (0.7–2.5)	1.2 (0.6–2.7)
23–26	58 (50.4)	3.1 (1.6–5.9)**	3.1 (1.4–6.7)**
27–30	10 (23.8)	0.9 (0.4–2.3)	1.0 (0.4–2.8)
Socioeconomic status			
High	16 (43.2)	1	1
Middle	67 (40.1)	0.9 (0.4–1.8)	1.0 (0.5–2.2)
Low	31 (24.8)	0.4 (0.2–0.9)*	0.5 (0.2–1.2)
Mental disorder			
No	60 (27.6)	1	1
Yes	62 (46.3)	2.3 (1.4–3.5)***	1.8 (1.1–3.1)*
Irritation (8–56)	/	1.04 (1.02–1.06)**	1.02 (1.00–1.05)
Job satisfaction (0–100)	/	0.98 (0.97–0.99)**	0.99 (0.97–1.01)
Mental disorder			
Independent variables	Mental disorder n (%)	Crude OR (95 % CI)	Adjusted OR[a] (95 % CI)
Apprenticeship trade			
General healthcare and nursing	44 (31.0)	1	1
Geriatric nursing	50 (38.5)	1.4 (0.8–2.3)	1.4 (0.8–2.7)
Early childhood education	40 (50.0)	2.2 (1.3–3.9)**	2.9 (1.4–6.0)**
Socioeconomic status			
High	9 (24.3)	1	1
Middle	73 (43.7)	2.4 (1.1–5.4)*	2.2 (0.9–5.4)
Low	43 (34.7)	1.7 (0.7–3.8)	1.5 (0.6–4.1)
MSD			
No	72 (31.4)	1	1
Yes	62 (50.8)	2.3 (1.4–3.5)***	2.1 (1.2–3.7)**
Self-efficacy (10–40)	/	0.89 (0.85–0.94)***	0.93 (0.87–0.99)*
Irritation (8–56)	/	1.07 (1.05–1.10)***	1.05 (1.02–1.08)**
Job satisfaction (0–100)	/	0.98 (0.97–0.99)**	0.98 (0.97–1.00)

Multivariate logistic regression analysis to determine variables associated with MSD was performed with $n = 318$ participants (Nagelkerke's Pseudo $R^2 = 0.18$).
Multivariate logistic regression analysis to determine variables associated with mental disorder was performed with $n = 310$ participants (Nagelkerke's Pseudo $R^2 = 0.25$)
[a]Adjusted for the other variables in the model
OR odds ratio, *CI* confidence interval; *p <0.05, **p <0.01, ***p <0.001

measured significantly higher irritation among apprentices in the second than in the first year of education. However, we did not control for academic performance in our study.

Kindergarten teachers/assistants had a 2.9-fold chance of experiencing mental disorder compared to hospital nurses. As the apprenticeship of early childhood education is provided by vocational schools without any reimbursement, a high financial burden is placed on apprentices. This could negatively affect their mental health status. However, differences observed between occupational groups could also be related to the SES. Individuals with a high SES have a lower risk of suffering from mental illnesses [41]. Hospital nurses had a significantly higher SES than the other groups, which could explain their better mental health status. In general, the dependency between SES and apprenticeship trade might have influenced the relationship between SES and mental disorder. In contrast to the literature, no association could be proven for the latter by logistic regression.

MSD and mental disorder were significantly associated in our study, although the direction of causality is unclear. Lewinsohn et al. [42] showed that physical illness was a significant risk factor for depression in older adolescents. There is also strong evidence for the coexistence of physical and mental illnesses in the general population [43].

Strengths and limitations

The use of heterogeneous instruments to measure health behaviour and status makes a comparison of literature difficult, and also limits the generalisability of the results of this study. Because of the cross-sectional design, no conclusions on causal relationships can be drawn. In addition, results are based on self-reports of participants. When validating the food frequency index, Winkler and Döring [30] pointed out that participants tend to overestimate intake of foods with a healthy image. Furthermore, frequencies of overweight in adolescents are underestimated by studies relying on self-report [44]. For that reason, unfavourable dietary patterns as well as overweight and obesity are likely to be even more prevalent than identified by this study. It was not feasible to draw a random sample of apprentices from the participating schools. The decisions of schools on which classes could take part in the study could not be influenced, as these depended on the upcoming practical periods and exams. Since a convenience sampling strategy had to be used, the study sample might not be representative. We calculated ORs to identify factors associated with MSD and mental disorders. However, these ORs should not be interpreted as estimates of relative risks, as the outcomes were frequent and because of the temporal ambiguity due to the cross-sectional design of our study (Table 4).

Limitations due to a non-response bias can be excluded because of the high response rate of 99 %. The number of missing values was under 5 % for nearly all variables. Extensive socio-demographic information on participants was collected in order to identify possible confounders.

Conclusions

According to the results of the study, it seems to be necessary to develop didactically sound teaching units aimed at strengthening the apprentices' health and avoiding risk factors. Among geriatric nurses, a high smoking rate indicates that more information on the consequences of smoking, individual support in stopping smoking and explicit anti-smoking policies at vocational schools are required [9]. Ergonomic working practices should be actively propagated during vocational training to prevent work-related MSD. Adequate financial support during the apprenticeship might help kindergarten teachers/assistants in reducing stress. Good concepts of health promotion at nursing schools in Germany could already be identified through an ideas competition. Examples are an in-house training in kinaesthetics and a regular running training, accompanied by lessons on anatomy, physiology and nutrition [45]. Such concepts still have to be developed for the field of early childhood education.

Due to the small sample size, the results of this study should be verified. By including a population-based comparison group, it could be possible to distinguish whether apprentices or young adults in general are at higher risk of the investigated disorders. Furthermore, it should be examined whether health status and health behaviour influence the choice of a particular apprenticeship or whether the particular working and learning conditions influence the health status and behaviour of the young adults. In addition to age, apprenticeship trade, self-efficacy and irritation, which were identified as the most important factors associated with MSD or mental disorder, future studies could evaluate muscle activity and endurance, academic performance, major life events and social support for their association with the health status in apprentices [18, 40, 42].

Leaving aside temporal ambiguity, future projects should concentrate on planning and implementing health promotion measures in the three occupational fields, taking into account the particular circumstances of an apprenticeship. Scientific evaluation can ensure the methodological and content-related quality of these measures.

Acknowledgements

The authors would like to thank all the apprentices who participated in the study and the vocational schools for their support. We also thank Prof. Dr. Zita Schillmöller for assistance with statistical analyses and interpretation of data.

Sources of funding

No external funding.

Authors' contributions

TW was responsible for the conception and design of the study, acquisition, analysis and interpretation of data, and was in charge of writing the article. AK participated in the conception and design of the study, analysis and interpretation of data, and the revision of the article for important intellectual content. GS contributed to the conception and design of the study and the revision of the article. AN participated in the conception and design of the study, interpretation of data and the revision of the article. All authors read and approved the final manuscript.

Competing interests

The authors declare that they have no competing interests.

Author details

[1]Institution for Statutory Accident Insurance and Prevention in the Health and Welfare Services, Department for the Principle of Prevention and Rehabilitation, Pappelallee 33/35/37, 22089 Hamburg, Germany. [2]University Medical Centre Hamburg-Eppendorf, Institute for Health Services Research in Dermatology and Nursing, Martinistraße 52, 20246 Hamburg, Germany.

References

1. Rothgang H, Müller R, Unger R. Themenreport "Pflege 2030" - Was ist zu erwarten - Was ist zu tun? Bertelsmann Stiftung. 2012. https://www.bertelsmann-stiftung.de/fileadmin/files/BSt/Publikationen/GrauePublikationen/GP_Themenreport_Pflege_2030.pdf. Accessed 15 Dec 2015.
2. Dathe D, Paul F, Stuth S. Soziale Dienstleistungen: Steigende Arbeitslast trotz Personalzuwachs. WZBrief Arbeit. 2012;12.

3. McGrath BJ, Huntington AD. The health and wellbeing of adults working in early childhood education. AJEC. 2007;32:33–8.
4. Simon M, Tackenberg P, Hasselhorn HM, Kümmerling A, Büschner A, Müller BH. Auswertung der ersten Befragung der NEXT-Studie in Deutschland. Bergische Universität Wuppertal; Universität Witten/Herdecke. 2005. http://www.next.uni-wuppertal.de/index.php?artikel-und-berichte-1. Accessed 21 May 2015.
5. Remschmidt H. Adoleszenz - seelische Gesundheit und psychische Krankheit. Dtsch Arztebl Int. 2013;110:423–4.
6. Hapke U, von der Lippe E, Gaertner B. Alcohol consumption, at-risk and heavy episodic drinking with consideration of injuries and alcohol-specific medical advice. Bundesgesundheitsbl. 2013;56:809–13. doi:10.1007/s00103-013-1699-0.
7. Lampert T, von der Lippe E, Müters S. Prevalence of smoking in the adult population of Germany. Bundesgesundheitsbl. 2013;56:802–8. doi:10.1007/s00103-013-1698-1.
8. Mensink GBM, Schienkiewitz A, Haftenberger M, Lampert T, Ziese T, Scheidt-Nave C. Overweight and obesity in Germany. Bundesgesundheitsbl. 2013;56:786–94. doi:10.1007/s00103-012-1656-3.
9. Smith DR. A systematic review of tobacco smoking among nursing students. Nurse Educ Pract. 2007;7:293–302. doi:10.1016/j.nepr.2006.09.003.
10. Hirsch K, Voigt K, Gerlach K, Kugler J, Bergmann A. Tabak-, Alkohol- und Drogenkonsum sowie Impfverhalten von Gesundheits- und KrankenpflegeschülerInnen in Sachsen-Anhalt. HeilberufeSCIENCE. 2010;1:127–32.
11. Kolleck B. Smoking among nursing students. Pflege. 2004;17:98–104. doi:10.1024/1012-5302.17.2.98.
12. Lehmann F, von Lindeman K, Klewer J, Kugler J. BMI, physical inactivity, cigarette and alcohol consumption in female nursing students: a 5-year comparison. BMC Med Educ. 2014;14. doi:10.1186/1472-6920-14-82.
13. von Lindeman K, Kugler J, Klewer J. Ernährungsgewohnheiten, BMI und Diätversuche von Auszubildenden in Gesundheitsfachberufen. HeilberufeSCIENCE. 2011;2:67–70.
14. Schwanke A, Bomball J, Schmitt S, Stöver M, Görres S. Gesundheitsförderung und Prävention in Pflegeschulen - Ergebnisse einer Studie zur bundesweiten Vollerhebung in Pflegeschulen. Pflegewissenschaft. 2011;4:205–12.
15. Neumann P, Klewer J. Health behaviour of trainees in the socially nursing field – A survey at vocational training schools in Saxony. Pflegewissenschaft. 2010;12:672–7.
16. Watson H, Whyte R, Schartau E, Jamieson E. Survey of student nurses and midwives: smoking and alcohol use. Br J Nurs. 2006;15:1212–6. doi:10.12968/bjon.2006.15.22.22557.
17. Singleton EK, Bienemy C, Hutchinson SW, Dellinger A, Rami JS. A pilot study: a descriptive correlational study of factors associated with weight in college nursing students. ABNF J. 2011;22:89–95.
18. Mitchell T, O'Sullivan PB, Burnett A, Straker L, Smith A, Thornton J, et al. Identification of modifiable personal factors that predict new-onset low back pain: a prospective study of female nursing students. Clin J Pain. 2010;26:275–83. doi:10.1097/AJP.0b013e3181cd16e1.
19. Rudman A, Gustavsson JP. Burnout during nursing education predicts lower occupational preparedness and future clinical performance: a longitudinal study. Int J Nurs Stud. 2012;49:988–1001.
20. Hoffmann SW, Tug S, Simon P. Obesity prevalence and unfavorable health risk behaviors among German kindergarten teachers: cross-sectional results of the kindergarten teacher health study. BMC Public Health. 2013;13:927.
21. Baldwin D, Gaines S, Wold JL, Williams A, Leary J. The health of female child care providers: implications for quality of care. J Community Health Nurs. 2007;24:1–17.
22. Mohr G, Müller A, Rigotti T. Normwerte der Skala Irritation: Zwei Dimensionen psychischer Beanspruchung. Diagnostica. 2005;51:12–20.
23. Nübling M, Stößel U, Hasselhorn H, Michaelis M, Hofmann F. Methoden zur Erfassung psychischer Belastungen. Erprobung eines Messinstrumentes (COPSOQ). Bremerhaven: Wirtschaftsverlag NW; 2005.
24. Schwarzer R, Jerusalem M. Skalen zur Erfassung von Lehrer- und Schülermerkmalen. Dokumentation der psychometrischen Verfahren im Rahmen der Wissenschaftlichen Begleitung des Modellversuchs Selbstwirksame Schulen. 1999. http://userpage.fu-berlin.de/~health/self/skalendoku_selbstwirksame_schulen.pdf. Accessed 20 Sept 2015.
25. Lange M, Kamtsiuris P, Lange C, Schaffrath Rosario A, Stolzenberg H, Lampert T. Messung soziodemographischer Merkmale im Kinder- und Jugendgesundheitssurvey (KiGGS) und ihre Bedeutung am Beispiel der Einschätzung des allgemeinen Gesundheitszustands. Bundesgesundheitsbl. 2007;50:578–89.
26. Geis A. Handbuch für die Berufsvercodung. GESIS. 2011. http://www.gesis.org/fileadmin/upload/dienstleistung/tools_standards/handbuch_der_berufscodierung_110304.pdf. Accessed 07 Jan 2016.
27. Ganzeboom H, Treiman D. Internationally comparable measures of occupational status for the 1988 International Standard Classification of Occupations. Soc Sci Res. 1996;25:201–39.
28. Thomas S, Heinrich S, Kühnlein A, Radon K. The association between socioeconomic status and exposure to mobile telecommunication networks in children and adolescents. Bioelectromagnetics. 2010;31:20–7. doi:10.1002/bem.20522.
29. Krug S, Jordan S, Mensink GBM, Müters S, Finger JD, Lampert T. Physical activity: results of the German Health Interview and Examination Survey for Adults (DEGS1). Bundesgesundheitsbl. 2013;56:765–70. doi:10.1007/s00103-012-1661-6.
30. Winkler G, Döring A. Kurzmethoden zur Charakterisierung des Ernährungsmusters: Einsatz und Auswertung eines Food-Frequency-Fragebogens. Ernahrungs-Umschau. 1995;42:289–91.
31. Bush K, Kivlahan DR, McDonell MB, Fihn SD, Bradley KA. The AUDIT Alcohol Consumption Questions (AUDIT-C): an effective brief screening test for problem drinking. Arch Intern Med. 1998;158:1789–95.
32. Reinert DF, Allen JP. The alcohol use disorders identification test: an update of research findings. Alcohol Clin Exp Res. 2007;31:185–99. doi:10.1111/j.1530-0277.2006.00295.x.
33. Hasselhorn HM, Freude G. Der Work Ability Index - ein Leitfaden. Bremerhaven: Wirtschaftsverlag NW; 2007.
34. Kristensen TS, Hannerz H, Hogh A, Borg V. The Copenhagen Psychosocial Questionnaire-a tool for the assessment and improvement of the psychosocial work environment. Scand J Work Environ Health. 2005;31:438–49.
35. Hosmer DW, Lemeshow S. Applied logistic regression. New York: John Wiley & Sons; 2000.
36. Kaminski A, Nauerth A, Pfefferle PI. Gesundheitszustand und Gesundheitsverhalten von Auszubildenden im ersten Lehrjahr - Erste Ergebnisse einer Befragung in Bielefelder Berufskollegs. Gesundheitswesen. 2008;70:38–46.
37. Bot SD, van der Waal JM, Terwee CB, van der Windt DA, Schellevis FG, Bouter LM, et al. Incidence and prevalence of complaints of the neck and upper extremity in general practice. Ann Rheum Dis. 2005;64:118–23. doi:10.1136/ard.2003.019349.
38. de Zwart BC, Broersen JP, Frings-Dresen MH, van Dijk FJ. Musculoskeletal complaints in the Netherlands in relation to age, gender and physically demanding work. Int Arch Occup Environ Health. 1997;70:352–60.
39. McBeth J, Jones K. Epidemiology of chronic musculoskeletal pain. Best Pract Res Clin Rheumatol. 2007;21:403–25.
40. Lakke SE, Soer R, Takken T, Reneman MF. Risk and prognostic factors for non-specific musculoskeletal pain: a synthesis of evidence from systematic reviews classified into ICF dimensions. Pain. 2009;147:153–64.
41. Busch M, Maske U, Ryl L, Schlack R, Hapke U. Prevalence of depressive symptoms and diagnosed depression among adults in Germany - Results of the German Health Interview and Examination Survey for Adults (DEGS1). Bundesgesundheitsbl. 2013;56:733–9. doi:10.1007/s00103-013-1688-3.
42. Lewinsohn PM, Rohde P, Seeley JR. Major depressive disorder in older adolescents: prevalence, risk factors, and clinical implications. Clin Psychol Rev. 1998;18:765–94.
43. Hogg-Johnson S, van der Velde G, Carroll LJ, Holm LW, Cassidy JD, Guzman J, et al. The burden and determinants of neck pain in the general population. Results of the Bone and Joint Decade 2000–2010 Task Force on Neck Pain and Its Associated Disorders. Spine. 2008;3:39–51.
44. Sherry B, Jefferds ME, Grummer-Strawn LM. Accuracy of adolescent self-report of height and weight in assessing overweight status: a literature review. Arch Pediatr Adolesc Med. 2007;161:1154–61. doi:10.1001/archpedi.161.12.1154.
45. Görres S, Stöver M, Bomball J, Schwanke A, Bremer M, Adrian C. Bundesweiter Ideenwettbewerb "Gesunde Pflegeausbildung". Anwendungsbeispiele für die Praxis Universität Bremen: IPP Schriften. 2012;10.

9

Total and respirable dust exposures among carpenters and demolition workers during indoor work in Denmark

Lilli Kirkeskov[1,2*], Dorte Jessing Agerby Hanskov[1] and Charlotte Brauer[1]

Abstract

Background: Within the construction industry the risk of lung disorders depends on the specific professions probably due to variations in the levels of dust exposure, and with dust levels depending on the work task and job function. We do not know the extent of exposure in the different professions or the variation between the different work tasks. The purpose of this study was therefore to assess if there were differences in dust exposure between carpenters and demolition workers who were expected to have low and high dust exposure, respectively.

Methods: Through interviews of key persons in the construction industry the most common work tasks were selected, and the concentration of dust during these tasks (indoors) were measured by personal sampling varying between 4 and 6 h of a working day. In total 38 measurements of total dust, and 25 of respirable dust on seven different work tasks were carried out for carpenters and 20 measurements of total dust, 11 of respirable dust and 11 of respirable crystalline silica dust on four different works tasks for demolition workers. Dust measurements were tested for differences using linear regression, t-test and one-way ANOVA.

Results: For carpenters the geometric mean for all the measurements of total dust was 1.26 mg/m^3 (geometric standard deviation 2.90) and the respirable dust was 0.27 mg/m^3 (geometric standard deviation 2.13). For demolition workers the geometric mean of total dust for all the measurements was 22.3 mg/m^3 (geometric standard deviation 11.6) and the respirable dust was 1.06 mg/m^3 (geometric standard deviation 5.64).
The mean difference between total dust for demolition workers and carpenters was 11.4 (95 % confidence interval 3.46–37.1) mg/m^3. The mean difference between respirable dust for demolition workers and carpenters was 3.90 (95 % confidence interval 1.13–13.5) mg/m^3.
Dust exposure varied depending on work task for both professions. The dustiest work occurred during demolition, especially when it was done manually.
Only few workers used personal respiratory protection and only while performing the dustiest work.

Conclusions: This study confirmed that the exposure to dust and especially total dust was much higher for demolition workers compared to carpenters.

Keywords: Total dust, Respirable dust, Respirable crystalline silica dust, Construction workers, Exposure assessment

* Correspondence: lilli.kirkeskov@regionh.dk
[1]Department of Occupational and Environmental Medicine, Bispebjerg Hospital, Copenhagen, Denmark
[2]Department of Occupational and Environmental Medicine, Unit of Social Medicine, Frederiksberg Hospital, Nordre Fasanvej 57, 2000 Copenhagen F, Denmark

Background

Workers in the construction industry represent 6 % of employees in Denmark and are still daily or regularly exposed to dust. Different kinds of dust exposure including crystalline silica dust exposure occur commonly in the construction industry and are known causes for developing lung disorders.

Dust exposure in the workplace can be associated with chronic obstructive pulmonary disease (COPD) and an increased risk of COPD for workers exposed to dust has been found [1].

Earlier studies have shown differences in the risk to be hospitalised due to diseases in the lower respiratory system among different professions within the construction industry in Denmark [2, 3] which may be caused by differences in dust exposures. A cross-sectional study of demolition workers found an increased prevalence of self-reported lung symptoms (cough and sputum daily for three month per year for two years) for demolition workers (Odds ratio, OR 2.0, 95 % confidence interval, CI 1.0–3.9) and carpenters (OR 1.7, 95 % CI 0.9–3.3) compared to a group of non-exposed hospital porters and an increased OR 2.7, 95 % CI 1.3–2.7 for forced expiratory volume in one second below lower limit of normal (($FEV_1 < LLN$) for demolition workers compared to carpenters [4].

The construction industry includes many professions and many different work tasks for each profession, and the transient nature of construction sites makes it more difficult to accurately characterize exposures among construction workers. The best way to determine an adverse effect on the respiratory system due to dust exposure for individual workers is to directly measure the dust exposure and relate it to the lung function parameter for the individual worker over long periods (years). However, it is expensive and time-consuming to measure prospectively, especially for diseases that take more than a decade to develop.

The purpose of this study was to assess whether there were differences in dust exposure between two types of construction workers: carpenters and demolition workers. Based on previous studies and practical knowledge carpenters and demolition workers were chosen because these professions in the construction industry would probably have low and high exposures to dust, respectively [5–7].

In Denmark, carpenters are skilled construction workers. Their primary work tasks include installation of gypsum, doors, windows, rafters and roofs, floorings made of wood, ceilings and insulation. Demolition workers are unskilled construction workers. Their job includes manual and mechanical demolition tasks on whole or large parts of buildings, including management of waste (building material) and cleaning after demolition.

Methods

Measurements of exposure

Interviews of key persons from the trade union in the construction sector were performed to identify the most common work tasks. The work tasks were categorized as installation of gypsum, ceilings, floorings, windows and doors, insulation, and 'other work tasks' for carpenters. For demolition workers the work tasks were categorized as manual demolition, mechanical demolition, waste management and 'other work tasks'.

The measurements were only carried out on indoor work tasks because of the outdoor measurement-uncertainties due to changing wind conditions. The working environment council of the construction industry participated in finding construction companies performing the requested tasks in two areas of Denmark (Copenhagen and Aarhus). Among companies accepting to participate we selected companies of different sizes and different work places.

A total of 11 companies (and 11 workplaces) were selected for carpenters. Measurements of total dust (TD) were carried out on 38 carpenters (1 measurement per worker) and of respirable dust (RD) on 17 carpenters (25 measurements) (1–2 measurements per worker).

Measurements of TD, RD and respirable crystalline silica dust (RCS) were carried out in 5 companies (5 workplaces) for demolition workers. Measurements of TD were carried out on 16 demolition workers. For seven workers RD was measured at the same time.

The measurements were made after identification of the most relevant work tasks, included measurements for each work task. Furthermore the measurements were conducted over an entire working day (excluding pauses) or as long as the task was done. Workplaces were not selected by level of dust (worst cases) but chosen if the work task was carried out.

The measurements were spread throughout the year: 11 % (winter), 22 % (spring), 30 % (summer), and 34 % (autumn).

In connection with the dust measurements it was registered if the workers used personal respiratory protective equipment, the use of local exhaust or other dust-reducing measures.

Performed measurements corresponded to a total of 255 working hours for carpenters and 113 working hours for demolition workers (pauses excluded).

Work place monitoring of airborne dust

The concentration of TD was measured by personal sampling during 4 to 6 h of a working day. Sampling was performed using 37 mm Millipore filter cassettes mounted with 0.8 μm Mixed Cellulose Ester Membrane filters (fa. Millipore AAWOP) mounted in closed face Millipore field monitors with a 5.6-mm inlet at 1.9 L/

min (inlet velocity = 1.25 m/s) (SKS Inc. Pennsylvania, U.S). The field monitor was placed in the breathing zone just below the collarbone. The inlet pointed downward. Flow rates were adjusted and controlled in the field before and after sampling by Porter Flow Meters (Porter Air Flow meters, model F65, measurement range 0.5-3 L/min.) calibrated against certified primary references. Air velocity in inlet was adjusted to 1.25 m/s according to Danish legislation. Each series of sampling were controlled and corrected towards two blank field samples. Conditioning of filters were performed prior and after sampling under controlled climatic conditions (temperature 22–28 °C and humidity 40–52 % RH). We used sampling pumps SKC 224 and SKC SideKick.

RD was sampled with modified Higgins and Dewell cyclones [8]. The 50 % aerodynamic diameter cut-point for collection efficiency was 5 μm, and the volumetric air sampling rate 2 L/min according to the Danish Working Environment Authority Guidelines [9]. The respirable fraction was collected on 37-mm diameter 1-μm membrane filters.

The collected mass of dust on the filters was determined gravimetrically. The limit of detection, LOD was calculated as three times the standard deviation (SD) of the blanks (30 μg) and the relative standard deviation of the method was 10 %.

Respirable crystalline silica dust (RCS) was analysed according to National Institute of Occupational Safety and Health (NIOSH) method 7602 (modified, accredited) [10]. The limit of detection was 5 μg. Both sampling and gravimetric analysis were carried out by Eurofins Miljø A/S. (Eurofins Miljø are accredited by The Danish Accreditation Fund); DANAK and testing was performed in accordance with the national and international standards as approved by DANAK, (DANAK Reg. No. 168 (sampling) and Reg. No. 522 (gravimetry)).

Data analysis

Statistical analyses were conducted using SPSS software (IBM SPSS Statistics, version 22, IBM Corp. 2013). We used a logarithmic scale for the graphic presentation because the distribution was skewed with a long right trail, and normalized by log-transformation. For measurements below the lowest limit of detection and above maximum quantification the detection limit/the maximum quantification values were used in the calculations. These values account for 4.8 and 1.9 % of the measurements, respectively.

The exposure levels were described by arithmetic means (AM), geometric means (GM), and geometric standard deviations (GSD) for each occupation and for each task.

The average exposure over an eight hour time period (normal work shift), 8-h TWA was calculated as: 8-h TWA = $\Sigma_{i=1}^{n}$ $CiTi/8$ h, where Ci = concentration during the ith interval, and Ti= duration of the ith interval.

Histograms, QQ-plots, and tests of skewness showed lognormal distribution and the dust concentrations were therefore lognormal transformed before statistical analysis. Differences in TD and RD between the two occupations, between work task measurements within the two occupations and across occupations were tested using t-test, one-way ANOVA and linear regression. Log(TD) and log(RD) were used in the models. Correlations between TD and RD for the two professions were tested (Spearman's correlation).

The relationship between dust concentration and occupation was also investigated using linear regression analysis with carpenters used as reference category and adjusted for seasonal variations. Season was in the analysis divided in winter/spring and summer/autumn with summer/autumn used as reference category. Analyses were made on log-transformed data.

Results

Carpenters

The GM of all the measurement of TD was 1.26 mg/m^3 ranging from minimum 0.08 mg/m^3 when installing material of iron to maximum 8.40 mg/m^3 when stiffening of beams. Within the work task installation of gypsum the concentration of TD varied between 1.40 mg/m^3 and 7.00 mg/m^3 (Table 1). The main reasons for dust exposure among carpenters was especially use of hand-held high-speed tools, grinding, lack of local exhaust ventilation, lack of cleaning during a work task, lack of cleaning before the next occupation started their work and dust exposure from other occupations who worked at the same time. None of the carpenters used airway protection during the work.

The calculated 8-h-TWA for TD was 1.07 mg/m^3 for all the measurements. None of the calculated 8-h-TWA for the individual measurements (0.04 to 4.27 mg/m^3) exceeded the Occupational Exposure Limit (OEL) of 10 mg/m^3 for TD.

The GM of RD was 0.27 mg/m^3 ranging from no detectable RD during wood work to a maximum of 1.50 mg/m^3 when installing gypsum on walls. The calculated 8-h-TWA for RD was 0.16 mg/m^3 for all the measurements. None of the calculated 8-h-TWA for the individual measurements (0.01 to 0.33 mg/m^3) exceeded the OEL of 5 mg/m^3 for RD.

Figure 1a shows the dust concentrations for TD and RD for carpenters divided in different work task. The dust concentrations differed comparing the work tasks for carpenters ($F = 2.39$, $df = 37$, $p = 0.05$) for TD, and ($F = 5.47$, $df = 24$, $p = 0.003$) for RD (Fig. 2a). The difference between the work tasks for RD disappeared when the job tasks: 'installing gypsum' and 'other work tasks' (stiffening of

Table 1 Measurements of dust for carpenters (GM, GSD, and AM)

	Number of measurements	Average sampling time (min)	Sampling time (min-max) (min)	Number of <LOD	GM mg/m³	GSD	AM mg/m³	min-max
Total dust								
Gypsum, installation	8	346	296–401	0	2.22	1.77	2.63	1.40–7.00
Ceilings, installation	12	281	211–292	0	0.86	3.92	1.56	0.08–4.00
Installation of windows, doors	5	308	262–433	0	0.61	1.78	0.69	0.32–1.00
Installation of floors	4	240	233–245	0	1.00	1.80	1.14	0.52–1.70
Insulation	5	232	100–289	0	1.59	1.13	1.60	1.30–1.80
Wood work	2	219	101–336	0	1.57	1.31	1.60	1.30–1.90
Other (stiffening of beams)	2	206	167–244	0	5.50	1.82	6.00	3.60–8.40
Total	38	280	100–401	0	1.26	2.90	1.94	0.08–8.40
Respirable dust								
Gypsum, installation	8	213	185–250	0	0.57	1.75	0.67	0.27–1.50
Ceilings, installation	0	-	-	0	-	-	-	-
Installation of windows, doors	5	205	196–239	1	0.18	1.75	0.20	<0.07–0.31
Installation of floors	2	244	239–249	0	0.24	1.22	0.25	0.20–0.30
Insulation	3	200	177–247	1	0.15	1.67	0.17	<0.09–0.30
Wood work, milling and cutting	5	198	187–248	1	0.16	1.42	0.17	<0.09–0.24
Other	2	202	196–208	0	0.42	1.85	0.46	0.27–0.65
Total	25	210	177–250	3	0.27	2.13	0.37	<0.09–1.50

Notes: *GM* geometric mean, *GSD* geometric standard deviation, *AM* arithmetic mean, *<LOD* below level of detection

beams) were excluded from the analysis (F = 0.48, df = 14, $p = 0.70$).

TD was moderate correlated with RD (Spearman's correlation $r_s = 0.64$), Fig. 2.

Demolition workers

The measurements showed GM of all the measurements of TD of 22.3 mg/m³ ranging between 0.30 mg/m³ for installation of scaffolding and support of ceilings and > 460 mg/m³ for manual demolition (Table 2). In general, mechanical demolition showed lower dust concentrations (4.4 mg/m³) compared to manual demolition (177 mg/m³). The concentrations were lowest during mechanical demolition, good ventilation, and/or use of water. During manual demolition using high-speed tools, dry-cutting, waste management and working indoors without sufficient ventilation the exposure was high. Waste management led to a high exposure to TD, RD and RCS. Demolition workers only used respiratory protection during manual demolition.

The calculated 8-h-TWA for TD was 17.8 mg/m³ for all the measurements. For 40 % of the measurements the calculated 8-h-TWA (0.06 to >86 mg/m³) exceeded the OEL of 10 mg/m³ for TD.

In total 11 measurements of RD and RCS were made. The measurements showed GM for RD concentrations of 1.06 mg/m³ (0.10–10 mg/m³), and for RCS of 0.12 mg/m³ [<0.01 (no detectable crystalline silica) to 0.92 mg/m³]. The lowest concentrations were shown for mechanical demolition and the highest for manual demolition.

The calculated 8-h-TWA for RD was 1.40 mg/m³ for all the measurements. Only one of the calculated 8-h-TWA for the individual measurements (management of waste) (range 0.06–5.02 mg/m³) exceeded the OEL of 5 mg/m³ for RD.

The calculated 8-h-TWA for RCS was 0.08 mg/m³ for all the measurements. In total 45 % of the calculated 8-h-TWA for the individual measurements (<0.02 to 0.24 mg/m³) exceeded the OEL of 0.1 mg/m³ for RCS.

Figure 1b shows the dust concentrations for TD and RD for demolition workers divided in different work task. When comparing the four work tasks differences in dust concentrations were found for TD (F = 18.9, df = 19, $p < 0.001$), but not for RD (F = 3.16, df = 10, $p = 0.10$). The difference between the work tasks for TD disappeared when the job tasks: 'manual demolition' and waste management were excluded from the analysis (F = 4.03, df = 10, $p = 0.09$).

TD was moderate correlated with RD (Spearman's correlation $r_s = 0.69$), Fig. 2.

Demolition workers compared to carpenters

The mean difference between TD for demolition workers and carpenters was 11.4 (95 % CI 3.46–37.1) mg/m³ (t = 4.26, df =56, $p < 0.001$). The mean difference

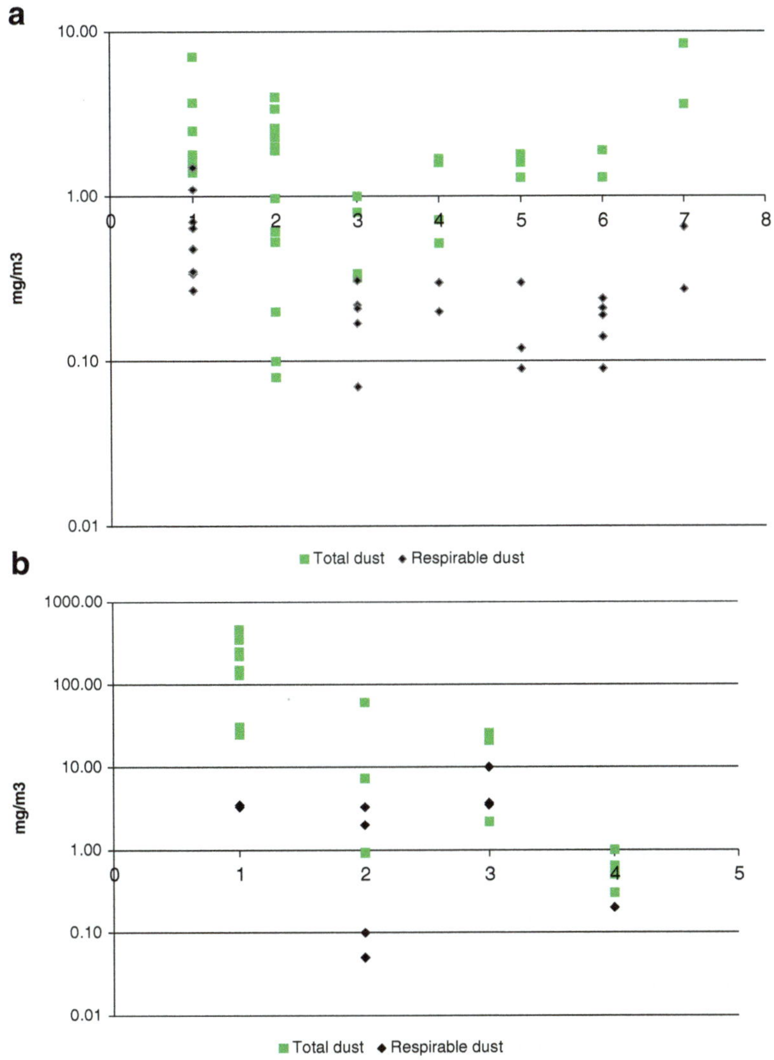

Fig. 1 a. Task-specific measurements of total and respirable dust among carpenters (mg/m^3). Note: 1: installation of gypsum; 2: installation of ceilings; 3: installation of windows and doors; 4: installation of floors; 5: insulation; 6: woodwork; 7: other work tasks. **b**. Task-specific measurements of total and respirable dust among demolition workers (mg/m^3). Note: 1: manual demolition; 2: mechanical demolition; 3: waste management; 4: other work tasks

between RD for demolition workers and carpenters was 3.90 (95 % CI 1.13–13.5) mg/m^3 (t = 2.40, df =34, p = 0.03).

In linear regression models, TD was exp(2.43) = 11.4 (95 % CI 4.58–28.2) in demolition workers compared to carpenters unadjusted and exp(2.20) = 9.03 (95 % CI 4.00–20.3) adjusted for season. TD was exp(1.71) = 5.53 (95 % CI 2.39–12.7) in winter/spring compared to summer/autumn. Written in equation: logTD = - 4.12 + 2.20 * occupation + 1.71 * season.

RD was exp(1.36) = 3.90 (95 % CI 1.65–9.23) for demolition workers compared to carpenters unadjusted and exp(1.24) = 3.46 (95 % CI 1.52–7.83) adjusted for season. RD was exp(1.08) = 2.94 (95 % CI 1.13–2.03) in winter/spring compared to summer/autumn.

Written in equation: logRD = - 3.79 + 1.24 * occupation + 1.08 * season.

Discussion

The results showed a more than ten-fold higher exposure to TD and four to five-fold higher exposures to RD for demolition workers compared to carpenters. The dust level depended on the work tasks and was highest for demolition workers during manual demolition and waste management and for carpenters during installing gypsum.

The calculated 8-h TWA of TD and RD were low for carpenters and below the OEL regardless of the work task (OEL are 10 mg/m^3 for TD and 5 mg/m^3 for RD in Denmark). The measurements showed very high concentrations especially of TD for demolition workers where the calculated 8-h TWA exceeded the OEL for 40 % of the measurements.

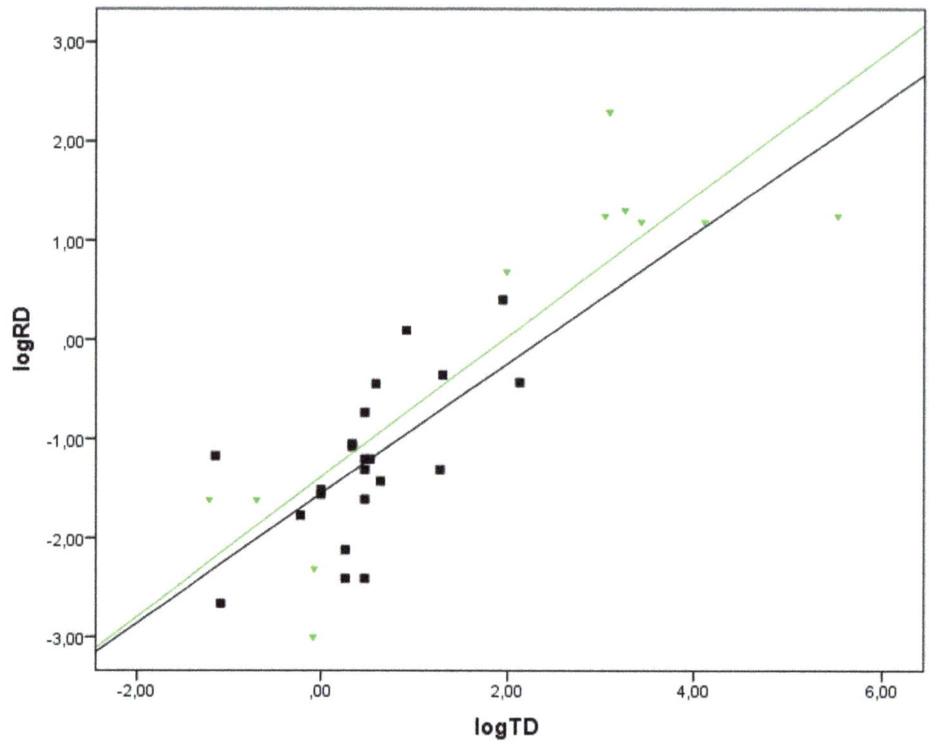

Fig. 2 Correlation between total dust (log TD) and respirable dust (log RD) for carpenters ($N = 21$, black square), Spearman correlation, $r_s = 0.64$ and demolition workers ($N = 11$, green triangle), Spearman correlation, $r_s = 0.69$

Wiebert et al. [11] assessed the exposure to dust for construction workers in Nordic countries by using job-exposure matrices and used levels of RCS of 0.01 mg/m^3, inhalable dust of 1 mg/m^3 and inhalable wood dust of 0.2 mg/m^3 for all construction workers. In the present study we found much higher dust concentrations, but only for demolition workers, and large variations in dust exposure for the two occupations depending on work tasks.

Bagschik et al. [5] collected 100,000 measurements recorded by the German Institution for Statutory Accident Insurance and Prevention. The measurements were carried out from 1972 onwards and were divided into occupations of construction and different work tasks. The average exposure of RD was 0.96 mg/m^3 (0.19–2.13 mg/m^3) for installing gypsum. The dust concentrations varied according to the type of material, the strength of the material and the local conditions. They showed demolition work to be among the most dust-intensive of all work tasks in the construction industry. The average concentration of RD during mechanized demolition was 1.15 mg/m^3 (0.25–2.67 mg/m^3) and of RCS 0.12 mg/m^3 (0.01–0.23 mg/m^3). For manual demolition the concentration of RCS was 0.26 mg/m^3. The highest concentrations occurred during demolition of concrete and reinforced concrete components, and when using high-speed handheld tools. Chrisholm [12] showed concentrations of RD due to demolition work between 1.3 mg/m^3 when using a jack hammer and 4.7 mg/m^3 when using a grinder. Karlsson and Christensson [7] reported concentration of RD of 7 mg/m^3 for demolition work in 1975 to 1988 and 3 mg/m^3 in 2005. Lumens and Spee [13] found concentrations of RD 10.8 to 14.4 mg/m^3 when working with dry saw cutting. The concentration was reduced to 1.1 mg/m^3 during wet cutting. The previous studies thus supported our findings of significant differences in the measured concentrations of RD depending on the profession, the work task and preventive measures.

The strength of this study was that the measurements were made after identification of the most relevant work tasks, included measurements for each work task and in different workers. Furthermore the measurements were conducted over an entire working day (excluding pauses) or as long as the task was done. The measurements also have been carried out on more workers performing the same work task at the same time and at the same workplace. Workplaces were not selected by level of dust (worst cases) but chosen if the work task was carried out.

The weakness of the study was no outdoor measurements which may result in an overestimation of the estimated dust exposure since the exposure outdoors are generally lower. Another weakness is a limited number of measurements especially for demolition workers.

Table 2 Measurements of dust for demolition workers (GM, GSD, and AM)

	Number of measurements	Average sampling time (min)	Sampling time (min-max) (min)	Number of <LOD	GM mg/m^3	GSD	AM mg/m^3	min-max
Total dust								
Manual demolition	8	119	90–264	0	138	2.42	227	31.0–> 460
Mechanical demolition	4	207	117–287	0	4.42	7.41	17.5	0.92–61.0
Waste management	4	163	123–257	0	22.9	3.24	23.0	21.0–26.0
Other	4	181	108–255	0	0.39	1.44	0.40	0.30–0.50
Total	20	158	90–287	0	22.3	11.6	108	0.92–> 460
Respirable dust								
Manual demolition	2	118	117–118	0	3.40	1.03	3.40	3.30–3.50
Mechanical demolition	4	207	117–287	0	0.43	6.18	1.40	0.05–3.30
Waste management	3	131	123–257	0	5.06	1.62	5.73	3.50–10.0
Other	2	116	108–124	0	0.20	1.00	0.20	-
Total	11	143	108–287	0	1.06	5.64	2.71	0.05–10.0
Respirable silica dust								
Manual demolition	2	118	117–118	0	0.69	1.03	0.69	0.67–0.71
Mechanical demolition	4	207	117–287	0	0.09	6.04	0.23	0.02–0.45
Waste management	3	131	123–257	0	0.15	4.77	0.35	0.06–0.92
Cleaning	2	116	108–124	2	nd.	-	nd.	-
Total	11	143	108–287	2	0.12	5.25	0.31	nd.–0.92

Notes: *GM* geometric mean, *GSD* geometric standard deviation, *AM* arithmetic mean, *nd* not detectable, *<LOD* below level of detection

Seasonal variations may cause a bias in the dust measurements if the performed work tasks and the ventilation through windows and doors changes during the seasons. In the analysis we therefore adjusted for eventually seasonal variations divided in winter/spring and summer/autumn. After adjustment for seasonal variations the results were only changed to a minor degree. Unfortunately, we had too few measurements to carry out statistical analysis in relation to each of the seasons which therefore may be a possible bias in this study.

The measurements showed only the current and not the previous level of dust exposure, where the level may have been higher, but most likely there have also previously been differences in the dust exposure between carpenters and demolition workers.

The literature has shown that prolonged exposure to high concentrations of RCS can cause silicosis, and studies have shown that COPD is associated with exposure to RCS [14, 15]. The risk of developing COPD depends, in general, on the level of dust exposure, on the duration of dust exposure per day and the number of years of exposure, in total. We do not know the level of exposure that affects the respiratory system or if there is a 'no effect level'. Studies suggest that exposure beyond OEL may also result in an increased risk of COPD [14, 15]. In this study 45 % of the 8-h-TWA of RCS for demolition workers exceeded OEL (up to 2.4 times the Danish OEL of 0.1 mg/m^3). The concentrations of RCS exceeded the OEL even though the RD level was below the OEL for RD. This emphasizes the importance of not only measuring the TD and RD but also supplementing these measurements with RCS if there is dust from concrete, mortar, gypsum or granite. It also supports the importance of using preventive measures such as water, local exhaust ventilation or respiratory protection. The measurements in this study support the practical experience and earlier measurements showing that different prevention strategies reduce the exposure and thus the risk of developing respiratory diseases [6].

Different sized particles deposit in different areas of the lung, nose and throat and may result in irritative symptoms including cough and COPD. The measurements of TD and RD concentrations are not directly comparable and there is no conversion factor to calculate the respirable fraction of dust by using measured TD concentrations. Studies report four times higher 'total' dust concentration compared to the respirable dust concentration among high-exposed cement workers [16, 17]. In a study from the cement industry RD, TD, and inhalable fractions were compared to thoracic fractions. The median ratios between the parameters' were 0.51, 2.4 and 5.9, respectively. They found therefore that the cement industry would be able to predict the health related dust level by future measurements of just one of the fractions [18]. In this study the dust measurements for carpenters and demolition workers, showed a correlation between TD and RD but with large differences in the measured concentrations of TD compared to RD and RCS. Even at high concentrations of TD the concentration of RD was low, and despite relatively low concentrations of RD concentration of RCS was high and exceeded the OEL. In the construction industry it is therefore not enough in future measurements to measure one of the fractions to predict the health related dust level.

In the current study carpenters did not use respiratory protection and the demolition workers used respiratory protection in less than 1/3 of the dusty work processes and they may thus have been considerably exposed to dust at some of the work tasks. The current measurements represent the workers' exposure to dust without using personal respiratory protection. Use of different types of personal equipment would reduce their exposure depending on the personal respiratory protection used (protection factor 5 to 50) [19].

Our study supports the importance to include different measurements of dust (e.g. TD, RD and RCS), for specific occupations and for work tasks where a dust exposure are expected, to use personal respiratory protection and other prevention measures.

Conclusions

This measurement study showed differences in dust exposure between two professions within the construction industry. As expected, demolition workers were exposed to a much higher extent than carpenters. There was difference in dust exposure depending on profession, but also depending on work task for both occupations.

Acknowledgments

Thanks to senior consultant Peter Vinzents, EUROFINS, who contributed to the collection of current measurements of dust.

Funding

The project is supported by the Danish Work Environment Research Fund Grant no. 21-2010-09.

Authors' contributions

LK prepared the manuscript. All authors contributed with text and critical revisions. All authors have reviewed and approved the final draft.

Competing interests

The authors declare that they have no competing interests.

References

1. Omland Ø, Würtz ET, Aasen TB, et al. Occupational chronic obstructive pulmonary disease: a systematic literature review. Scand J Work Environ Health. 2014;40(1):19–35.
2. Molgaard EF, Hannerz H, Tuchsen F, et al. Chronic lower respiratory diseases among demolition and cement workers: a population-based register study. BMJ Open. 2013;3(1):e001938. doi:10.1136/bmjopen-2012-001938.
3. Tuchsen F, Hannerz H, Molgaard EF, et al. Time trend in hospitalised chronic lower respiratory diseases among Danish building and construction workers, 1981–2009: a cohort study. BMJ Open. 2012;2(6):e001761. doi:10.1136/bmjopen-2012-001761.
4. Hanskov D, Brauer C, Breinegaard N, et al. Respiratory symptoms and lung function among Danish construction workers. A cross-sectional study. Int J Respir Pulm Med. 2015;2(4):1–6.
5. Bagschik U, Böckler M, Chromy W, et al. Exposure to quartz at the work place. BGIA-Report 8/2006e 2008:1–154.
6. Christensson B, Ostlund G, Alvarez E, et al. Effektiva åtgärder mot damm på byggarbetsplatser. Etapp 2. [Effective measures aganst dust at construction sites] [in Swedish]. IVL. Stockholm: Svenska Miljöinstitutet; 2012.
7. Karlsson A, Christensson B. Effektiva åtgärder mot damm på byggarbetsplatser. Etapp 1 [Effective measures against dust at construction sites stage 1] [in Swedish]. Stockholm: Svenska Miljöinstitutet; 2008. p. 1–47.
8. Higgins R, Dewell P. A gravimetric size selecting personal dust sampler. In: Davies CN, editor. Inhaled Particles and Vapours II. Oxford: Pergamon Press; 1967. p. 575–86.
9. Anonymous. Working Environment Authoritues Guidelines. Substances and Materials. C.0.1. Danish Working Environment Authority 2007;C.1.0.:1–84.
10. Silica. Crystalline by IR: Method 7602. NIOSH Manual of Analytical Methods (NMAM) 2003 (3):1–6.
11. Wiebert P, Lönn M, Fremling K, et al. Occupational exposure to particles and incidence of acute myocardial infarction and other ischaemic heart disease. Occup Environ Med. 2012;69:651–7.
12. Chrisholm J. Respirable dust and respirable silica concentrations from construction activities. Indoor Built Environ. 1999;8:94–106.
13. Lumens M, Spee T. Determinants of exposure to respirable quartz dust in the construction industry. Ann Occup Hyg. 2001;45(7):585–95.
14. Rushton L. Review of literature on chronic obstructive pulmonary disease and occupational exposure to Silica. London: Imperial College London; 2007. p. 1–53.
15. Rushton L. Chronic obstructive pulmonary disease and occupational exposure to silica. Rev Environ Health. 2007;22(4):255–72.
16. Mirzaee R, Kebriaei A, Hashemi S, et al. Effects of exposure to Portland and cement dust on lung function in Portland cement factory workers in Kash, Iran. Iran J Environ Health Sci Eng. 2008;5:201–6.
17. Mwaiselage J, Moen B, Bråtveit M. Acute respiratory health effects among cement factory workers in Tanzania: an evaluation of a simple health surveillance tool. Int Arch Occup Environ Health. 2006;79:49–56.
18. Notø HP, Nordby K-C, Eduard W. Relationships between personal measurements of 'total' dust, respirable, thoracic, and inhalable aerosol fractions in the cement production industry. Ann Occup Hyg. 2016;60(4): 453–66.
19. OSHA. Assigned protection factors for revised respiratory protection standard. OSHA, Occupational Safety and Health Administration U S Department of Labor 2009;OSHA 3352–02:1–47.

10

Work-related exposures and disorders among physical therapists: experiences and beliefs of professional representatives

Maria Girbig[1*†], Alice Freiberg[1†], Stefanie Deckert[1], Diana Druschke[1], Christian Kopkow[1], Albert Nienhaus[2] and Andreas Seidler[1]

Abstract

Background: According to international study results, physical therapists are afflicted with work-related musculoskeletal, psychosocial and dermal disorders as well as infections. The few existing studies in German-speaking regions focus mainly on dermal and psychosocial exposures and resulting complaints. An overview of all relevant work-related exposures and complaints of physical therapists is currently lacking.
We sought to identify work-related exposures based on the subjective experiences and beliefs of physiotherapeutic representatives, in order to identify relevant work-related complaints and diseases. Likewise we aimed to compare the international evidence with the actual situation of physical therapists in Germany.

Methods: Two complementary qualitative approaches were used: 1) a focus group discussion with representatives of professional physiotherapy associations as well as health and safety stakeholders and 2) qualitative semi-structured telephone interviews incorporating currently employed physical therapists. The group discussion was conducted applying a moderation technique, and interviews were analyzed using the content analysis approach by Mayring.

Results: The focus group discussion with five participants and the 40 semi-structured interviews with physical therapists identified comparable results. The main exposures of physiotherapeutic work were considered to be musculoskeletal (e.g., awkward body postures during treatment, patient transfers, passive mobilization), psychosocial (e.g., statutory audit of prescriptions and the associated conflicts with doctors and health insurance providers) and partly dermal and infectious (e.g., wet work and risk of infection) factors. Diseases of the spine, wrist or finger joints, burnout syndrome and infections were mentioned as possible consequences.

Conclusions: The subjective data generated by both groups (focus group discussion and interviews) were comparable and consistent with the current state of research. The results provide new insight regarding work-related exposures and diseases of physical therapists working in Germany. These findings aided the design of a German-wide representative survey of practicing physical therapists.

Keywords: Physical therapist, Occupational diseases, Occupational health, Qualitative research

* Correspondence: maria.girbig@tu-dresden.de
†Equal contributors
[1]Institute and Policlinic of Occupational and Social Medicine, Faculty of Medicine Carl Gustav Carus, TU Dresden, Fetscherstr 74, 01307 Dresden, Germany
Full list of author information is available at the end of the article

Background

Work-related complaints and disorders of physical therapists have been researched consistently since the mid-1980s. International studies of physical therapists identified musculoskeletal diseases, skin diseases and infections as well as mental complaints and diseases to be relevant, with most studies observing increased risks of *musculoskeletal complaints and diseases* involving, in particular, the upper back, lumbar spine, neck, shoulders, wrist/hands, knees and thumbs [1–7]. Studies focusing on *mental complaints*, also found a low to moderately increased prevalence of burnout syndrome among physical therapists [8–11]. Concerning *work-related skin diseases* of physical therapists, only single reports [12–14] and an overview about potentially harmful substances [15] exist in the literature. However, contact with patients' open wounds (e.g., risk of hepatitis C, hepatitis B or HIV infection) or with infectious patients (e.g., tuberculosis and Methicillin-Resistant Staphylococcus aureus (MRSA)) is associated with an increased *risk of infection* [16, 17].

In Germany, scientific research of workload among non-physician health care professionals has focused mainly on caregivers and nurses [18–20], although physical therapists, with currently about 228 000 employees in Germany [21], represent a significant occupational group within the health care sector. The few existing articles focusing on physical therapists in Germany indicate that the physiotherapeutic work is associated with psychosocial [22, 23] and dermal exposures [24] as well as diseases [15]. However, a comprehensive national or international overview of all relevant work-related complaints and diseases among physical therapists is missing to date.

The main objectives of this work are, to give a first overview of perceived work-related exposures and disorders among physical therapists in Germany from the perspective of experts, and to determine if the results are consistent with international research on this the topic.

Methods

Using an exploratory approach, two qualitative methods with purposive sampling strategies were applied simultaneously to identify experiences, attitudes and knowledge of professionals regarding physiotherapeutic work-factors (including workload and resources) and work-related complaints and diseases as well as possible associations between them:

1. A focus group discussion with experts of German professional physiotherapy associations as well as health and safety stakeholders,
2. Semi-structured interviews with physical therapists currently working in Germany.

Subsequently, the results of both methods were analyzed and compared.

The study is reported according to the consolidated criteria for reporting qualitative studies (COREQ) [25].

Focus group discussion

The aim of this approach was to assess the professional policy perspective. Therefore, experts from German professional physiotherapy associations as well as health and safety stakeholders were included, and a focus group discussion was conducted to utilize group dynamic processes and the participants' discussion as a source of knowledge [26]. In addition, this method allows the direct representation of information about similar and different opinions of participants [27] and reasons for individual statements [28].

Setting and participants

One representative of each German professional physiotherapy association *(Bundesverband selbstständiger Physiotherapeuten (IFK) e. V.; Physiotherapieverband e. V. (VDB); Verband Physikalische Therapie (VPT); Deutscher Verband für Physiotherapie (ZVK) e. V.)* and one representative of the Institution for Statutory Accident Insurance and Prevention in the Health and Welfare Services *(Berufsgenossenschaft für Gesundheitsdienst und Wohlfahrtspflege, BGW)* were invited to participate in the focus group discussion. The focus group discussion was conducted at the Institute and Policlinic of Occupational and Social Medicine, Technical University Dresden.

Material and analysis

An a priori defined semi-standardized guideline, based on the international state of research on work-related exposures (with reference to the work area and/or employment status) and diseases of physical therapists was utilized. To achieve a structured and consensus based discussion result, the whole focus group discussion was conducted by applying the moderation method [29]. Two moderators (scientists with expertise in physical therapy and psychology) (M.G. and D.D.) involved all participants equally and were responsible for a structured group discussion. First, participants were asked about individual perceptions concerning typical work-related exposures. The second part of the discussion contained questions regarding characteristics of work-related complaints and diseases, and the third part focused on perceptions of work-related resources. The guideline was used by the moderators as orientation for the course of the discussion, nevertheless, thematic digressions were allowed.

Flipcharts and magnet boards were used to illustrate consensus results. The discussion was recorded visually by two persons and the results were documented with photos. Group discussion results were summarized based on a cluster building process of the work-related exposures, complaints and diseases as well as resources. In addition, the final protocol was mailed to the participants for their acceptance.

Semi-structured interviews

Semi-structured interviews were performed to identify physiotherapeutic work-related exposures as well as main complaints and diseases from the perspective of working physical therapists themselves.

Setting and participants

Interviewees were selected from different employment settings to represent as many work-related facets as possible, and to obtain a heterogeneous group of German physical therapists. We attempted to include professional physical therapists with as many combinations of the following criteria as possible:

- gender,
- region: north, south, east and west of Germany,
- professional experience (entrants and professionally experienced) and
- work area: hospital/rehabilitation (inpatient) and ambulance (outpatient).

Selection also guaranteed that physical therapists working in different disciplines (orthopedics/surgical ward; neurology; internal medicine and other) were represented. The recruitment was realized using the Yellow Pages®, where businessmen and -women in Germany – including self-employed physical therapists – offer their services. A list of all physiotherapy practices from three German federal states (Saxony, Baden- Wurttemberg and Berlin) was generated to include different regions. These therapists were contacted per email and/or telephone and asked to participate in our study. Physical therapists were interviewed at their workplace or home by telephone.

Table 1 Interview guideline for semi-structured telephone interviews

1.What does a typical day in your practice/on your station look like?
Important points that should be answered within this question:
▪ What are your main activities at work?
▪ How many patients do you treat every day on average?
▪ How much time do you have on average for one treatment?
▪ How many breaks do you take per day? How long are these?
▪ Do you have additional time slots for scheduling and documentation tasks?
▪ Is tidying and cleaning a part of your responsibilities? If so, do you do this within working hours?
2.Do you have the feeling that your work as physiotherapist has an impact on your health in any way (positive or negative)?
Important points that should be answered within this question:
▪ In what area of your health do you think your work has a special influence and how does this manifest itself? – With respect to e.g.,: physical health; mental health; skin complaints/disorders or infections
▪ Do you think that the physiotherapy knowledge and the work in this area are beneficial to your health?
▪ Do you have complaints/diseases, which are associated with your work as a physiotherapist?
3.What factors (activities, circumstances etc.) do you see in your work as physiotherapist as particularly stressful?
▪ If symptoms/diseases exist that originate from the physiotherapy work:
- What do you think are the specific working conditions/factors that have led to these complaints/diseases?
▪ How do you deal with the designated strain? What do you do for compensation? – e.g., leisure activities (sports etc.) or compensation with additives within the stressful activity
4.How do you feel when you go to work in the morning or come back home in the evening?
Important points that should be answered within this question:
▪ Do you look forward to your work and the contact with patients?
▪ What do you like/do you not like about your job?
▪ With your current knowledge, would you absolve qualification as a physiotherapist once again?
▪ Have you ever thought about leaving your job? Why?
▪ Are you planning to attend any further training/study? What?

Material and analysis

Standardized semi-structured telephone interviews were pilot-tested and conducted using an interview guideline developed by two physical therapists and a psychologist (M.G., C.K., D.D.) (Table 1). The guideline was based on the current international state of research regarding work-related exposures, complaints and diseases of physical therapists. The guideline provided orientation for the interviewer, but still allowed for thematic digressions. Demographic and occupational data were also collected from all participants. Basically, the questions were open-ended to promote as unaffected an exchange of opinions and attitudes as possible. In addition, minor questions were provided to be used when detailed explanations of the initial questions were necessary or when only parts of the corresponding subject area were addressed. Data collection continued until the research team agreed that no new themes were being generated and data saturation had been achieved. Each semi-structured interview was recorded digitally, transcribed and anonymized. Consent was obtained verbally prior to the start of interviews. Interviews were analyzed using Mayrings' qualitative content analysis [30]. To achieve an understanding of the data, a coding system was developed for categorizing participants' answers, which allowed for the reduction of statements and detecting groups of answers. A mixed inductive-deductive approach was used, meaning that, on the one hand, already existing international knowledge was integrated; on the other hand, new categories were formed based on the interview material. The finalized coding frame was systematically applied to all transcripts by one data coder using quali.xls [31]. Citations were translated into the English language by a native speaker for the purpose of publication.

Each participant of both qualitative approaches was offered the results of the study.

Results

The focus group discussion [32] involved five participants (see aforementioned affiliations) aged between 30 and 73 years. The age of the 40 interviewed working physical therapists ranged between 25 and 56 years. Participant characteristics are summarized in Table 2. The focus group discussion continued four hours and the interviews lasted an average of 35 min.

The results of both qualitative approaches were first considered separately and subsequently compared.

Focus group discussion

Work-related exposures

Musculoskeletal and psychosocial factors were identified as the two main exposure categories afflicting German physical therapists (Fig. 1). Especially awkward postures during treatments, patient transfers, exertion and passive joint mobilizations were named as the most relevant *musculoskeletal exposures* of this profession. Participants also believed that underpayment, obligations to check prescriptions and dealing with death are the most important *psychosocial exposures* faced by physical therapists.

Table 2 Demographic characteristics of participants

	Focus group discussion	Semi-structured interviews
Total respondents (number)	5	40
Sex – Female (number (%))	4 (80%)	22 (55%)
Age – Range (years)	30-73	25-56
Clinical Setting	N.A.	
Inpatient (number (%))		5 (12.5%)
Outpatient (number (%))		25 (62.5%)
Both (number (%))		10 (25.0%)
Employment status[a]	N.A.	
Full time (≥39 h/ week)		24 (60.0%)
Part time		15 (37.5%)
Professional experience[b]	N.A.	
1 – 10 years (number (%))		12 (30.0%)
11 – 20 years (number (%))		14 (35.0%)
21 – 30 years (number (%))		5 (12.5%)
31 – 40 years (number (%))		4 (10.0%)

Notes: N.A. not applicable, [a]missing value of one person, [b]missing value of five persons

Based on the current state of research, the moderators pointed out additional factors requiring discussion. The experts were asked to vote on whether they believed dermal, infectious or physical working conditions might play a role within physiotherapeutic work. In this context, *dermal exposures*, especially wet work and risk of infections, were appraised as important for the occupation. Even though work-related *infections* are more frequent among caregivers and nurses, they are also considered relevant for physical therapists. Regarding physical work factors related to shortwave and microwave treatments, participants were discordant on how to classify these special kinds of work-related factors. The reason for inconsistent opinions was the fact that physical therapists in Eastern Germany applied elements of electrotherapy more often than their colleagues in Western Germany. As a consequence, thermic factors like burns and scalding were unanimously voted as being partially relevant for physical therapists.

According to the predefined consensus, participants discussed the relevance of the named work-related exposures of physical therapists in the context of work setting and employment status. As a result, the existence of physical exposures seems to be particularly associated with the respective work area. In contrast, psychosocial exposures were more strongly associated with employment status. Thus, physical therapists in the outpatient sector are especially confronted with increased physical exertion, while the self-employed are particularly exposed to psychosocial strain due to economic stress and existential fears.

Work-related complaints and diseases

Following the discussion of work-related exposures, focus group participants discussed if complaints and diseases (including occupational diseases) could possibly be connected with the pertinent exposures. According to the experts, among the diseases included in the German list of occupational diseases, the following are potentially relevant for physical therapists:

- Severe or recurrent skin diseases (No. 5101), e.g., by use of massage lotion, salve or gloves and wet work;
- Disc-related diseases of the lumbar spine (No. 2108), e.g., by patient transfer (including partial body transfer);
- Infectious diseases (No. 3101) and Obstructive diseases of the respiratory tract (No. 4301 & 4302) e.g., by working with ill patients and allergenic substances (especially in inpatient and/or elderly care).

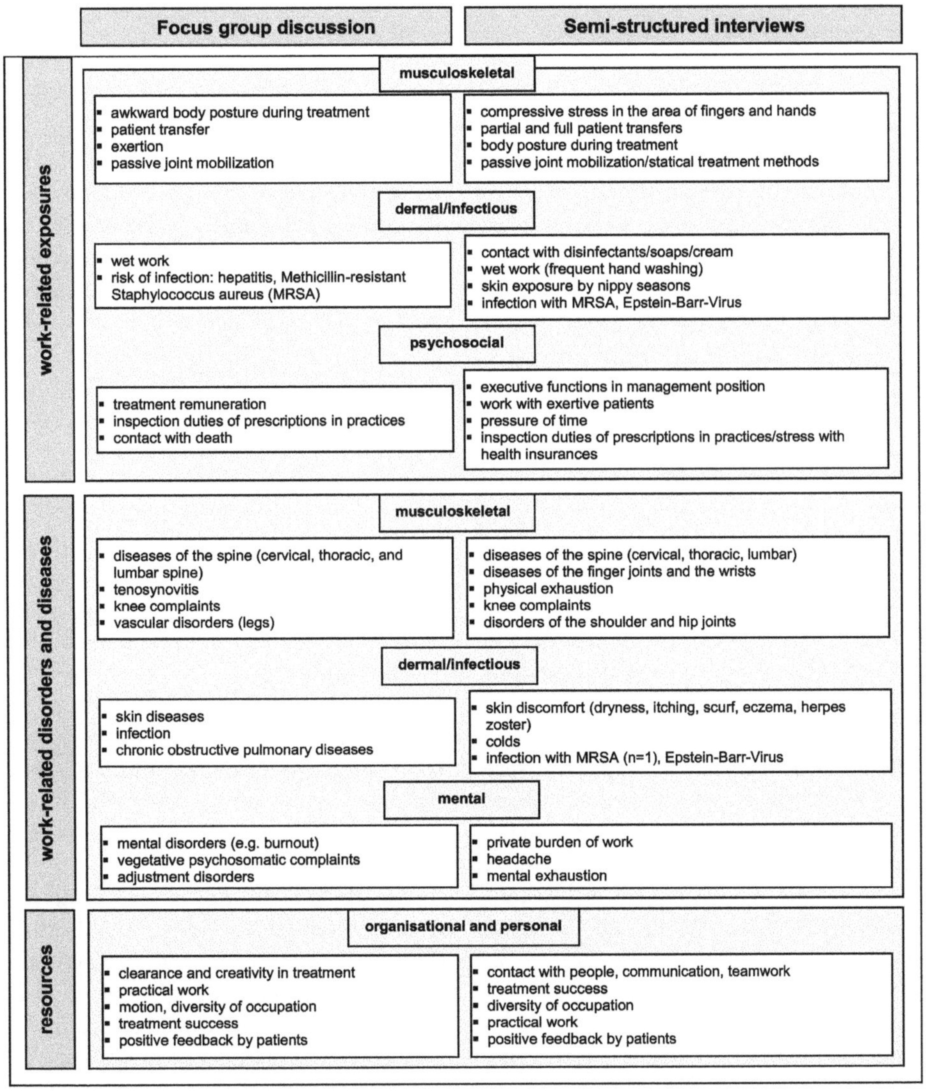

Fig. 1 Complementary juxtaposition of results of both qualitative approaches

In addition, other complaints/diseases were named which might be (in part) due to the work as a physical therapists. These include further complaints of the spine (cervical spine and thoracic spine), tenosynovitis, knee complaints and circulatory disorders (e.g., varices). Within the area of mental complaints and disorders, burnout syndrome, vegetative-psychosomatic complaints and adjustment disorders were proposed as most important.

Resources

The experts pointed out that the physiotherapeutic work also includes health promoting aspects; consequently, resources were considered. In particular, the participants highlighted the independence and creativity involved in selecting and implementing treatments, practical work, occupational diversity, treatment success and positive feedback from patients as having a beneficial effect on the health of physical therapists.

Semi-structured interviews

The results of the interviews are listed below according to frequency of nomination. In addition, some particularly concise quotations of individual people are presented.

Work-related exposures

The most commonly reported *musculoskeletal exposures* were pressure loads in the area of fingers and hands, partial and full patient transfers, awkward body postures during treatments, non-ergonomic working conditions and prolonged standing at the treatment table.

"Knowing what I know now, I wouldn't choose the profession again – because of the physical exertion."

Regarding psychosocial conditions, the main *psychosocial exposures* considered were executive functions (in management positions), working with difficult patients, time pressure and problems with the administrative processing of prescriptions in private-practices (stress with health insurance providers).

"It bothers me when patients are rude."

"I don't like being treated like a "waste bin" for some patients."

"I don't like the trouble with the health insurance companies- incorrectly completed prescriptions, no money for services performed, messed around with like a dancing bear."

"Due to prescriptions being returned by a particular health insurance company... I regularly explode on the phone."

The most frequently mentioned *dermal exposures* were contact with disinfectants, soaps and creams and frequent hand washing (wet work). Contact with infected patients was rarely considered by the respondents as an exposure. In this regard only infections with Methicillin-Resistant Staphylococcus aureus (MRSA) and the Epstein-Barr Virus were specified.

Work-related complaints and diseases

The main *musculoskeletal complaint* named by the interviewees was discomfort of the spine. Eight of these therapists could not further specify their problems. Among the remaining therapists, complaints were located in the cervical spine, lumbar spine and thoracic spine. Other frequently affected body areas mentioned in the interviews were wrist and finger joints, knees, shoulders and hips. Some of the respondents perceived physical exhaustion at the end of the day. Slightly more than a quarter of the consulted physical therapists had not yet experienced any work-related impacts on their physical health or well-being. According to the respondents, work-related *psychosocial exposures* are particularly transferred into the private life, and in this regard, were associated with headache ($n = 4$) and mental fatigue.

"At the end of the day I have the feeling that my brain is full of knots."

"I don't want to talk in the evening."

"To me, the psychological burden is greater than the physical."

Work-related *complaints of the skin*, such as skin dryness, itching, peeling, eczema and herpes zoster were rated by one quarter of the physical therapists as relevant to their work. With respect to possible *risks of infection*, two physical therapists working with outpatients reported that they suffer from influenza infection more often due to work. Two others had already undergone an infection with MRSA and Epstein-Barr virus, respectively.

Resources

The most frequently named work-related resources by the interviewed therapists were contact with people, communication and teamwork. In addition, treatment success, occupational diversity, the practical work as well as positive feedback from the patients were considered as benefits.

"If the payment would be better, it would be almost a dream job"

The subjective data of both groups of professional representatives were assimilable and consistent with the current state of research. A comparison of the main results of both qualitative approaches can be found in Fig. 1.

Awkward body postures during treatments, patient transfers and passive joint mobilization were specified as the *main work-related exposures* of musculoskeletal complaints and diseases. Professionals also often mentioned stress due to compressive load from working tasks on fingers and hands. In the area of work-related psychosocial stress factors, particularly the existing statutory audit of prescriptions and the associated conflicts with physicians and health insurance providers was considered as a burden. Wet work and the risk of infection with methicillin-resistant Staphylococcus aureus (MRSA) were considered to be the main dermal and infectious problems by both groups. *Work-related complaints and diseases* in the whole area of the spine were described by both groups as the main existing musculoskeletal disorders. Results of semi-structured interviews additionally indicated that complaints of the fingers and wrists as well as general physical exhaustion are potential problems. Both, the political experts and the professionals named skin disorders and diseases as common work-related problems. The participants of the focus group mentioned mental and psychosomatic symptoms as well as autonomic adjustment disorders as the foremost occurring mental disorders. The working professionals named headache, mental fatigue and private strain because of their occupation as particularly important. Both political experts and working professionals identified the practical work of physical therapists, the existing scope for professional development, the diversity of activities, the positive feedback from patients and the possibilities of teamwork, as essential *resources of the occupation.*

Discussion

Using the two qualitative approaches presented (focus group discussion and semi-structured interviews), the entire spectrum of work-related exposures and diseases of physical therapists in Germany was investigated for the first time. According to the results, work-related musculoskeletal, mental, dermal and infectious complaints and diseases may compromise the health of physical therapists. Basically the specifications of both qualitative approaches are very similar or complement each other very well (see Fig. 1). However – particularly in the field of psychosocial exposures - the prioritization of the named factors appears to be different (the order of the points listed in the boxes indicates their priority). The participants of the focus group discussion were more concerned with current political topics such as remuneration of treatment and inspection duties of prescriptions in practices. In comparison, the participants of the interviews (mostly physical therapists in outpatient settings) were more focused on the strain of the daily practical work as physical therapist, like the work with difficult patients and time pressure. We think these differences are due to the diverse current working activities of the participants (focus group discussion: mostly management positions/interviews: practical working German physical therapists) and the resulting differences in the importance of specific stress areas.

There were also slight differences in the data on mental disorders and diseases. For example the burnout syndrome as a possible mental disorder of physical therapists was – consistent with existing national [22] and international studies [33–37] – specifically mentioned within the focus group discussion (not by the interviewees). This, together with the other data in this area allows the assumption that the participants of the focus group discussion were more concerned with this field of study, or had more points of contact with the issue of work-related disorders/diseases in general (one participant was a representative of the Institution for Statutory Accident Insurance and Prevention in the Health and Welfare Services). Likewise, the results provide the first evidence for the transferability of international research on work-related exposures and disorders to physical therapists working in Germany.

Until now, neither national nor comparable international qualitative studies reflecting the experiences and beliefs of physiotherapeutic experts comprehensively examined all important work-related exposures, complaints and diseases. For the first time, the present study summarizes all work-related exposures and health outcomes of physical therapists in Germany considered relevant by experts. The few existing international qualitative studies focused only on musculoskeletal exposures and complaints as central themes [38–40]. German-speaking studies with qualitative approaches dealing with work-related exposures or complaints of physical therapists mainly focused on psychosocial exposures and diseases [23, 41] or job satisfaction in general [42].

Within our study new aspects were specified in the field of psychosocial exposure of physical therapists which have not been mentioned in the international literature so far, for example obligations to check prescriptions and conflicts with health insurance providers and/or physicians. In particular, self-employed physical therapists reported being concerned by economic stress and existential fears while physical therapists working as employees are often confronted with underpayment, time pressure and significant exertion. These issues appear to be typical for the situation of German physical therapists. For example, within the German healthcare system, patients in need of physiotherapy services have to first obtain a prescription for the treatment from a physician (i.e., patients do not have direct access to physiotherapy like in other countries, such as Australia, the Netherlands, Sweden, Norway, Great Britain and Canada etc.). These prescriptions will be only acknowledged (and paid) by the according health insurance if all data are complete and filled in correctly. The verification of the data is the responsibility of the attending physical therapist. If there are any problems, the therapist (or the patient) has to deal with the treating physician or the health insurance. This requires considerable administrative effort and can lead to existential fears in the affected practices. The remuneration of physiotherapy services by the health insurances in Germany is considered to be too low. This results in the frequently discussed low payment of physical therapists (especially in East Germany), and in an increased turnover rate of professionals [23, 43].

Concerning the most important musculoskeletal exposures (e.g., patient transfer, awkward body postures and passive joint mobilization) as well as the body areas mainly affected by musculoskeletal complaints (spine, fingers and wrists as well as knees), the findings of the present study are consistent with the current state of international research described above [1–7]. Occupational skin diseases (specific diagnoses were not mentioned) and corresponding exposures within the physiotherapeutic work were named, but considered to be less relevant by both expert groups. This is in line with the current state of international research but in contrast to the fact that work-related skin diseases (No. 5101) were the most reported ($n = 311$) and recognized ($n = 15$) occupational diseases for physical therapists in Germany according to data of the German Institution for Statutory Accident Insurance and Prevention in the Health and Welfare Services (BGW) in 2014 (personal information of the BGW, 2015). The discrepancy might be a result of participant selection, and subjects with only few or no skin problems may have been selected by chance or subjects with skin problems might have been on sick leave due to their skin diseases. Subsequently, this may have yielded less consideration of work-related skin diseases within the focus group discussion as well as the interviews. However, the recognition incidence of musculoskeletal occupational diseases in Germany is generally low. Therefore, the recognition of occupational diseases is not necessarily directly associated with the actual prevalence of these disorders among professionals in this field. International studies of infections among physical therapists are rare and focus mainly on hepatitis B infections [16] and tuberculosis [17]. In contrast, infections with MRSA and Epstein-Barr-Virus were named in our assessment.

The present study addresses for the first time the entire spectrum of possible work-related exposures and complaints as well as diseases of physical therapists in Germany. A qualitative approach was chosen to gain a first impression of this research area and to screen to what extent the results of past international research applies to Germany.

The greatest *strength* of this study is the use of two different qualitative methods. This enables the different perspectives of two groups of physiotherapeutic profession experts to be captured. Through the focus group discussion, a wide spectrum of knowledge and opinions could be gained because a representative of each existing professional physiotherapy association in Germany participated. In addition, the study sample of the semi-structured interviews was relatively large and the participants were recruited from a wide geographical area of Germany with varying professional backgrounds and experiences. This was very important because the work as physical therapist in Germany varies greatly depending on the work area (inpatient or outpatient), discipline (e.g., surgery, neurology, internal medicine etc.) and acquired advanced training (e.g., manual therapy, manual lymphatic drainage, sports physical therapy etc.).

General *limitations* of qualitative research, which also pertain to this study, are the missing generalizability of the knowledge gained to other people or settings and the possibility that the results were influenced by the researcher (data collection and categorization) [44]. The results of the present study are consistent with the international literature, suggesting these limitations did not greatly impact the study results. One additional potential limitation of focus group discussions can be that the group itself may influence the produced data, and a classical problem is the influence of the group interaction on the individual contribution of each participant in the group discussion [45]. However, any resulting distortion of results could be compensated by the individual interviews.

Conclusions

The results of our study indicate that physical therapists in Germany generally have an increased risk of musculoskeletal and psychosocial exposures, and to a lesser degree dermal and infectious exposures. Furthermore, a possible association between musculoskeletal and mental complaints was indicated. To verify these potential relationships, a representative study of physical therapists is necessary. For this reason, the results of our described exploratory method was used to design a comprehensive study to investigate the detected variety of work-related exposures, complaints and diseases [46].

Abbreviations

BGW: Berufsgenossenschaft für Gesundheitsdienst und Wohlfahrtspflege; COREQ: Consolidated criteria for reporting qualitative studies; IFK: Bundesverband selbstständiger Physiotherapeuten; MRSA: Methicillin-Resistant Staphylococcus aureus; VDB: Physiotherapieverband e. V.; VPT: Verband Physikalische Therapie; ZVK: Deutscher Verband für Physiotherapie e. V.

Acknowledgements

The authors gratefully acknowledge all German professional physiotherapy associations for participation in focus group discussion as well as all interviewees. We also thank Dr. Janice Hegewald (Institute and Policlinic of Occupational and Social Medicine, TU Dresden) for careful linguistic revision of this article.

Funding

The research project is sponsored by the Institution for Statutory Accident Insurance and Prevention in the Health and Welfare Services (BGW).

Authors' contributions

MG: drafting/revising of the manuscript, study concept and design, study coordination. AF: drafting/revising of the manuscript, analysis of the interviews. SD: drafting/revising of the manuscript, concretion of study design, support of the focus group discussion. DD: preparation of the interview guidelines, moderation of the focus group discussion, realization of the interviews. CK: realization of the interviews. AN: external quality control. AS: study concept and design, study supervision. All authors approved and critically reviewed the final version of the manuscript.

Competing interests

The authors report no competing interests. The funder has no role in the collection, analysis, and interpretation of data; on the writing of the report; and on the decision to submit the paper for publication.

Author details

[1]Institute and Policlinic of Occupational and Social Medicine, Faculty of Medicine Carl Gustav Carus, TU Dresden, Fetscherstr 74, 01307 Dresden, Germany. [2]Institute for Health Services Research in Dermatology and Nursing, Hamburg Center for Health Economics, University Hamburg, Hamburg, Germany.

References

1. Molumphy M, Unger B, Jensen GM, Lopopolo RB. Incidence of work-related low back pain in physical therapists. Phys Ther. 1985;65:482–6.
2. Alrowayeh HN, Alshatti TA, Aljadi SH, Fares MF, Alshamire MM, Alwazan SS. Prevalence, characteristics, and impacts of work-related musculoskeletal disorders: a survey among physical therapists in the State of Kuwait. BMC Musculoskelet Disord. 2010;11:116.
3. Cromie JE, Robertson VJ, Best MO. Work-related musculoskeletal disorders in physical therapists: prevalence, severity, risks, and responses. Phys Ther. 2000;80:336–51.
4. West D, Gardner D. Occupational injuries of physiotherapists in North and Central Queensland. Aust J Physiother. 2001;47:179–86.
5. Campo MA, Weiser S, Koenig KL, Nordin M. Work-Related musculoskeletal disorders in physical therapy: A prospective cohort study with 1-year follow-up. Phys Ther. 2008;88(5):608–19.
6. Glover W, McGregor A, Sullivan C, Hague J. Work-related musculoskeletal disorders affecting members of the Chartered Society of Physiotherapy. Physiotherapy. 2005;91:138–47.
7. Wajon A. Prevalence of thumb pain in physical therapists practicing spinal manipulative therapy. J Hand Ther. 2003;16:237–44.
8. Wandling BJ, Smith BS. Burnout in Orthopaedic Physical Therapists. J Orthop Sports Phys Ther. 1997;26:124–30.
9. Donohoe E, Nawawi A, Wilker L, Schindler T, Jette DU. Factors associated with burnout of physical therapists in Massechusetts rehabilitation hospitals. Phys Ther. 1993;73:750–6.
10. Mandy A, Rouse S. Burnout and work stress in junior physiotherapists. BJTR. 1997;4:597–603.
11. Pavlakis A, Raftopoulos V, Theodorou M. Burnout syndrome in Cypriot physiotherapists: a national survey. BMC Health Serv Res. 2010;10:63–10.
12. Sanchez-Perez J, Garcia-Diez A. Occupational allergic contact dermatitis from eugenol, oil of cinnamon and oil of cloves in a physiotherapist. Contact Dermatitis. 1999;41:346–7.
13. Loughney E, Harrison J. Irritant contact dermatitis due to 1-bromo-3-chloro-5,5-dimethylhyddantoin in a hydrotherapy pool. Risk assessments: the need for continous evidence-based assessments. Occup Med. 1998;48(7):461–3.
14. Girbig M, Hegewald J, Seidler A, Bauer A, Uter W, Schmitt J. Type-IV sensitizations in physical therapists: Patch test results of the Information Network of Departments of Dermatology (IVDK) 2007–2011. JDDG. 2013;8:1185–93.
15. Weßbecher R, Schrägle J, Buhles N. Hautbelastungen bei Masseuren, medizinischen Bademeistern und Physiotherapeuten. Aktuelle Datenlage und sozialmedizinische Überlegungen ArbeitsmedSozialmedUmweltmed. 2009;44(9):471–7.
16. Hadler SC, Doto IL, Maynard JE, Smith J, Clark B, Mosley J, et al. Occupational risk of hepatitis B infection in hospital workers. Infect Control. 1985;6:24–31.
17. Hill A, Burge A, Skinner C. Tuberculosis in National Health Service hospital staff in the west Midlands region of England, 1992–5. Thorax. 1997;52:994–7.
18. Galatsch M, Iskenius M, Muller BH, Hasselhorn HM. A comparison of general health and potential predictors of general health among nurses in different age groups in Germany. Pflege. 2012;25:23–32.
19. Schulz M, Damkroger A, Voltmer E, Lowe B, Driessen M, Ward M, et al. Work-related behaviour and experience pattern in nurses: impact on physical and mental health. J Psychiatr Ment Health Nurs. 2011;18:411–7.
20. Simon M, Tackenberg P, Nienhaus A, Estryn-Behar M, Conway PM, Hasselhorn HM. Back or neck-pain-related disability of nursing staff in hospitals, nursing homes and home care in seven countries-results from the European NEXT-Study. Int J Nurs Stud. 2008;45:24–34.
21. Destatis (Statistisches Bundesamt): Gesundheit. Personal 2000 bis 2014. Wiesbaden: Statistisches Bundesamt; 2016: Fachserie 12 Reihe 7.3.2].
22. Gröbel S. Psychosoziale Belastungen von PhysiotherapeutInnen. Querschnittsstudie zur Arbeitsbelastung mittels des Copenhagen Psychosocial Questionnaire. pt_Zeitschrift für Physiotherapeuten. 2008;60:1068–137.
23. Burtchen I. Berufsbedingte Belastungen von Physiotherapeuten und ihre Bewältigung! Z f Physiotherapeuten. 2006;58:2–5.
24. Weßbecher R, Straube M, Szliska C, Schwanwitz HJ. Anamneseauxilium und gewerbedermatologische Beurteilung bei medizinischen Bademeistern, Masseuren und Physiotherapeuten. Hautarzt. 1998;49:912–9.
25. Tong A, Sainsbury P, Craig J. Consolidated criteria for reporting qualitative research (COREQ): a 32-item checklist for interviews and focus groups. Int J Qual Health Care. 2007;19:349–57.
26. Bortz J, Döring N. Forschungsmethoden und Evaluation für Human- und Sozialwissenschaftler., 4. Auflage edn. Heidelberg: Springer Medizin Verlag; 2006.
27. Morgan DL. Focus Groups as Qualitative Research. 2nd ed. London: Sage; 1997.
28. Kitzinger J. Introducing focus groups. BMJ. 1995;311:299–302.
29. Klebert K, Schrader E, Straub W. Moderations-Methode. Gestaltung der Meinungs- und Willensbildung in Gruppen, die miteinander lernen und leben, arbeiten und spielen. Rimsting: Preisinger; 1984.
30. Mayring P. Qualitative content analysis. Forum: Qual Social Res. 2000;1(2):20.
31. Stauche H. PC-Hilfe bei der Auswertung semistandardisierter Interviews. 2005
32. Girbig M, Deckert S, Druschke D, Nienhaus A, Seidler A. Arbeitsbedingte Belastungen, Beschwerden und Erkrankungen von Physiotherapeuten in Deutschland. Ergebnisse einer Fokusgruppendiskussion [Work-related strains, complaints and diseases of Physiotherapists in Germany. Results of a Focus Group Discussion]. Physioscience. 2013;9:66–71.
33. Balogun JA, Titiloye V, Balogun A, Oyeyemi A, Katz J. Prevalence and determinants of burnout among physical and occupational therapists. J Allied Health. 2002;31(3):131–9.
34. Martinussen M, Borgen PC, Richardsen AM. Burnout and engagement among physiotherapists. IJTR. 2011;18:80–8.
35. Ogiwara S, Hayashi H. Burnout amongst physiotherapists in Ishikawa prefecture. J Phys Ther Sci. 2002;14:7–13.
36. Schuster ND, Nelson DL, Quisling C. Burnout among physical therapists. Phys Ther. 1984;64(3):299–303.
37. Serrano Gisbert MF, de Los Fayos EJ. Hidalgo Montesinos MD: [Burnout in Spanish physiotherapists]. Psicothema. 2008;20(3):361–8.
38. Graham L, Gray H. Recently qualified physiotherapists' perceptions of work-related musculoskeletal disorders. Int J Ther Rehabil. 2005;12:299–307.
39. Gropelli TM, Corle K. Nurses' and Therapists' Experience with occupational musculoskeletal Injuries. AAOHN J. 2010;58:159–66.
40. Passier L, McPhail S. Work related musculoskeletal disorders amongst therapists in physically demanding roles: qualitative analysis of risk factors and strategies for prevention. BMC Musculoskelet Disord. 2011;12:24.
41. Gröbel S. Fühlen Sie sich heute erschöpft? Wenn Arbeitsanforderungen zur Belastung werden. pt_Zeitschrift für Physiotherapeuten. 2008;60:1134–7.
42. Neubauer I. Arbeitszufriedenheit von Physiotherapeuten. Physioscience. 2005;1:72–80.
43. Hügler S: Traumberuf zu Albtraumlöhnen. Physiopraxis 2013;4:10-3.
44. Choy LT. The strengths and weaknesses of research methodology: comparison and complimentary between qualitative and quantitative approaches. IOSR-JHSS. 2014;19(4):99–104.
45. Janis IL. Groupthink. In: Psychological Studies of Policy Decisions and Fiascos. 2nd ed. Boston: Houghton-Mifflin; 1982.
46. Girbig M, Deckert S, Kopkow C, Latza U, Dulon M, Nienhaus A, et al. Work-related complaints and diseases of physical therapists – protocol for the establishment of a "Physical Therapist Cohort" (PTC) in Germany. J Occup Med Toxicol. 2013;8:34.

11

Potential exposure to endocrine disrupting chemicals and selected adverse pregnancy outcomes: a follow-up study of pregnant women referred for occupational counselling

Jessica Bengtsson[1*†], Pernille Søgaard Thygesen[1†], Linda Kaerlev[2,3], Lisbeth E. Knudsen[4] and Jens Peter Bonde[1,4]

Abstract

Background: Experimental evidence indicates that fetal exposure to xenobiotics with the potential to interfere with the endogenous steroid hormone regulation of fetal development may reduce birth weight. However, epidemiological studies are limited. The aim of the study was to investigate whether potential occupational exposure to endocrine disrupting chemicals (EDC) of the mother during pregnancy is associated with preterm birth and low birth weight.

Methods: Pregnant women referred to an Occupational Health Clinic (OHC) in two Danish regions (Copenhagen or Aarhus) between 1984 and 2010, suspected of being exposed to occupational reproductive hazards were included in the study. A job exposure matrix enabled estimation of potential occupational exposure to EDC on the basis of job title. Births by women potentially exposed to EDC ($n = 582$) were compared to births by women referred to an OHC on the suspicion of other exposures than EDC ($n = 620$), and to a sample of births by all occupationally active women in the same geographical regions ($n = 346{,}544$), including 1,077 births of the referred women's non-referred pregnancies.

Results: No indications of reduced birth weight or increased risk of preterm birth were found among women potentially exposed to EDC. Women potentially exposed to EDC had children with a higher birth weight compared to the sample of occupationally active women but not compared to other women referred to an OHC.

Conclusions: Potential maternal exposure to EDC at Danish workplaces is not related to low birth weight or preterm birth among women referred to occupational counselling. Occupational exposures might be too weak on the average to cause these adverse effects or counselling at the OHCs is effective in preventing them.

Keywords: Endocrine disrupting chemicals, Birth weight, Gestational age, Job exposure matrix, Occupational health clinic, Work health, Prospective study, Epidemiology, Public health

Background

Endocrine disrupting chemicals (EDC) are exogenous substances that cause adverse health effects through interference with the endocrine system [1, 2]. EDC may affect the endocrine system by mimicking or blocking the action of an endogenous hormone or bind to transport proteins. Furthermore, EDC may interfere with the normal endocrine system by changing the normal hormone level through stimulation or inhibition of the production of hormones [1, 2]. Several epidemiological studies suggest that a range of EDC may actually cause preterm birth and/or low birth weight [3, 4]. Many of these studies are concerned with specific substances, such as phthalates [5], some pesticides [6, 7] and poly-chlorinated biphenyls (PCB) [8]. For example, exposure to PCB is believed, with increasing evidence, to inhibit fetal growth [8]. Due to methodological restrictions, the complexity of these chemical substances,

* Correspondence: jebe@sund.ku.dk
†Equal contributors
[1]Department of Occupational and Environmental Medicine, Frederiksberg and Bispebjerg Hospitals, Bispebjerg Bakke 23, Copenhagen, NV DK-2400, Denmark
Full list of author information is available at the end of the article

and due to preventive measures, the effects are often limited and the results inconsistent [9, 10]. Therefore, it is difficult to determine whether associations between EDC and preterm birth and/or low birth weight are causal [11, 12].

Denmark has had regulation on worker protection since 1873. According to the Danish Working Environment Act, the employer is responsible for ensuring a safe and sound working environment (Executive Order no. 1072 of 7 Sept. 2010). If a potentially harmful reproductive risk is present at the workplace, including exposure to EDC, pregnant women may be referred to an Occupational Health Clinic (OHC) by their general practitioner or midwife for reproductive risk assessment. This usually happens between 8 and 12 weeks of gestation. The clinics perform a risk assessment based upon available evidence in order to assess if the pregnant woman may continue in her job or whether there is a case for intervention in terms of actions to reduce or eliminate hazardous exposures, restructuring of job tasks, reassignment of job functions or – as the ultimate and least desirable solution - maternity leave due to reproductive risks that could not be resolved otherwise [13, 14]. Referred pregnant women are relocated or granted sick leave until the potential risk has been determined. However, keeping the pregnant women in their job, if possible, may be beneficial for the women in order to maintain income and attachment to the labor market.

Assuming that pregnant women referred to an OHC have a more hazardous occupational setting compared to pregnant women in general, since they are referred on the basis of a concrete suspicion of a harmful risk factor, these women constitute a relevant population to investigate. The national and complete coverage of the Danish Birth Register enable comparison of birth weight and gestational age of births by women referred to these clinics to all births in the same geographical regions. The aim of the present study was to examine if potential occupational exposure to EDC during pregnancy is related to preterm birth and/or low birth weight.

Methods

Study population

The study population consists of pregnant women referred to an OHC for occupational counselling in two Danish regions (Copenhagen and Aarhus) in the 26 year period from 1984 to 2010. A sample of all occupationally active women giving birth in the same time period and the same geographical regions, constitute an external reference group. We made restrictions as to those who were working at the onset of their pregnancy, mother's age at delivery 16–45 years, birth weight 1,000–7,000 g and gestational age 154–310 days. Furthermore, one birth was chosen by random sampling among women with two or more deliveries in each of the groups, which left 1,202 women referred to an OHC (261 from Copenhagen, 941 from Aarhus), and 346,544 in the external reference group including 1,077 births of the referred women's non-referred pregnancies.

Among women receiving occupational counselling, 582 were referred on the basis of suspected exposure to EDC (defined below) and 620 were referred due to other exposures. These 620 pregnancies constitute an internal reference group.

Information about the study population obtained from the OHCs was linked to data from *Statistics Denmark* [15] and *the Medical Birth Registry* [16]. These links enabled comparison of gestational age and birth weight between the women referred to an OHC and the external reference group.

Exposure assessment

Exposure status of referred women was determined by using a job-exposure matrix (JEM) developed by van Tongeren et al. [1]. The JEM includes 348 job titles according to the Categories of Occupation from 1980 (CO80). When developing the JEM, three occupational hygienists classified the likelihood of exposure to seven different substance groups with suspected endocrine disrupting properties (pesticides, polychlorinated organic compounds, phthalates, alkyl-phenolic compounds, biphenolic compounds, heavy metals and other substances) for all job titles independently. The authors defined the likelihood of exposure as *unlikely*, *possible* or *probable* [1].

Women referred to an OHC have been assigned a Danish occupational code. The code for each woman was translated into one of the job titles in the JEM. All women possibly or probably exposed to EDC in their occupation, according to the JEM, were combined into one group labelled potentially exposed. The seven substance categories in the JEM were combined into one overall group of EDC.

Every person with permanent residence in Denmark is given a unique 10-digit Personal Identification Number (PIN) [17]. In the present study, the PIN enabled linkage between data from the OHCs with data from Statistics Denmark, which provided information on the mothers' age, year of births, PIN of their children, country of origin, and socioeconomic status (SES) [15]. Linkage to The Medical Birth Registry enabled access to information on birth weight, gestational age, previous pregnancies and smoking status during pregnancy [16].

Outcome and confounder assessment

We examined the following outcomes: gestational age and birth weight, birth weight at week 40, preterm birth (<37 weeks) and low birth weight (<2500 g). The limits of preterm birth and low birth weight were set according to the WHO definition [18].

To classify the mothers into four groups of SES, DISCO-88 codes were used [19]. DISCO-88 is the Danish version of the International Standard Classification of Occupation (ISCO) and is divided into 10 main categories based on level of skills. *Group 1* (D1-2) refers to top leaders, managers and employees with skills at the highest level. Employees with skills at medium level are classified into *group 2* (D3). *Group 3* (D4-8) contains employees with skills at basic level, and *group 4* (D9-0) contains employees with unspecified working skills. Since the DISCO-88 codes were first registered in our data from 1991, only mothers giving birth hereafter are included in this variable.

Strategy of statistical analysis

We performed linear regression analyses of the effects of potential exposure to EDC (yes/no) on gestational age (days) and birth weight (grams) respectively while adjusting for a fixed set of potential confounding variables defined a priori: maternal age (*16–24, 25–34*

Table 1 Characteristics of women with potential occupational exposure to endocrine disrupting chemicals (EDC), women unexposed to EDC (internal references) and all occupationally active women in Copenhagen and Aarhus in the time period from 1984 to 2010 (external references)

	Exposed to EDC ($n = 582$)		Internal references ($n = 620$)		External references ($n = 346,544$)	
	n	%	n	%	n	%
Maternal age						
16–24 years	106	18.2	115	18.6	44,414	12.8
25–34 years	422	72.5	417	67.3	243,236	70.2
35–45 years	54	9.3	88	14.2	58,894	17.0
Year of birth						
1984–1989	90	15.5	65	10.5	76,423	22.1
1990–1994	92	15.8	57	9.2	62,752	18.1
1995–1999	138	23.7	120	19.4	60,723	17.5
2000–2004	141	24.2	193	31.1	64,324	18.6
2005–2010	121	20.8	185	29.8	82,322	23.8
Parity						
First birth	342	59.3	329	53.8	175,945	51.0
Second birth	173	30.0	206	33.7	122,148	35.4
Third or more births	62	10.8	77	12.6	46,926	13.6
Missing	1,538					
Socioeconomic status[a]						
Group 1	31	5.3	62	10.1	49,973	14.4
Group 2	87	15.0	92	14.9	64,780	18.7
Group 3	220	37.8	274	44.5	98,666	28.5
Group 4	97	16.7	47	7.6	14,162	4.1
Unknown	147	25.3	141	22.9	118,657	34.3
Missing	310					
Ethnicity						
Danish	501	86.2	556	90.3	313,238	91.1
Foreign	80	13.8	60	9.7	30,741	8.9
Missing	2,570					
Smoking habits during pregnancy[b]						
No	364	77.9	410	76.2	206,286	80.1
Yes	103	22.1	128	23.8	51,242	19.9
Missing	89,213					

[a] = Does only include information from 1991–2010
[b] = Does only include information from 1996–2010

Table 2 Crude gestational age (days) with 95% confidence intervals (CI) among referred women potentially exposed to endocrine disrupting chemicals (EDC), and among the internal and the external reference group

	n	Median	Mean	95% CI	Mean difference (95% CI)	
					Exposed versus internal reference	Exposed versus external reference
Exposed to EDC	582	280	277.5	276.4 – 278.7	−1.21 (−2.82 – 0.39)	−0.27 (−1.4 – 0.90)
Internal references	620	280	278.7	277.7 – 279.9	.	.
External references	346,544	280	277.8	277.8 – 277.8	.	.

and *35–45* years), year of birth (*1984–1989, 1990–1994, 1995–1999, 2000–2004* and *2005–2010)*, parity (*first, second* and *third or more)*, SES (*group 1, group 2, group 3, group 4* and *unknown)*, ethnicity (*Danish/non-Danish*) and smoking at any time during pregnancy (yes/no).

In addition to linear regression of continuous outcomes we computed odds ratios (OR) for preterm birth and low birth weight according to exposure status by logistic regression analyses. We adjusted for maternal age, year of birth, parity, SES, ethnicity and smoking habits during pregnancy.

All calculations were made by the statistical program SAS version 9.3 (SAS Institute Inc, Cary, NC, USA).

Results

Table 1 provides the descriptive characteristics of the study population including the women potentially exposed to EDC, the internal reference group of women referred to an OHC due to exposures other than EDC, and the women in the external reference group of gainfully employed persons. The three groups are similar with respect to characteristics except that mothers referred to an OHC are younger than the external references, and tend to belong to a lower SES group.

Gestational age was approximately equal across the three groups (Table 2) and linear regression analysis with adjustment for the potential confounders showed no significant effect of potential exposure to EDC on gestational age (data not shown).

The mean birth weight of the children born to women in the external reference group was marginally lower than the mean birth weight of the births given by women referred to an OHC, while the mean birth weight in the 40th week of pregnancy was marginally lower in the group potentially exposed to EDC compared to the external references. However, the confidence intervals overlap, indicating no significant difference in mean birth weight (Table 3).

In analyses adjusting for gestational age and potential confounders, women potentially exposed to EDC had children with a higher birth weight when compared to the external references (in average 63 g higher, 95% CI: 22–101), but not when compared to internal referents (in average 37 g higher, 95% CI: -19–93).

The proportion of preterm births among the women potentially exposed to EDC was marginally larger than the proportion of preterm births among the women in the internal reference group (Table 4), but the difference was not statistically significant. There were no difference in the proportion of preterm births between the women potentially exposed to EDC and the external references.

There was no difference in the proportion of children with low birth weight born to the women potentially exposed to EDC compared to the internal references (Table 5). Compared to the external references, the proportion of children with low birth weight was marginally lower among the women potentially exposed to EDC. This lower risk of low birth weight was likewise not statistically significant.

A sensitivity analysis only including first births did not show any differences of importance for gestational age and birth weight between the three exposure groups (data not shown).

Table 3 Crude birth weight and birth weight at week 40 (grams) with 95% confidence intervals (CI) among referred women potentially exposed to endocrine disrupting chemicals (EDC), and among the internal and the external reference group

		n	Median	Mean	95% CI	Mean difference (95% CI)	
						Exposed versus internal references	Exposed versus external references
Birth weight	Exposed to EDC	582	3,553	3,531	3,479–3,583	−5.42 (−76,9 – 66,1)	35.0 (−17,2 – 87,2)
	Internal reference	620	3,500	3,537	3,487–3,586	.	.
	External reference	346,544	3,500	3,496	3,494–3,499	.	.
Birth weight at week 40	Exposed to EDC	117	3,580	3,566	3,462–3,671	−3.2 (−141 – 136)	−21.5 (−126,4 – 83,5)
	Internal reference	118	3,565	3,570	3,479–3,660	.	.
	External reference	76,277	3,550	3,588	3,584–3,592	.	.

Table 4 Odds ratio with 95% confidence interval (CI) for preterm birth among women potentially exposed to endocrine disrupting chemicals (EDC) compared to the internal and external references respectively

	Preterm birth		Term birth					
	n	%	n	%	OR	95% CI	OR	95% CI
Exposed to EDC	46	7.9	536	92.1	1.53[a]	0.91–2.57	1.02[b]	0.73–1.43
Internal references	36	5.8	584	94.2	1	.	.	.
External references	27,815	8.0	318,729	92.0	.	.	1	.

[a]Exposed compared to internal references
[b]Exposed compared to external references

Discussion

In this prospective follow-up study of pregnant women referred to an OHC for counselling, we found no indications of reduced birth weight or increased risk of preterm birth among women potentially exposed to EDC. Women potentially exposed to EDC had children with a higher birth weight when compared to the external references. This might reflect an anabolic effect of EDC (for instance an estrogenic effect), but without consistent findings in analyses using the internal references, we consider this a chance or spurious result.

Women referred to an OHC are presumed to represent a high risk group, and constitute thereby a preferable basis for investigation compared to a population based study. The present study design enables comparison between women referred to an OHC potentially exposed to EDC and women referred to an OHC but unexposed to EDC. These two groups are highly comparable, since they are expected to be similar in most aspects except exposure status. Furthermore, use of register data provides a large study population contributing to enhanced statistical power.

These reassuring results can be understood in several ways. First of all, Denmark has a long tradition of worker protection regulation and the Danish Working Environment Authorities regularly performs inspections at Danish workplaces. Thus, potentially harmful chemical exposures of pregnant women at Danish workplaces are in general considered well controlled and chemically induced birth defects are rarely notified to the National Board of Industrial Injuries [20]. Therefore, the women defined as potentially exposed to EDC in the present study might not have been exposed to EDC to an extent that is strong enough to cause detectable adverse effects on gestational age and birth weight. A second explanation of the findings might be that the risk imposed by EDC is reduced by occupational risk assessment and counselling. If the risk assessment indicates a harmful exposure, actions to reduce or eliminate the exposure are recommended. Finally, awareness of potential harmful exposure, induced by the referral to an OHC, might cause a behavior change to a more protective lifestyle during pregnancy [13]. However, human embryo development is most vulnerable to toxic substances and endocrine disruption in the early embryonic period during the first 8 weeks of gestation, while counselling at an OHC usually takes place between 8 and 12 weeks of gestation.

One limitation of this study concerns the determination of exposure to EDC. The risk of EDC might go undetected in the present study due to misclassification associated with determination of exposure status. Using a JEM does not necessarily give an accurate picture of exposure since exposure might vary within job titles [7].

The JEM of van Tongeren et al. divides the chemical substances into seven substance categories [1]. In the present study all substances were combined into one group of EDC. By doing so, some accuracy in relation to potential differences between substances is lost. However, these reductions of categories were made to address the purpose of the present study - to investigate the general potential effects of EDC on gestational age and birth weight.

Finally and importantly, EDC are also found in many consumer products and the exposure besides the occupationally induced might be profound which would diminish the association in the present study. We know very little about what factors pregnant women are exposed to at home [21].

Table 5 Odds ratio with 95% confidence intervals (CI) for low birth weight among women potentially exposed to endocrine disrupting chemicals (EDC) compared to the internal and external references respectively

	Low birth weight		Normal birth weight					
	n	%	n	%	OR	95% CI	OR	95% CI
Exposed to EDC	21	3.6	561	96.4	0.98[a]	0.40–2.39	0.76[b]	0.41–1.37
Internal references	22	3.6	598	96.4	1	.	.	.
External references	16,330	4.7	330,214	95.3	.	.	1	.

[a]Exposed compared to internal references
[b]Exposed compared to external references

Conclusion

Pregnant women with potential occupational exposure to EDC were not at increased risk of delivering preterm or low birth weight babies. Findings may reflect that exposure levels are low without impact on the studied reproductive outcomes or that occupational counseling result in effective preventive actions.

Abbreviations

CI: Confidence intervals; CO80: Categories of occupation; EDC: Endocrine disrupting chemicals; ISCO: International standard classification of occupation; JEM: Job-exposure matrix; OHC: Occupational health clinic; OR: Odds ratio; PCB: Polychlorinated biphenyls; PIN: Personal identification number; SES: Socioeconomic status

Acknowledgements

Not applicable.

Funding

This study has no external funding.

Authors' contributions

JB and PST have contributed equally to the analysis of data and in writing the manuscript. All authors read and approved the final manuscript.

Competing interests

The authors declare that they have no competing interests.

Author details

[1]Department of Occupational and Environmental Medicine, Frederiksberg and Bispebjerg Hospitals, Bispebjerg Bakke 23, Copenhagen, NV DK-2400, Denmark. [2]Research Unit of Clinical Epidemiology, Institute of Clinical Research, University of Southern Denmark, Odense, Denmark. [3]Center for Clinical Epidemiology, Odense University Hospital, Odense, Denmark. [4]Department of Public Health, Section of Environmental Health, University of Copenhagen, Copenhagen, Denmark.

References

1. Van Tongeren M, Nieuwenhuijsen MJ, Gardiner K, Armstrong B, Vrijheid M, Dolk H, et al. A job-exposure matrix for potential endocrine-disrupting chemicals developed for a study into the association between maternal occupational exposure and hypospadias. Ann Occup Hyg. 2002;46:465–77.
2. Schug TT, Janesick A, Blumberg B, Heindel JJ. Endocrine disrupting chemicals and disease susceptibility. J Steroid Biochem Mol Biol. 2011;127:204–15.
3. Triche EW, Hossain N. Environmental factors implicated in the causation of adverse pregnancy outcome. Semin Perinatol. 2007;31:240–2.
4. Caserta D, Mantovani A, Marci R, Fazi A, Ciardo F, La Rocca C, et al. Environment and women's reproductive health. Hum Reprod Update. 2011;17:418–33.
5. Wolff MS, Engel SM, Berkowitz GS, Ye X, Silva MJ, Zhu C, et al. Prenatal phenol and phthalate exposures and birth outcomes. Environ Health Perspect. 2008;116:1092–7.
6. Wohlfahrt-Veje C, Main KM, Schmidt IM, Boas M, Jensen TK, Grandjean P, et al. Lower birth weight and increased body fat at school age in children prenatally exposed to modern pesticides: a prospective study. Environ Health Glob Access Sci Source. 2011;10:79.
7. Burdorf A, Nieuwenhuijsen MJ. Endocrine disrupting chemicals and human reproduction: fact or fiction? Ann Occup Hyg. 1999;43:435–7.
8. Govarts E, Nieuwenhuijsen M, Schoeters G, Ballester F, Bloemen K, de Boer M, et al. Birth weight and prenatal exposure to polychlorinated biphenyls (PCBs) and dichlorodiphenyldichloroethylene (DDE): a meta-analysis within 12 European Birth Cohorts. Environ Health Perspect. 2012;120:162–70.
9. Figà-Talamanca I. Occupational risk factors and reproductive health of women. Occup Med Oxf Engl. 2006;56:521–31.
10. Suárez-Varela MMM, Kaerlev L, Zhu JL, Bonde JP, Nøhr E-A, Llopis-González A, et al. Hospital work and pregnancy outcomes: a study in the Danish national birth cohort. Int J Occup Environ Health. 2009;15:402–9.
11. Meeker JD. Exposure to environmental endocrine disruptors and child development. Arch Pediatr Adolesc Med. 2012;166:952–8.
12. DiVall SA. The influence of endocrine disruptors on growth and development of children. Curr Opin Endocrinol Diabetes Obes. 2013;20:50–5.
13. Kaerlev L, Jacobsen LB, Olsen J, Bonde JP. Long-term sick leave and its risk factors during pregnancy among Danish hospital employees. Scand J Public Health. 2004;32:111–7.
14. Bonde JP, Johansen JP. [The occupational environment and pregnancy. Occupational medicine advice to pregnant women in potentially high-risk occupational environments]. Ugeskr. Laeger. 1987;149:677–80.
15. Statistics Denmark [Internet]. [cited 2015 Apr 22]. Available from: http://dst.dk/en
16. Knudsen LB, Olsen J. The Danish medical birth registry. Dan Med Bull. 1998; 45:320–3.
17. Pedersen CB. The Danish civil registration system. Scand J Public Health. 2011;39:22–5.
18. WHO | Preterm birth [Internet]. WHO. [cited 2015 Apr 3]. Available from: http://www.who.int/mediacentre/factsheets/fs363/en/
19. DISCO-88. Statistics Denmark's standard classification of occupation. Copenhagen: Statistics Denmark; 1996.
20. Arbejdsskader - årsopgørelser - Arbejdstilsynet [Internet]. [cited 2017 Feb 7]. Available from: http://arbejdstilsynet.dk/da/statistik/arbejdsskader/arbejdsskader-arsopgorelser
21. Morales-Suárez-Varela M, Kaerlev L, Zhu JL, Bonde JP, Nohr EA, Llopis-González A, et al. Unemployment and pregnancy outcomes: a study within the Danish national birth cohort. Scand J Public Health. 2011;39:449–56.

12

Short Questionnaire for Workplace Analysis (KFZA): factorial validation in physicians and nurses working in hospital settings

Patricia Appel[1*], Michael Schuler[1], Heiner Vogel[1], Amina Oezelsel[2] and Hermann Faller[1]

Abstract

Background: In recent years, there has been an increasing interest in psychosocial workplace risk assessments in Germany. One of the questionnaires commonly employed for this purpose is the Short Questionnaire for Workplace Analysis (KFZA). Originally, the KFZA was developed and validated for office workers. The aim of the present study was to examine the factorial validity of the KFZA when applied to hospital settings. Therefore, we examined the factorial structure of a questionnaire that contained all the original items plus an extension adding 11 questions specific to hospital workplaces and analyzed both, the original version and the extended version.

Methods: We analyzed questionnaire data of a total of 1731 physicians and nurses obtained over a 10-year period. Listwise exclusion of data sets was applied to account for variations in questionnaire versions and yielded 1163 questionnaires (1095 for the extended version) remaining for factor analysis. To examine the factor structure, we conducted a principal component factor analysis. The number of factors was determined using the Kaiser criterion and scree-plot methods. Factor interpretation was based on orthogonal Varimax rotation as well as oblique rotation.

Results: The Kaiser criterion revealed a 7-factor solution for the 26 items of the KFZA, accounting for 62.0% of variance. The seven factors were named: "Social Relationships", "Job Control", "Opportunities for Participation and Professional Development", "Quantitative Work Demands", "Workplace Environment", "Variability" and "Qualitative Work Demands". The factor analysis of the 37 items of the extended version yielded a 9-factor solution. The two additional factors were named "Consequences of Strain" and "Emotional Demands". Cronbach's α ranged from 0.63 to 0.87 for these scales.

Conclusions: Overall, the KFZA turned out to be applicable to hospital workers, and its content-related structure was replicated well with some limitations. However, instead of the 11 factors originally proposed for office workers, a 7-factor solution appeared to be more suitable when employed in hospitals. In particular, the items of the KFZA factor "Completeness of Task" might need adaptation for the use in hospitals. Our study contributes to the assessment of the validity of this popular instrument and should stimulate further psychometric testing.

Keywords: KFZA, Mental health, Work-related stress, Hospital, Psychosocial workplace risk assessment, Validation

* Correspondence: patricia.appel@uni-wuerzburg.de
[1]Department of Medical Psychology and Psychotherapy, Medical Sociology and Rehabilitation Sciences, University of Würzburg, Klinikstrasse 3, 97070 Würzburg, Germany
Full list of author information is available at the end of the article

Background

Analyses and monitoring of risks and hazards at the workplace are important tools to achieve and maintain healthy working conditions. In recent years, there has been a growing awareness of mental health aspects, which in Germany is also reflected by an amendment to the Safety and Health at Work Act (cf. section 5 of the Occupational Health and Safety Act, number 6). This has led to an increasing interest in Psychosocial Workplace Risk Assessments i.e., a systematic evaluation of health risks caused by workplace conditions. However, they are not often put into practice [1] resulting in a significant lack of experience [2]. Therefore, the practical aspects as the selection of suitable tools that capture all relevant psychosocial factors as defined below [3] and their implementation are gaining importance.

Tools for psychosocial workplace risk assessments

Psychosocial factors in the workplace, such as work intensity, job control, emotional demands or social support, may influence mental health and have an impact on staff turnover and sickness absence rate. A guideline that describes all the relevant factors and acts as a compass for the relevant authorities has been published by the Joint German Occupational Safety and Health Strategy (GDA) [3]. As a first step, it is often recommended to use standardized written staff surveys to obtain a rough analysis. It has proven practical to employ an instrument with a maximum number of 40 questions, which take no longer than 20 min to be completed [4].

One of the questionnaires that fulfil these recommendations is the Short Questionnaire for Workplace Analysis (KFZA) developed by Prümper et al. [5]. It is listed in the toolbox of the Federal Institute of Work Safety and Occupational Medicine (BAuA). Originally, the KFZA was developed and validated for the analysis of working conditions at office workplaces, but it has been described as a universal tool applicable to all types of workplaces, industries and occupations [6, 7]. Both, the KFZA as such and modified versions that were integrated in a larger set of assessments, have been used in several previous studies in hospital workplaces [8–10].

Working conditions in hospitals

About 10% of the workforce in Germany are employed in the health care system [11]. Analyses by health care insurances show that health care professionals tend to have the highest rates of health-related incapacity for work [12]. Multiple studies have shown that stress-related working conditions, such as time pressure, workload, interruptions of workflow, difficulties with patients or conflicts with co-workers and supervisors, are common in hospital workplaces [13–15] and may lead to reduced psychological and physical well-being [16, 17]. In addition, it is worth recalling that these working conditions can have negative consequences for patient outcome [16, 18].

As hospital workplaces are often characterized by stress-related working conditions and an increasingly challenging financial situation [19], it is especially important to choose a survey that is short, economic and practical. We therefore aimed to examine the suitability of the KFZA for this purpose by analyzing the factorial validity when applied to hospital settings. In the present study we used an extended version of the questionnaire with additional questions specific to hospital workplaces. The factorial structure of both the original and the extended versions were examined.

Methods

The legally mandated Psychosocial Workplace Risk Assessments were conducted by a center for occupational medicine over a 10-year period between 2004 and 2014 and yielded questionnaire data of a total of 1731 hospital employees. As anonymous data collected as part of routine practice were analyzed, ethical approvement was not deemed necessary by the local ethics committee.

Sample and procedure

The participating hospitals were located in northern Germany and the employees worked at regular wards, intensive care, intermediate care, emergency rooms and surgical departments.

Physicians and nurses from different disciplines were surveyed representing surgery, internal medicine, pediatrics, gynecology, urology, anesthesiology, neurology, orthopedics, ophthalmology, ENT, psychiatry and palliative care.

In preparation of the survey the employees were informed about purpose and procedure of the Psychosocial Workplace Risk Assessment and were given the opportunity to ask questions. These informative meetings were held by occupational psychologists and occupational physicians and were complemented by information letters. Participation was voluntary.

Please note, given that the data was collected in small group samples, demographic data was often not collected to protect the anonymity of the respondents due to requests by the work council or by data protection officers.

Questionnaire

The self-administered questionnaire applied was based on the Short Questionnaire for Workplace analysis (KFZA), which consists of 26 items and 11 scales [5], and was extended adding 11 items that covered aspects lacking in the original KFZA and that are either of general importance or specific to hospital workplaces. The 11 scales of the KFZA are assigned to four aspects of work: "Job Content", "Resources", "Stressors" and "Organizational Culture". An additional table shows work aspects,

KFZA scales and items including additional items (see Additional file 1: Table S1).

The scales that focus on "Job Content" are *Variability* and *Completeness of Task*. The scale *Variability* contains three items (VS1-VS3), one example is "I can fully apply my knowledge, skills and abilities at work". *Completeness of Task* is covered by two items (GH1/GH2), for example "My work allows me to complete products from beginning to end".

Three of the scales cover "Resources": *Job Control, Social Support* and *Cooperation*, each embracing three items. One example for the items of *Job Control* (HS1-HS3) is "I can determine the sequence of my job tasks", for *Social Support* (SR1-SR3) "In difficult work situations I can rely on my co-workers" and for *Cooperation* (ZU1-ZU3) "My work requires close cooperation with other people in the department", respectively.

Four scales focus on "Stressors", including two items each. One example for *Qualitative Work Demands* (QL1, QL2) is "The demands that are made on my concentration are usually too high", for *Quantitative Work Demands* (QN1, QN2) "I frequently work under time pressure", for *Work Disruptions* (AU1, AU2) "I am repeatedly interrupted during my actual work" and for *Workplace Environment* (UB1, UB2) "There are unfavorable environmental conditions at my workplace, such as noise, air, dust", respectively.

The remaining two scales embracing two items each cover the aspect "Organizational Culture". One of the items of *Information and Participation* (IM1, IM2) is "We are sufficiently informed about important things and events that concern our department", one example for *Benefits* (BL1, BL2) is "Our department provides good training opportunities".

For the extended version the items of the KFZA were complemented by 11 items which add one item to the domain *Cooperation* (ZU4, "The various professional groups cooperate well") and address the 3 additional domains *Work Equipment* (AM, "I have sufficient and adequate work equipment"), *Emotional Demands* (EB1-EB3, for example "My work is emotionally taxing") and *Consequences of Strain* (FB1-FB6, for example "Due to work-related issues, I experience disordered sleep"), i.e. effects of psychosocial factors.

Each item was rated on a 5-point Likert scale.

Statistical analysis

All analyses were performed with SPSS Statistics 23 and MS Office Excel 2013.

Means and standard deviations of the items were calculated. Regarding missing data, the effect of the variation in questionnaire versions was reported. Data sets with missing data were excluded listwise. We tested the effect of exclusion by comparing the group of analyzed data sets to the group of deleted data sets concerning the distribution of profession, gender, age and duration of department affiliation.

Due to the fact that the items ZU1, ZU3 and QL1 were only presented to a part of the sample, the responses to these questions were missing remarkably often. In some questionnaire versions item ZU1 ("My work requires close cooperation with other people in the department") was deliberately left out because these circumstances apply to the majority of workplaces in a hospital. Item ZU3 ("I always receive feedback *by my supervisors and co-workers* about the quality of my work") and item QL1 ("In my work, there are things that are too complicated") were sometimes replaced by variations which divided these questions into two sub-questions: ZU3a ("I always receive feedback *by my supervisors* ..."), ZU3b ("I always receive feedback *by my co-workers* ..."), QL1a ("In my work, there are things that are too complicated due to *ambiguous process procedures*") and QL1b ("... due to *insufficient training*").

Thus, the accumulation of missing data was caused by variations in questionnaire versions instead of refusal to reply.

To examine the factor structure of the 26 items (37 items in the extended version), we conducted an exploratory factor analysis through principal component factoring method. The number of factors was determined using both the Kaiser criterion and scree-plot methods. Factor interpretation was based on the orthogonal Varimax rotation method as well as a direct oblimin method with an oblique rotation. Correlation coefficients among the extracted factors based on oblique rotation were calculated. The internal consistency of the scales was analyzed through Cronbach's α coefficient of reliability.

Results

Sample characteristics

The data set of 1731 hospital employees included 476 physicians and 1255 nurses. A listwise exclusion of data sets with missing data left the data of 1163 questionnaires (1095 for the extended version) remaining for factor analysis. The following sociodemographic characteristics are listed in valid percent: 76.5% of the respondents were female, 23.5% male (n = 490 missing values). Regarding the age of the respondents 16.3% were 20-29 years old, 31.9% 20-39, 31.3% 40-49 and 20.4% 50-65 years old (n = 347 missing values). The duration of department affiliation amounted to 1-5 years in 39.6%, 5-10 years in 24.6% and >10 years in 35.8% (n = 392 missing values).

Comparing the analyzed sample to the deleted one, we found that the analyzed sample contained significantly more nurses, male and younger participants as well as more participants with a department affiliation of 1-5 years or more than 10 years.

Factor analysis of the KFZA

The value of the Kaiser-Meyer-Olkin measure of sampling adequacy (0.87) and a significant Bartlett's test of sphericity ($p < 0.001$, df = 325, chi-square = 10,603.331) indicated a high factoriability for the sample.

Principal component factor analysis was performed. The Kaiser criterion revealed a 7-factor solution for the 26 items of the KFZA, accounting for 62.0% of variance, whereas Cattell's scree-plot indicated a 4-factor solution accounting for 49.0% of variance. As extracting too few factors is considered to be a more serious error than extracting too many [20], we opted for the 7-factor solution.

First, we applied Varimax orthogonal rotation enabling us to compare our results with the empirical scales obtained by Prümper et al. [5], which were based on a two-step factor analytical procedure. Table 1 shows the rotated matrix of components. As all factor loadings for item GH2 were below 0.40, it was assigned to factor II on which it showed the highest loading (0.36). An additional oblique rotation yielded a comparable factorial structure (data not shown).

Substantive considerations supported the number of seven factors: The first factor (24.6% of total variance) contained the complete set of items from the KFZA factors *Social Support* (SR1-SR3) and *Cooperation* (ZU1-ZU3) and thus was labeled ***Social Relationships***. The second factor (10.1%) included all items from the KFZA factor *Job Control* (HS1-HS3) and one additional item from *Completeness of Task* (GH2) "My work allows me to complete products from the beginning to the end". Item GH2 is not precisely fitting to a hospital workplace and loaded on various factors with loadings lower than

Table 1 Factor loadings (orthogonal solution)

KFZA items	Component (% of variance)						
	I (24.6)	II (10.1)	III (7.4)	IV (6.9)	V (4.6)	VI (4.4)	VII (4.0)
SR1 Social support by co-workers	*0.77*	0.05	0.11	−0.07	0.11	0.06	0.22
SR3 Social cohesion within the department	*0.73*	0.11	0.31	−0.01	0.09	0.09	0.06
SR2 Social support by supervisors	*0.70*	0.03	0.38	−0.03	0.10	0.06	0.13
ZU2 Opportunity for social exchange with co-workers	*0.63*	0.24	0.03	0.29	−0.05	0.03	−0.11
ZU3 Feedback from supervisors and co-workers	*0.61*	0.17	0.24	0.24	−0.04	0.09	−0.17
ZU1 Necessity of cooperation	*0.53*	−0.05	−0.07	−0.30	0.04	0.31	0.23
HS1 Influence on sequence of activities	0.10	*0.86*	0.13	0.01	0.00	0.07	0.12
HS3 Influence on work load and procedures	0.10	*0.85*	0.19	0.03	0.05	0.11	0.08
HS2 Influence on work content	0.09	*0.84*	0.14	0.03	0.05	0.16	0.05
GH2 Completeness of product	0.33	0.36	0.08	0.20	0.20	0.31	−0.04
IM2 Consideration of employee input	0.22	0.12	*0.74*	0.05	0.04	0.12	0.00
IM1 Information about organizational developments	0.26	0.14	*0.73*	0.00	0.17	0.01	−0.03
BL1 Continuous education	0.08	0.10	*0.71*	0.03	0.11	0.24	0.08
BL2 Opportunities for advancement	0.11	0.12	*0.64*	0.09	−0.02	0.16	−0.09
QN2 Workload	0.04	0.06	0.05	*0.82*	0.14	0.08	0.19
QN1 Time pressure	0.10	0.09	0.01	*0.79*	0.14	0.07	0.22
AU2 Interruptions of workflow	−0.03	−0.06	0.11	*0.62*	0.41	0.07	−0.17
UB2 Insufficient work space and equipment	0.08	0.08	0.03	0.07	*0.83*	0.01	0.09
UB1 Unfavourable physicochemical conditions	0.11	0.06	0.07	0.20	*0.76*	0.06	0.04
AU1 Lack of information, work materials or equipment	0.00	0.01	0.20	0.34	*0.47*	−0.05	0.13
VS3 Variety of tasks	−0.03	0.01	0.13	−0.03	−0.05	*0.78*	−0.01
VS2 Use of knowledge, skills and ability	0.20	0.24	0.27	0.12	0.08	*0.58*	0.07
VS1 Learning new skills	0.16	0.18	0.39	0.17	−0.04	*0.56*	−0.06
GH1 Visibility of task accomplishment	0.25	0.35	0.07	0.07	0.13	*0.48*	0.03
QL1 Excessive complexity of tasks	0.06	0.14	−0.04	0.03	0.08	−0.01	*0.83*
QL2 Excessive demands on concentration	0.12	0.08	0.00	0.35	0.10	0.03	*0.74*

Abbreviations: KFZA Kurzfragebogen zur Arbeitsanalyse (Short Questionnaire for Workplace Analysis)
Note: Factor loadings >0.4 are presented in italics

0.40. This question seems to cover the ability to perform nursing measures or medical interventions from the beginning to the end. Therefore, item GH2 can be assigned to aspects that concern control over demands and tasks at work and the second factor was named ***Job Control***. Factor III (7.40%) contained all items from the KFZA factors *Information and Participation* (IM1, IM2) and *Benefits* (BL1, BL2) and thus was labeled ***Opportunities for Participation and Professional Development***. The fourth factor (6.91%) included all items from the KFZA factor *Quantitative Work Demands* (QN1, QN2) and one additional item from *Work Disruptions* (AU2). As the number of interruptions can be subsumed under the aspect of quantitative work demands, we kept the label ***Quantitative Work Demands***. Factor V (4.64%) included all items from the KFZA factor *Workplace Environment* (UB1, UB2) and one item from *Work Disruptions* (AU1) "I often do not have the required information, materials, or tools at my disposal". Lack of information and equipment can also be assigned to aspects of workplace environment which is why the factor was labeled ***Workplace Environment***. The sixth factor (4.38%) revealed a picture somewhat similar to that of the second factor. It contained all items from the KFZA factor *Variability* (VS1-VS3) and the other item from *Completeness of Task* (GH1). Again, item GH1 is not precisely fitting a hospital workplace. On account of the predominant variability component of most items of this factor, the label ***Variability*** was maintained. Lastly, factor VII (4.00%) included both items from the KFZA factor *Qualitative Work Demands* (QL1, QL2). Therefore, the label ***Qualitative Work Demands*** was retained. In summary, the seven determined factors correspond quite well with the original KFZA factors.

Table 2 shows correlations among the seven extracted factors based on the additional oblique rotation. Correlation coefficients tend to be low and range from $r = |0.04|$ (Factor III vs. Factor VII) to $r = |0.29|$ (Factor IV vs. Factor V).

Reliability

We estimated the reliability of the scales on the basis of Cronbach's α. The scales had 2 to 6 items each and Cronbach's α reliability coefficient ranged from 0.63 to 0.80 (Table 3). The internal consistency of the scales *Social Relationships, Job Control, Opportunities for Participation and Professional Development* and *Quantitative Work Demands* can thus be regarded as satisfying. For the scales *Workplace Environment, Variability* and *Qualitative Work Demands* values of Cronbach's α ranged only from 0.63 to 0.70. However, application is still acceptable for the use in larger samples to investigate scientific questions [21].

Factor analysis of the extended version

In a second step, we conducted a factor analysis as described above of the 37 items of the extended version including 11 additional items specific to hospital workplaces. Again, the value of the Kaiser–Meyer–Olkin measure of sampling adequacy (0.88) and a significant Bartlett's test of sphericity ($p < 0.001$, df = 666, chi-square = 14,472.214) indicated a high factoriability.

The Kaiser criterion yielded a 9-factor solution accounting for 59.5% of the variance. Using Varimax orthogonal rotation, all factor loadings were above 0.40.

As Factor I included the one additional item of the original domain *Cooperation* (ZU4) and the six items (ZU1-ZU3, SR1-SR3) of the previously determined factor ***Social Relationships,*** this label was maintained. The second factor contained the additional items from the domain *Consequences of Strain* (FB1-FB6) and was therefore named ***Consequences of Strain***. Factor III – contrary to the previously determined factor II – included only the complete set of items from the KFZA factor *Job Control* (HS1-HS3) and was labeled ***Job Control***. Factor IV (IM1, IM2, BL1, BL2) and factor V (QN1, QN2, AU2), respectively, match the factors identified before, ***Opportunities for Participation and Professional Development*** and ***Quantitative Work Demands***. The sixth factor contained the additional item of the domain *Work Equipment* (AM) and the three items (UB1, UB2, AU1) of the previously determined factor ***Workplace Environment***. As the availability of adequate working equipment is also part of the environment of a workplace, this name was kept. Factor VII included the additional items from the domain *Emotional Demands* (EB1-EB3) and item GH2 "My work allows me to complete products from the beginning to the

Table 2 Correlations among extracted factors (oblique solution)

	SR	JC	OPPD	QNWD	WE	VAR	QLWD
Social Relationships (SR)	–						
Job Control (JC)	0.26	–					
Opportunities for Participation and Professional Development (OPPD)	−0.28	−0.26	–				
Quantitative Work Demands (QNWD)	−0.05	−0.16	0.14	–			
Workplace Environment (WE)	−0.15	−0.12	0.19	0.29	–		
Variability (VAR)	−0.26	−0.28	0.27	0.05	0.08	–	
Qualitative Work Demands (QLWD)	−0.14	−0.07	−0.04	0.01	0.16	0.04	–

Table 3 Descriptive statistics and internal consistency of the scales of the KFZA (orthogonal solution)

Scales	Eigenvalues	M	SD	Cronbach's α	Number of items
Social Relationships	3.10	3.53	0.46	0.80	6
Job Control	2.72	3.17	0.24	0.80	4
Opportunities for Participation and Professional Development	2.69	2.84	0.57	0.76	4
Quantitative Work Demands	2.28	2.34	0.19	0.76	3
Workplace Environment	1.87	2.92	0.29	0.65	3
Variability	1.87	3.63	0.22	0.68	4
Qualitative Work Demands	1.59	3.62	0.17	0.63	2

Abbreviations: KFZA Kurzfragebogen zur Arbeitsanalyse (Short Questionnaire for Workplace Analysis)

end" which before was assigned to the second factor *Job Control.* As this item seems to cover the aspect that an employee has the possibility to accompany patients from the beginning to the end of their stay and witness their recovery it might operate as relief of strain. Therefore, factor VII was labeled ***Emotional Demands.*** Factor VIII (VS1-VS3, GH1) and Factor IX (QL1, QL2), respectively, match the previously determined factors ***Variability*** and ***Qualitative Work Demands.*** Thus, the nine factors of the extended version correspond well with the seven factors of the original KFZA version that emerged from our study.

Reliability of the extended version

Again, we estimated the reliability of the nine scales on the basis of Cronbach's α which ranged from 0.60 to 0.87 (Additional file 2: Table S2). The internal consistency of three scales (*Social Relationships, Consequences of Strain, Job Control)* can be regarded as good and of two scales (*Opportunities for Participation and Professional Development, Quantitative Work Demands)* as satisfying, respectively, while for four scales (*Workplace Environment, Emotional Demands, Variability, Qualitative Work Demands)* values of Cronbach's α ranged from 0.60 to 0.70.

Discussion

Our study examined the factorial validity of the KFZA, a questionnaire developed and validated for office workers [5], plus an extended version of this questionnaire, in hospital settings. Our results suggest a 7-factor solution instead of the 11 factors originally proposed by the authors of the KFZA. A comparison can be seen in Table 4.

The comparison of these two sets of factors shows that only the factor ***Qualitative Work Demands*** turned out to be an exact match. In addition to this factor, we found six factors instead of 10. The items of the original distinct factors *Social Support* and *Cooperation* combined to form a factor that was labeled ***Social Relationships.*** However, we acknowledge that this is based on our strictly empirical approach. Another approach might have been to retain the original factor structure based on theoretical constructs, that is, preserving the subscales found by Prümper et al. [5] instead of merging them, as the loadings of items from two specific scales in the original paper on one factor in our analysis may well be the result of these two scales being related in hospital settings. Likewise, the items of *Information and Participation* and *Benefits* built a factor which was named ***Opportunities for Participation and Professional Development.*** In this case, our results align with the empirical structure obtained by Prümper et al. [5].

The items of the original factors *Completeness of Task* and *Work Disruptions* did not load on independent factors but divided up to load on four other factors. One item of *Completeness of Task* was assigned to the factor ***Variability***, the other item to ***Job Control.*** The low factor loadings of 0.48 and 0.36, respectively, suggest that the wording of these items is not optimally suitable for the use in hospitals and they might have been interpreted in different ways. An example covered by item GH1 ("From the outcomes of my work I can tell whether I did a good job or not") might be that despite a correctly performed chemotherapy a patient may develop metastases. Likewise, item GH2 can be interpreted differently and covers various aspects as described above in the results section. One of the two items of *Work Disruptions* (AU2) was assigned to ***Quantitative Work Demands***, the other one (AU1) to ***Workplace Environment.*** Given that quantitative demands are the biggest contributing factor to frequent work disruptions (e.g., patients calling, phones ringing) this factor solution has face validity. Therefore, item AU2 "Interruptions of workflow", with a factor loading of 0.62, seems to be a useful complement to the items of the factor ***Quantitative Work Demands.*** In contrast, item AU1 ("Lack of information, work materials or equipment") describes a form of work disruptions less commonly found in hospitals and loads merely at 0.47 on the factor ***Workplace Environment.*** A reason for this might be this item being similar to the item "Insufficient work space and equipment".

For the seven scales we obtained, Cronbach's α reliability coefficient ranged from 0.63 to 0.80, whereas values for the 11 scales in the original publication ranged from 0.40 to 0.76. When calculating Cronbach's α, it is important to keep in mind that it increases with the

Table 4 Comparison of original KFZA factors and factors determined in this study

Work aspects	KFZA factor	Items (item code)	Factors determined in this study
Job Content	Variability	Learning new skills (VS1)	VI Variability
		Use of knowledge, skills and ability (VS2)	
		Variety of tasks (VS3)	
	Completeness of Task	Visibility of task accomplishment (GH1)	
		Completeness of product (GH2)	II Job Control
Resources	Job Control	Influence on sequence of activities (HS1)	
		Influence on work content (HS2)	
		Influence on work load and procedures (HS3)	
	Social Support	Social support by co-workers (SR1)	I Social Relationships
		Social support by supervisors (SR2)	
		Social cohesion within the department (SR3)	
	Cooperation	Necessity of cooperation (ZU1)	
		Opportunity for social exchange with co-workers (ZU2)	
		Feedback from supervisors and co-workers (ZU3)	
Stressors	Qualitative Work Demands	Excessive complexity of tasks (QL1)	VII Qualitative Work Demands
		Excessive demands on concentration (QL2)	
	Quantitative Work Demands	Workload (QN2)	IV Quantitative Work Demands
		Time pressure (QN1)	
	Work Disruptions	Interruptions of workflow (AU2)	
		Lack of information, work materials or equipment (AU1)	V Workplace Environment
	Workplace Environment	Unfavourable physicochemical conditions (UB1)	
		Insufficient work space and equipment (UB2)	
Organizational Culture	Information and Participation	Information about organizational developments (IM1)	III Opportunities for Participation and Professional Development
		Consideration of employee input (IM2)	
	Benefits	Continuous education (BL1)	
		Opportunities for advancement (BL2)	

Abbreviations: KFZA Kurzfragebogen zur Arbeitsanalyse (Short Questionnaire for Workplace Analysis)

number of items, such that in our analysis the number of items per scale was 2-6, while in the original analysis with 11 scales this value was 2-3. However, Cronbach's α showed also an acceptable value for the scale ***Qualitative Work Demands,*** which consisted of the identical items as the original factor.

Most correlation coefficients among the seven factors turned out to be low, i.e. $r < |0.20|$. This is compatible with the high correspondence between the solutions based on Varimax rotation and on oblique rotation, respectively, with the former assuming statistical independence between the factors. Indeed, some of these correlations appear plausible, e.g., the highest positive correlation (0.29) for the scales ***Quantitative Work Demands*** and ***Workplace Environment,*** as environmental circumstances such as insufficient work space and equipment may lead to higher work demands like interruptions of workflow and time pressure. One of the highest negative correlations (−0.28) was found between the scales ***Variability*** and ***Job Control***. This might be due to the fact that a workplace that is characterized by a diverse and varied task profile may at the same time be quite unpredictable and difficult to plan. However, it should be noted that if scales correlate due to common causes, reaching scales with low coefficients may not be a goal in itself.

The factor analysis of the extended version of the questionnaire yielded a 9-factor solution (Additional file 3: Table S3). Of the seven previously determined factors, four were identified as consistent: ***Qualitative Work Demands***, ***Quantitative Work Demands***, ***Opportunities for Participation and Professional Development*** and ***Variability***. Some of the additional items produced two new factors: ***Consequences of Strain***, consisting of the six supplementary items from this domain, and ***Emotional Demands*** including the corresponding supplementary items and item GH2 of *Completeness of Task* that had been assigned to ***Job Control*** before. Again, this item showed a low factor loading of 0.46. Thus, the factor ***Job Control*** was reduced to the original three items of the KFZA. The factors ***Social Relationships*** and ***Workplace Environment*** were enhanced fittingly by one additional item each from the domains *Cooperation* respectively *Work Equipment.* Taken together, items that loaded on the same factor in our analysis of the KFZA remained assigned to this factor in the analysis of the extended version, except for item GH2. With a number of 2 to 7 items per scale, Cronbach's α ranged from 0.63 to 0.87, with the scale ***Job Control*** showing highest internal consistency.

In summary, we were able to replicate the overall content-related structure found by the authors of the KFZA quite well, despite the reduced number of factors. The differences in the factorial structure can be explained by the differences in the specific stress-related working conditions, as detailed below.

The working conditions of hospital staff are characterized by a general increase in workload, by shift work, time pressure and frequent overtime, a high degree of responsibility, work disruptions, only partially predictable amount of work, hierarchical structures with deficits in communication and impairment through increasing economic interests [22–24]. In contrast, the factor analysis conducted by the authors of the KFZA was based on a sample of office workers. Whereas the main focus of hospital staff is working with human beings and mistakes and failures can lead to vital consequences, the work in an office is focused on administrative and organizational tasks and is characterized by the overall use of a computer [25]. Office workers report to experience especially time pressure, work disruptions and, besides a general increase in workload, primarily an increase in the flood of information by email [26].

However, in spite of these differences, there are also a number of similarities between the two fields that might contribute to the similarities of the results. For example, in both fields female employees predominate, with a proportion of two thirds in offices and 85% among nursing staff [27, 28]. Even among hospital physicians, the percentage of female doctors is growing and amounted to 46 – 56% in 2013 [29]. Further similarities are – as mentioned above – the dominance of time pressure, work disruptions and a general increase in workload, which correspond to universal changes in working environment [30].

Recently, Keller et al. [31] have presented results from a factorial analysis of a questionnaire specifically designed for hospital settings, the "Instrument for stress-related job analysis for hospital physicians" (ISAK-K). The size of this questionnaire containing 30 items is similar to that of the KFZA. Comparison of our determined KFZA factors with the 14 factors of the ISAK-K shows the following consistencies:

The factors of the ISAK-K "Time pressure", "Problems in workflow due to supervisors and physicians", "Problems in workflow due to other professional groups", "Social support from direct supervisors", "Social support from medical colleagues", "Autonomy", "Participation", "Possibilities for further education" and "Possibilities for skill development" correspond well with our factors ***Quantitative Work Demands, Social Relationships, Job Control, Opportunities for Participation and Professional Development*** and ***Variability***, respectively.

Concerning the remaining factors, consistencies are less obvious. The ISAK-K factor "Uncertainty" contains items like "How often does it happen that you have to take a decision, where consequences are difficult to predict?" One might interpret this as complexity, which is included in the KFZA factor ***Qualitative Work Demands*** in terms of "In my work, there are issues that are too complicated". The ISAK-K factor "Frustration about how work needs to be done" contains items that describe a lack of time for patient care and for conversations with patients and relatives. The time aspect of this content is described by ***Quantitative Work Demands,*** the emotional aspect by ***Emotional Demands.*** Items of the ISAK-K factor "Social stressors with patients" such as "How often does it happen that patients or their families reproach you?" correspond most likely to the items of the KFZA factor ***Emotional Demands.*** However, factors consistent to the ISAK-K factors "Emotional dissonance" and "Justice" are not to be found in the KFZA, while in the ISAK-K there are no factors consistent to the KFZA factors ***Workplace Environment*** and ***Consequences of Strain.***

Comparison of our results with psychosocial factors that are listed in the guideline of the GDA [3] shows that except of the GDA factors "Responsibility", "Work time" and "Physical factors" all other psychosocial factors are covered by the extended version of the KFZA. Especially the GDA factors "Emotional demands" and "Work equipment", which were not covered by the original KFZA, are captured by the additional items of the factors ***Emotional Demands*** and ***Workplace Environment.*** For further development of the KFZA, it might be important to note that items of ***Completeness of Task*** were difficult to assign to factors and might not be appropriate for the use in hospitals. While the GDA recommends that this psychosocial factor should be analyzed, it might be necessary to design more specific questions for the hospital setting. Subsequently, these items should be evaluated e.g., using cognitive interviewing. Concerning the items of *Work Disruptions,* item AU1 might be omitted as it is similar to item AM which describes the GDA factor "Work equipment" more specifically. In addition, the newly determined KFZA-factor ***Quantitative Work Demands*** corresponds well with the GDA factor "Work process" that includes possible critical attributes such as time pressure, work intensity and frequent interruptions. The items of the factor

Consequences of Strain, which are not psychosocial factors but a result of distress, are relevant due to a currently developed GDA checklist that is used by the supervisory authorities. Regarding to this checklist a company receives an additional credit point in the audit by surveying information about consequences of strain such as physical impairments.

Limitations

Some limitations of this study should be noted. First, we had to exclude 568 questionnaires listwise (636 for the extended version) due to missing data as a result of varying questionnaire versions used. A comparison showed that the analyzed sample had a slightly but significantly different composition than the deleted one. Therefore, it cannot be ruled out that a factor analysis performed with the original sample would have yielded slightly different results. Another limitation might be that the content of the questionnaire is somewhat heterogeneous mixing psychosocial factors that may cause psychological distress and items representing consequences of strain. However, the latter items load on a distinct factor. Furthermore, the fact that sometimes items were left out due to the request by the work council might have led to selection bias, but we do not believe that any systematic effects were present in determining such decisions. In addition, the sample consisted of two occupational groups – physicians and nurses – whose specific working conditions have a lot in common but also show differences. The fact that the group of nurses outweighs the group of physicians may lead to bias, particularly as the ratio of nurses to physicians in our sample was higher than the national average. The factorial structure of our sample should be cross-validated in other samples of hospital workers. Furthermore, we only analyzed the aspect of the factorial validity. To complete the psychometric evaluation, further studies are necessary.

Practical implications

The KFZA and its extended version are currently implemented to conduct Psychosocial Workplace Risk Assessments in hospitals. The results of such surveys are generally presented through the means of the original KFZA factors. Our study shows that this may not be entirely adequate, since it yielded specific factors for the use in hospital settings. Therefore, we suggest that the factors found should now be used as the basis for future analyses. Furthermore, items which have been shown as not appropriate for the use in hospitals should be rephrased and additional items might be generated to cover the missing GDA factors "Responsibility", "Work time" and "Physical factors". Further psychometric evaluation including cross-validation of the factorial structure in other samples should be performed to achieve an instrument for the use in hospital workplaces.

Conclusion

Overall, our study shows the suitability of the KFZA, both in its original and in its extended version, for the use in hospital workers. However, instead of the 11 factors originally proposed by the authors of the KFZA on the basis of studies with office workers, a seven factor-solution appears to be a better fit when employed in hospitals. Even with the reduced number of factors we were able to replicate the overall content-related structure quite well. Some of the additional items of the extended KFZA version produced two additional factors whereas others were assigned to the existing factors. The extended version of the KFZA covers the psychosocial factors that are examined by the supervisory authorities to a greater extent but might be completed by further items. Our study contributes to the assessment of the validity of this popular instrument. It should be complemented by psychometric evaluation in further studies.

Abbreviations

BAuA: Federal Institute of Work Safety and Occupational Medicine (Bundesanstalt für Arbeitsschutz und Arbeitsmedizin); GDA: Joint German Occupational Safety and Health Strategy (Gemeinsame Deutsche Arbeitsschutzstrategie); ISAK-K: Instrument for stress-related job analysis for hospital physicians (Instrument zur stressbezogenen Arbeitsanalyse für Klinikärztinnen und –ärzte); JC: Job Control; KFZA: Short Questionnaire for Workplace Analysis (Kurzfragebogen zur Arbeitsanalyse); OPPD: Opportunities for Participation and Professional Development; QLWD: Qualitative Work Demands; QNWD: Quantitative Work Demands; SR: Social Relationships; VAR: Variability; WE: Workplace Environment

Acknowledgements

This study summarizies the research of the dissertation of Patricia Appel.

Funding

This publication was funded by the German Research Foundation (DFG) and the University of Wuerzburg in the funding programme Open Access Publishing.

Authors' contributions

PA was responsible for the conception and design of the study, analysis and interpretation of data and drafting and writing of the manuscript. MS was involved in the analysis and interpretation of data and supervision. HV was involved in the conception and design of the study and supervision. AO was involved in the conception and design of the study, acquisition and interpretation of data. HF was involved in the conception and design of the study, was responsible for its supervision and drafting of the manuscript as well as revising it critically. All authors read and approved the final manuscript.

Competing interests

The authors declare that they have no competing interests.

Author details

[1]Department of Medical Psychology and Psychotherapy, Medical Sociology and Rehabilitation Sciences, University of Würzburg, Klinikstrasse 3, 97070 Würzburg, Germany. [2]Center for Occupational Health and Psychology, hanza resources, Hammerbrookstr. 93, 20097 Hamburg, Germany.

References

1. Wittig P, Nöllenheidt C, Brenscheidt S. Grundauswertung der BIBB/BAuA-Erwerbstätigenbefragung 2012. Dortmund: Bundesanstalt für Arbeitsschutz und Arbeitsmedizin; 2013.
2. Beck D, Morschhäuser M, Einführung HHM. In: Bundesanstalt für Arbeitsschutz und Arbeitsmedizin, editor. Gefährdungsbeurteilung psychischer Belastung: Erfahrungen und Empfehlungen. Berlin: Erich Schmidt; 2014. p. 13–8.
3. Beck D, Berger S, Breutmann N, Fergen A, Gregsen S, Morschhäuser M, Reddehase B. Recommendations for implementing psychosocial risk assessment. Berlin: Management of the GDA Mental Health Working Programme; 2014. http://www.gda-psyche.de/SharedDocs/Publikationen/EN/Recommendations%20for%20implementing%20psychosocial%20risk%20assessment.pdf?__blob=publicationFile&v=2. Accessed 7 Dec 2016
4. Holm M, Geray M. Integration der psychischen Belastungen in die Gefährdungsbeurteilung. Berlin: Geschäftsstelle der Initiative Neue Qualität der Arbeit; 2012.
5. Prümper J, Hartmannsgruber K, Frese M. KFZA – Kurzfragebogen zur Arbeitsanalyse. Zeitschrift für Arbeits- und Organisationspsychologie. 1995;39:125–32.
6. Prümper J. KFZA- Kurzfragebogen zur Arbeitsanalyse. In: Sarges W, Wottawa H, Roos C, editors. Handbuch wirtschaftspsychologischer Testverfahren: Band II: Organisationspsychologische Instrumente. Lengerich: Pabst Science Publishers; 2010. p. 157–64.
7. Richter G. Toolbox Version 1.2: Instrumente zur Erfassung psychischer Belastungen; Forschung Projekt F 1965. 2nd ed. Dortmund: Bundesanstalt für Arbeitsschutz und Arbeitsmedizin; 2011.
8. Buddeberg-Fischer B, Klaghofer R, Buddeberg C. Die Motivation zur Weiterbildung in Psychiatrie und Psychotherapie: eine Untersuchung bei jungen Ärztinnen und Ärzten in der Deutschschweiz. Schweiz Arch Neurol Psychiatr. 2008;159:34–41.
9. Ehlbeck I, Lohmann A, Prümper J. Erfassung und Bewertung psychischer Belastungen mit dem Kurzfragebogen zur Arbeitsanalyse (KFZA) Praxisbeispiel Krankenhaus. Leitretter, editor. Düsseldorf: Arbeit in Krankenhäusern human gestalten; 2008. p. 32–58.
10. Eichert H-C. Supervision als Kompensation?: Eine Untersuchung zur supervision in der stationären Psychiatrie. Organisationsberatung - Supervision - Coaching. 2009;16:19–34.
11. Glaser J, Höge T. Probleme und Lösungen in der Pflege aus Sicht der Arbeits- und Gesundheitswissenschaften. Bundesanstalt für Arbeitsschutz und Arbeitsmedizin: Dortmund; 2005.
12. DAK – Deutsche Angestellten Krankenkasse. Gesundheitsreport 2013.: Analyse der Arbeitsunfähigkeitsdaten. Hamburg: Update psychische Erkrankungen – Sind wir heute anders krank ? 2013.
13. Ovd K, Klein J, Grosse Frie K, Blum K, Siegrist J. Psychosoziale Arbeitsbelastungen bei chirurgisch tätigen Krankenhausärzten: Ergebnisse einer bundesweiten Befragung. Dtsch Arztebl Int. 2010;14:248–53.
14. Bauer J, Groneberg DA. Ärztlicher Disstress - eine Untersuchung badenwürttembergischer Ärztinnen und Ärzte in Krankenhäusern. Dtsch Med Wochenschr. 2013;47:2401–6.
15. Schulz M, Damkröger A, Heins C, Wehlitz L, Löhr M, Driessen M, et al. Effort-reward imbalance and burnout among German nurses in medical compared with psychiatric hospital settings. J Psychiatr Ment Health Nurs. 2009;16:225–33.
16. Gothe H, Köster A-D, Storz P, Nolting H-D, Häussler B. Job Satisfation among doctors: a review of international literature. Dtsch Arztebl. 2007:1394–9.
17. Angerer P, Petru R, Nowak D, Weigl M. Arbeitsbedingungen und Depression bei Ärzten. Dtsch Med Wochenschr. 2008;133:26–9.
18. Wilkins K, Shields M. Correlates of medication error in hospitals. Health Rep. 2008;19:7–18.
19. Augurzky B, Krolop S, Hentschker C, Pilny A, Schmidt CM. Krankenhaus Rating Report 2013: Krankenhausversorgung zwischen Euro-Krise und Schuldenbremse. Heidelberg: medhochzwei; 2013.
20. Fabrigar LR, Wegener DT, MacCallum RC, Strahan EJ. Evaluating the use of exploratory factor analysis in psychological research. Psychol Methods. 1999;4:272–99.
21. Schermelleh-Engel K, Werner C. Methoden der Reliabilitätsbestimmung. In: Moosbrugger H, Kelava A, editors. Testtheorie und Fragebogenkonstruktion Heidelberg. Heidelberg: Springer; 2008. p. 114–33.
22. Baldwin DC Jr, Daugherty SR, Tsai R, Scotti MJ Jr. A national survey of residents' self-reported work hours: thinking beyond specialty. Acad Med. 2003;78:1154–63.
23. Iseringhausen O. Psychische Belastungen und gesundheitliches Wohlbefinden von Beschäftigten im Krankenhaus. In: Badura B, Klose J, Macco K, Schröder H, editors. Fehlzeiten-Report 2009: Arbeit und Psyche: Belastungen reduzieren - Wohlbefinden fördern; Zahlen, Daten, Analysen aus allen Branchen der Wirtschaft. Berlin: Springer; 2010. p. 117–28.
24. Glaser J, Höge T. Spezifische Anforderungen und Belastungen personenbezogener Krankenhausarbeit. In: Badura B, Schellschmidt H, Vetter C, editors. Fehlzeiten-Report 2004: Gesundheitsmanagement in Krankenhäusern und Pflegeeinrichtungen; Zahlen, Daten, Analysen aus allen Branchen der Wirtschaft. Berlin: Springer-Verlag; 2005. p. 51–64.
25. Bundesanstalt für Arbeitsschutz und Arbeitsmedizin. Moderne Bildschirmarbeit. 2017. https://www.baua.de/DE/Themen/Arbeitsgestaltung-im-Betrieb/Neue-Technologien-und-Arbeitsformen/Moderne-Bildschirmarbeit/Moderne-Bildschirmarbeit.html. Accessed 8 May 2017.
26. Grabbe Y, Berger J, Nolting H-D, Krämer K. Arbeitsplatz Büro. Arbeitsbedingungen und Gesundheit bei Bürofach- und Bürohilfskräften. DAK Zentrale: Hamburg; 2007.
27. Bundesamt S. 5,2 Millionen Beschäftigte im Gesundheitswesen im Jahr 2012: Pressemitteilung vom 5. März 2014 – 75/14. Wiesbaden: Statistisches Bundesamt Pressestelle; 2014.
28. Bundesamt S. Auf dem Weg zur Gleichstellung?: Bildung, Arbeit und Soziales – Unterschiede zwischen Frauen und Männern. Statistisches Bundesamt: Wiesbaden; 2014.
29. Bundesamt S. 46% des ärztlichen Personals in Krankenhäusern sind Frauen. Wiesbaden: Statistisches Bundesamt Pressestelle; 2015.
30. Morschhäuser M, Beck D, Lohmann-Haislah A. Psychische Belastung als Gegenstand der Gefährdungsbeurteilung. In: Gefährdungsbeurteilung psychischer Belastung: Erfahrungen und Empfehlungen, editor. Bundesanstalt für Arbeitsschutz und Arbeitsmedizin. Berlin: Erich Schmidt; 2014. p. 13–8.
31. Keller M, Bamberg E, Kersten M, Nienhaus A. Instrument for stress-related job analysis for hospital physicians: validation of a short version. J Occup Med Toxicol. 2013;8:10.

13

An evaluation of the protective role of vitamin C in reactive oxygen species-induced hepatotoxicity due to hexavalent chromium in vitro and in vivo

Xiali Zhong[1†], Ming Zeng[1†], Huanfeng Bian[2], Caigao Zhong[1] and Fang Xiao[1*]

Abstract

Backgroud: Drinking water contamination with hexavalent chromium [Cr (VI)] has become one of the most serious public health problems, thus the investigation of Cr (VI)-induced hepatotoxicity has attracted much attention in recent years.

Methods: In the present study, by determining the indices of hepatotoxicity induced by Cr (VI), the source of accumulated reactive oxygen species (ROS), and the protective effect of the antioxidant Vitamin C (Vit C), we explored the mechanisms involved in Cr (VI)-induced hepatotoxicity in vitro and in vivo.

Results: We found Cr (VI) caused hepatotoxicity characterized by the alterations of several enzymatic and cytokine markers including aspartate aminotransferase (AST), alanine aminotransferase (ALT), interleukine-1β (IL-1β), and tumor necrosis factor-α (TNF-α), etc. ROS production after Cr (VI) exposure was origins from the inhibition of electron transfer chain (ETC) and antioxidant system. Vit C inhibited ROS accumulation thus protected against Cr (VI)-induced hepatotoxicity in L-02 hepatocytes and in the rat model.

Conclusions: We concluded that ROS played a role in Cr (VI)-induced hepatotoxicity and Vit C exhibited protective effect. Our current data provides important clues for studying the mechanisms involved in Cr (VI)-induced liver injury, and may be of great help to develop therapeutic strategies for prevention and treatment of liver diseases involving ROS accumulation for occupational exposure population.

Keywords: Hexavalent chromium [Cr (VI)], Reactive oxygen species (ROS), Hepatotoxicity, Vitamin C (Vit C), Mitochondrial respiratory chain complex I (MRCC I)

Background

Chromium (Cr) is commercially used in various industrial processes such as leather tanning, stainless steel welding and chrome plating [1]. The pollution of hexavalent chromium [Cr (VI)] has become one of the most serious public health problems worldwide and the serious pollution incidents have dramatically increased in the last few years. The adverse health effects following occupational or accidental exposures of Cr (VI) and its compounds include a range of slight gastrointestinal reactions such as nausea and vomiting to more serious effects including hepatic damage, primary liver cancers, and even death [2]. Now we have to pay attention that not only the Cr-operating workers, but also the general population may also be at risk because Cr (VI) and the compounds are now widespread in our intimately related environment even in the food [3]. It is known that Cr (VI) enters the target cells and then undergoes metabolic reduction to pentavalent chromium [Cr (V], tetravalent chromium [Cr (IV)] and trivalent chromium [Cr (III)], causing the accumulation of reactive oxygen species (ROS) [4]. ROS, including hydroxyl radicals (OH·), hydrogen peroxide (H_2O_2), and superoxide anion radical ($O_2\cdot^-$), are the molecules that contain an odd number of electrons.

* Correspondence: fangxiao@csu.edu.cn
†Equal contributors
[1]Department of Health Toxicology, Xiangya School of Public Health, Central South University, NO. 238 Shangmayuanling Road, Kaifu District, Changsha 410078, Hunan, People's Republic of China
Full list of author information is available at the end of the article

The main sources of intracellular ROS are enzymatic reactions, nicotinamide adenine dinucleotide phosphate-oxidase (NADPH oxidase), and mitochondrial respiration [5]. Mitochondrial respiratory chain complexes (MRCCs), whose inhibition may cause the escape of electrons from electron transfer chain (ETC), are the most important source of heavy metal-induced ROS accumulation [6]. The major sites of ETC for ROS production remained controversial, and it is reported by others that MRCC III from the ETC is the major site for ROS production [7]. The members of antioxidant system including superoxide dismutase (SOD) and glutathione (GSH) are known as ROS scavenging enzymes whose function are associated with the elimination of excess ROS. ROS play an important role in various cellular signaling processes at low levels while exert a cytotoxic effect by damaging macromolecules such as proteins, lipids and nucleic acids. The reduction of Cr (VI) results in the formation of free radicals which induce a cascade of cellular events including apoptosis, genotoxicity and carcinogenicity, but the related mechanisms of the accumulated free radicals still remain unclear. In the present study we hypothesize that the accumulation of free radicals after Cr (VI) exposure is associated with both the burst generation and the decreased elimination of ROS.

Since there is accumulating evidence indicating a possible causative involvement of ROS in liver injury [8], the anti-oxidative therapy may be of great importance for the established Cr (VI)-associated liver diseases. Vitamin C (Vit C), also known as ascorbic acid, is necessary for the body and widely found in fruits and vegetables. Vit C plays a role as an essential coenzyme in the oxidative stress (OS) pathways, and is an important antioxidant and ROS scavenger. Therefore, Vit C is potentially useful as a therapeutic agent in the treatment of the disorders that associated with free radicals. The liver, an important body organ for its involvement in the biotransformation of various xenobiotics, plays crucial roles in metal homeostasis and detoxification. Although Cr (VI) has been reported to induce hepatotoxicity and natural and synthetic antioxidants have been shown to exert protective effects, the related molecular and cellular mechanisms as well as the potential anti-hepatotoxic protective effect of Vit C on Cr (VI)-induced hepatotoxicity both in vitro and in vivo remain to be fully elucidated. Therefore, we aimed to explore the underlying mechanism of Cr (VI)-induced hepatotoxicity and the possibility that the administration of Vit C would have a beneficial effect on Cr-induced hepatic injuries for the occupation exposure population. The present work was undertaken to study the liver injury by detecting the enzymatic and cytokine markers, to examine the possible sources of the elevated ROS, and to investigate the protective effect of Vit C on Cr (VI)-induced hepatotoxicity both in L-02 hepatocyte and in the rat model.

Materials and methods

Cell line

Human L-02 hepatocyte line was obtained from Type Culture Collection of Chinese Academy of Sciences, Shanghai, China. Cells were cultured as previously described [9].

Animals

The adult Sprague-Dawley (SD) rats aged about 2 months with the average body weight of 180 ± 20 g were purchased from the animal center of Central South University (Changsha, Hunan, China). All rats were housed at the temperature of 22 ± 2 °C and a humidity of 55 ± 5% in a 12h light/dark cycle in standard clear plastic cages with food and water. All animal experiments were performed in accordance with the guidelines of China Council on Animal Care and Use. All animal procedures carried out in this study were reviewed, approved, and supervised by the Animal Care and Use Committee of Central South University.

Animal experiment design

Sixty SD rats were randomly divided into 6 groups, each with 10 animals. Group 1 was the control group, and received normal saline (NS); group 2 was treated with low dose of Cr (VI) (8.84 mg/kg.Bw) (potassium dichromate ($K_2Cr_2O_7$) was dissolved in NS and then was configured to various test doses); group 3 received high dose of Cr (VI) (17.68 mg/kg.Bw); group 4 received Vit C alone (500 mg/kg.Bw); group 5 was treated with the combination of Vit C (500 mg/kg.Bw) plus Cr (VI) (8.84 mg/kg.Bw); group 6 was treated with the combination of Vit C (500 mg/kg.Bw) plus Cr (VI) (17.68 mg/kg.Bw). All rats were given the drugs by gavage at a dose of 0.5 ml/100 g body weight daily for a week (7 consecutive days). Group 1, 2 and 3 were firstly treated with NS by gavage, half an hour later, group 1 received NS and group 2 and 3 received Cr (VI); group 4, 5 and 6 were firstly treated with Vit C by gavage, half an hour later, group 4 received NS and group 5 and 6 received Cr (VI).

Sample collection and preparation

One week later and at the end of the experiment, the urine and stool of the last 24 h treatment of all rats were collected. The urine was precipitated to remove residue, and the stool was dried to constant weight. Blood samples (4 ml of each rat) collected from the femoral artery were allowed to coagulate for 30 min and centrifuged at 2500 rpm for 15 min to separate the serum for biochemical analysis as described below. The rats were sacrificed using ether anesthesia. For each rat, liver specimen (1 g) was collected and then was suspended in ice-cold NS and homogenized in a polytron homogenizer to obtain

10 ml liver tissue suspension. All the samples were stored at −80 °C for further analysis.

Materials

$K_2Cr_2O_7$ and Vit C were purchased from Sigma (St. Louis, MO, USA). RPMI-1640 culture medium, fetal bovine serum (FBS), and trypsin were obtained from Solarbio (Beijing, China). All chemicals and solvents were of analytical grade or the best pharmaceutical grade.

The detection of enzymatic makers of liver injury

The supernatant from treated hepatocytes and serum samples from rats in groups 1 to 6 were analyzed for aspartate aminotransferase (AST) and alanine aminotransferase (ALT) activities spectrophotometrically using the detection kits (Jiancheng Institute of Biological Products, Nanjing, China). The experiments were performed according to the manufacturer's protocols.

The detection of cytokines and LTB4 levels

The levels of leukotriene B4 (LTB4) and the cytokines including interleukine-1β (IL-1β), tumor necrosis factor-α (TNF-α), interferon-γ (IFN-γ), and interleukine-10 (IL-10) were examined using the enzyme linked immunosorbent assay (ELISA) detection kits (Huamei Institute of Biological Products, Wuhan, China). The experiments were performed according to the manufacturer's protocols.

ROS detection

ROS levels were evaluated using fluorescent probe 5-(and 6)-chloromethyl-2′, 7′-dichlorodihydrofluorescein diacetate (CM-H2DCFDA, Molecular Probers, USA). Briefly, after the treatment of various compounds as indicated in the legends to figures, cells of each group were incubated with 10 μM CM-H2DCFDA and analyzed by fluorescence microscope and flow cytometry (Ex 485 nm and Em 535 nm). 2′, 7′-dichlorofluorescein (DCF) is the oxidized product of CM-H2DCFDA. Intracellular ROS level was considered to be directly proportional to the fluorescence intensity of the oxidized product DCF after CM-H2DCFDA treatment. Three independent experiments were performed for each assay condition.

Superoxide anion production detection

Superoxide anion production was assessed by dihydroethidium (DHE) staining. The cells were cultured and treated as above. After rinsed twice with phosphate buffered saline (PBS), the cells were incubated in the dark with 5 μM DHE (Sigma-Aldrich, St Louis, MO) for 30 min. In the presence of superoxide anion, DHE can be oxidized to ethidium bromide (EtBr) (Ex 488 nm and Em 610 nm) which expressing red fluorescence. Thus the amount of EtBr is well correlated to the level of cellular superoxide anion. Superoxide anion in the cells was analyzed by flow cytometry and presented by the percentage of positively staining cells.

Mitochondria isolation

Mitochondria were isolated as described previously [10]. Cells were washed twice with cold PBS, and resuspended with 5 ml buffer A (250 mM sucrose, 20 mM 4-(2-hydroxyethyl)-1-piperazineethanesulfonic acid (HEPES), 10 mM KCl, 1.5 mM $MgCl_2$, 1 mM ethylene diaminetetra acetic acid (EDTA), 1 mM ethylene glycol-bis (2-aminoethylether)- N, N, N ′, N ′-tetraacetic acid (EGTA), 1 mM dithiothreitol, 0.1 mM phenylmethylsulfonyl fluoride, pH 7.5). Cells were homogenized and centrifuged twice at 750×*g* for 10 min. Mitochondria pellets were obtained after centrifugation at 10,000×*g* for 15 min. Isolated mitochondria were used immediately for the measurement of complexes activity. In order to confirm the purity and functionality of the purified mitochondria, transmission electron microscope was used to observe the ultra-structure at magnification of 300,000 times and Clark-type oxygen electrode was used to detect the respiratory function.

Measurement of MRCC activities

The activities of MRCC I-IV were determined using MRCC activity assay kits (Genmed Scientifics, shanghai, China) and were quantified using an UV-9100 spectrophotometer. MRCC I (Nicotinamide adenine dinucleotide (NADH) CoQ oxidoreductase) activity was measured following the oxidation of NADH at 340 nm and expressed as nmol oxidized NADH/min/mg prot; MRCC II (succinate: 2, 6-Dichloroindophenol (DCIP) oxireductase) activity was measured following the reduction of DCIP at 600 nm and expressed as nmol reduced DCIP/min/mg prot; MRCC III (ubiquinol: cytochrome c (Cyt c) reductase) activity was measured following the reduction of Cyt c at 550 nm and expressed as nmol reduced Cyt c /min/mg prot, and MRCC IV (Cyt c oxidase) activity was measured following the oxidation of Cyt c at 550 nm and expressed as nmol oxidized Cyt c/min/mg prot. All measurements were performed at least three times.

Real-time quantitative PCR

Total RNA was extracted from L-02 hepatocytes treated with different concentrations of Cr (VI) using the RNeasy Mini Kit (QIAGEN, Hilden, Germany). Then the total RNA (5 μg) from each treatment group was reverse-transcribed by the PrimeScript RT reagents kit (Takara, Dalian, China) according to the standard protocol. cDNAs were analyzed immediately for Real-time PCR assay using SYBR®Premix Taq™ (Takara, Dalian, China) with Applied Biosystems 7900HT Fast Real-Time PCR System (Applied Biosystems, Inc., Foster City, CA, USA) to observe the mRNA levels of targeted genes. The primer sequence of MRCC I [NADH dehydrogenase [ubiquinone] iron-sulfur protein 3 (NDUFS3)]: 5′- atgttgcc caaactggtctc –3 (forward primer), 5′- tcactgccttcccagagagt –3′ (reverse primer).

Measurement of GSH, SOD, Trx, MDA cellular levels and protein levels

The assessments of the GSH, SOD, and malondialdehyde (MDA) levels were conducted by using the standard kits (Jiancheng Bioengineering Institute, Nanjing, China). And the examination of thioredoxin (Trx) level was also using the kit (Huamei Bioengineering Institute, Wuhan, China). GSH level was examined by the amount of total non-protein sulfhydryl groups, SOD level was examined based on the inhibitory effect of SOD on nitro blue tetrazolium (NBT), Trx level was examined by a double antibody sandwich ELISA method, and MDA level was examined by thiobarbituric acid reactive substances (TBARS).

Protein levels were determined by Western Blotting. Cell lysate was prepared by lysing the cells and then the protein was electrophoretically transferred onto polyvinylidene difluoride (PVDF) membranes and immunoblotted with the antibodies GSH-1 (H-41) (sc-292,189), SOD-1 Antibody (FL-154) (sc-11,407), and Trx (FL-105) (sc-20,146) (Santa Cruz Biotechnology, USA). After incubated with second antibodies, the membranes were developed with the detection system and exposed to films.

Measurement for cell survival rate

Three-(4,5-dimethylthiazol-2yl-)-2,5-diphenyl tetrazolium bromide (MTT) assay was used to evaluate cell survival rate. Briefly, the hepatocytes were seeded at a density of 1×10^4 cells/well in the 96-well plate. Vit C of indicated final concentrations were added to the cultures. Control cells and medium controls without cells received DMSO. The cells were incubated at 37 °C in 5% CO_2 saturated atmosphere and then were washed twice with PBS. Cells were treated with 5 μl 5 mg/ml MTT solution for additional 4 h at 37 °C, and then were lysed in PBS containing 20% Sodium dodecyl sulfate (SDS) and 50% N, N-dimethylformamide (pH 4.5). MTT conversion was quantified by a multiwell ELISA reader Versamax (Molecular Devices, Sunnyvale, CA, USA) at 570 nm.

Histopathological examination of liver

Liver tissue samples were fixed overnight with 10% neutral buffered formalin and then were rinsed for 2 h using running water. The tissues were dehydrated with different concentrations of ethanol and dimethylbenzene and then were embedded in paraffin, sectioned at a thickness of 4 μm, and stained with hematoxylin and eosin (H&E). The specimens were then examined under light microscopy.

Measurement of Cr content

The chromium contents of the samples were determined using the flame atomic absorption spectrometry (F-AAS) method as described earlier [11]. Briefly, prepare chromium standard solution (10 μg/l) and add with 1% spectra pure HNO_3. Then determine the absorbance of different concentrations of standard chromium solution (0, 0.2, 0.5, 1.0, 2.0, 4.0 μg/l) and draw the standard curve. Cr contents of stool, urine, liver and plasma samples were then measured at a wavelength of 357.9 nm.

Measurement of free radical scavenging capacity

The assay was based on benzoic acid hydroxylation method with slight modification. Briefly, in a colorimetric tube, 20 μl $FeSO_4$ (20 mM) and 20 μl EDTA (3 mM) were added. Then, 100 μl sample solution and 1840 μl PBS (pH 7.4) and 20 μl benzoic acid (10 g/l) were added to give a total volume of 2 ml. The reaction mixture was incubated in 37 °C water bath for 90 min. Then the fluorescence was measured at excitation/emission wavelengths of about 305/410 nm. Free radical scavenging capacity % = 100% × [Fs-(Ft-Fc)]/(Fs-Fc). Fs is the fluorescence intensity of the colorimetric tube without the adding of liver sample solution, Ft is the fluorescence intensity of the colorimetric tube with the adding of liver samples from different treatment groups, and Fc is the fluorescence intensity of the colorimetric tube without the adding of $FeSO_4$ or liver sample solution.

Statistical analysis

The results are expressed as mean ± standard deviation (SD). Normal distribution test and Levene's test were performed for Equality of Variances. Significant differences were calculated by one-way analysis of variance (ANOVA) (data fitting normal distribution) or Kruskal-Wallis rank test (data not fitting normal distribution). All statistical analyses were performed using SPSS 19.0. The level of significance was set at $p < 0.05$.

Results

Cr (VI) induced hepatotoxicity in vitro

AST and ALT levels are widely used enzymatic markers of hepatotoxicity. The Cr (VI) treatment groups (8 and 16 μM) showed considerable increase in AST and ALT activities compared with that of the control group (Fig.1a). IL-1β is a potent pro-inflammatory cytokine and IL-10 is an anti-inflammatory cytokine. TNF-α and IFN-γ are also the members of cytokine family that involved in systemic inflammation. IL-10 possesses a hepatic protective effect on proliferation, and it has been shown to inhibit the production of pro-inflammatory

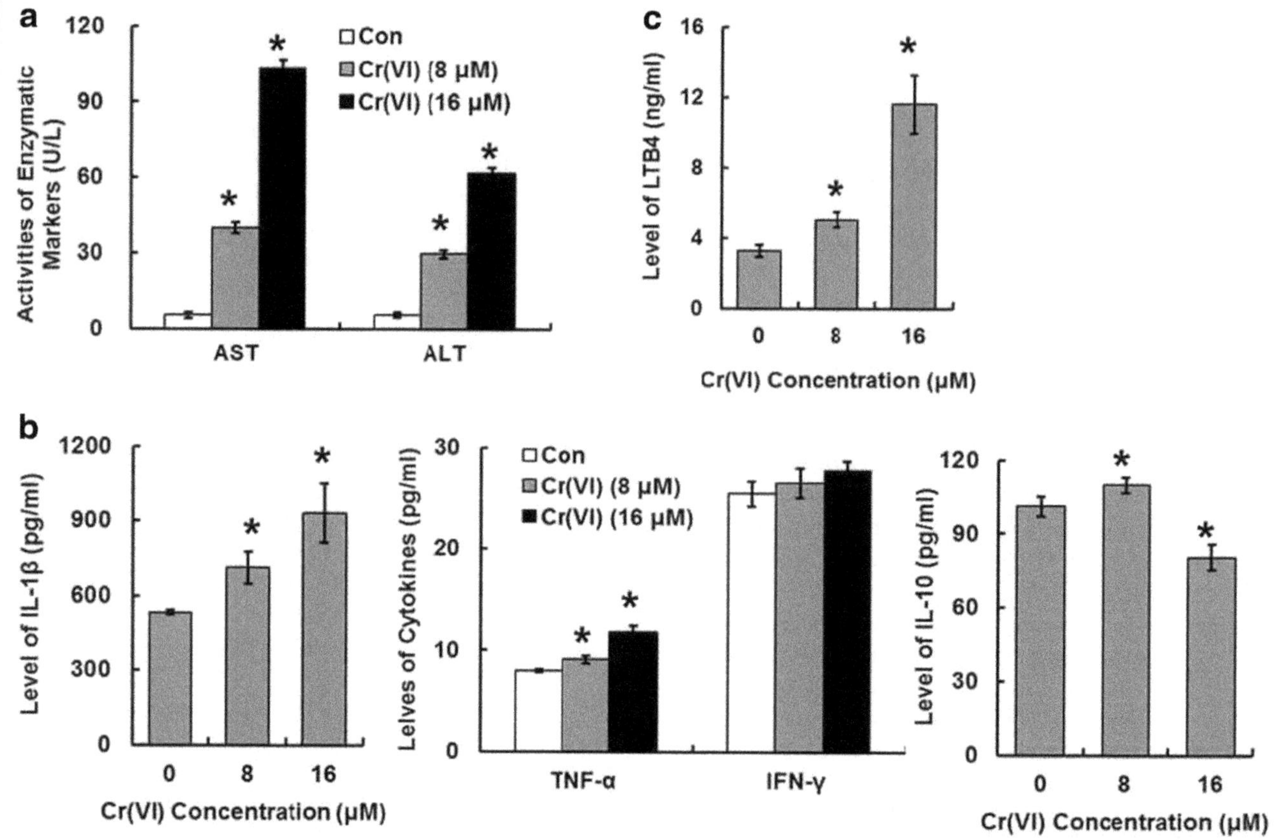

Fig. 1 Cr (VI) induced hepatotoxicity in vitro. L-02 hepatocytes were treated with Cr (VI) (8 and 16 μM) for 24 h, then the cells were collected and the indexes of hepatotoxicity were determined. **a** The changes of activities of enzymatic markers AST and ALT. **b** The production of pro-inflammatory cytokines (IL-1β, TNF-α, IFN-γ and IL-10) after Cr (VI) exposure. **c** Effect of Cr (VI) exposure on LTB4 level. Data represent mean ± SD. $^*p < 0.05$, compared with the control (untreated) group

cytokines, such as TNF-α and IL-1β during the acute inflammation. As shown in Fig. 1b, after Cr (VI) exposure, IL-1β and TNF-α production were increased obviously compared with control, while IFN-γ level showed no obvious change. IL-10 level was increased at the Cr (VI) treatment concentration of 8 μM and decreased at 16 μM. Fig. 1c revealed that Cr (VI) induced increased level of LTB4.

Cr (VI) induced ROS accumulation in the hepatocytes

ROS have been implicated in liver injury. To evaluate the effect of Cr (VI) treatment on intracellular ROS level, we performed the assay by utilizing fluorescent probe CM-H2DCFDA in L-02 hepatocytes treated with different concentrations of Cr (VI) (8 and 16 μM). We identified that compared with control group, Cr (VI) treatment induced higher level of fluorescence signals when observed under microscope (Fig. 2a, left panel). The values of the related DCF fluorescence of each group quantitated by flow cytometry were also shown (Fig. 2a, right panel). DCFH can be oxidized directly by Cr intermediates such as Cr (IV) and Cr (V), thus in the present study we also used DHE which is insensitive to Cr intermediates to monitor superoxide anion production. Superoxide anion is one of a group of molecules referred to as ROS. It has been confirmed that superoxide anion can be produced by both MRCCs and NADPH oxidase in a highly regulated manner and low amounts of superoxide anion plays critical roles in cell proliferation and apoptosis [12]. Superoxide anion production in the hepatocytes was assessed by DHE staining. We found that the percentage of positive staining cells was obviously higher in Cr (VI)-treated groups than that of the control group (Fig. 2b).

The inhibition of MRCC I and antioxidant system were associated with Cr (VI)-induced ROS accumulation

The enzyme complexes of the ETC locate in the mitochondrial inner membrane and play central roles in energy metabolism and other physiological activities. We inferred that the MRCCs in ETC may be responsible for ROS overproduction because the inhibition of MRCCs could induce increased electron leakage from ETC. We examined the alterations of MRCC I-IV activities in

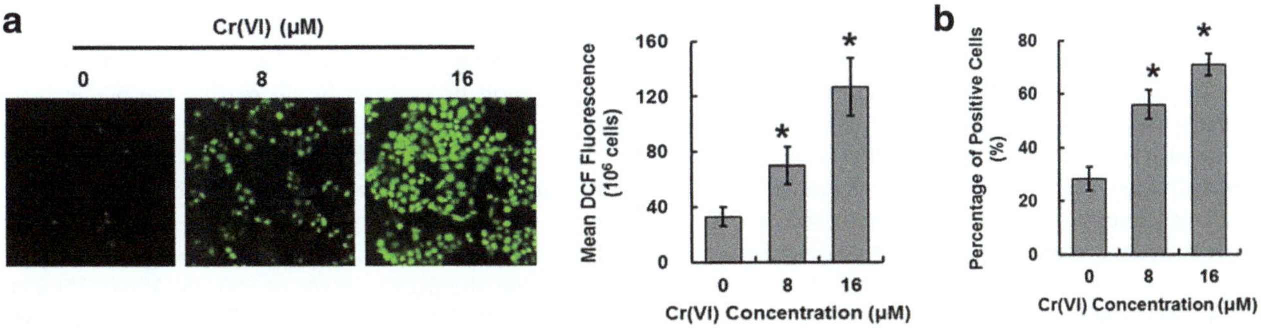

Fig. 2 Cr (VI) induced ROS accumulation in the hepatocytes. The cells were treated as described in Fig. 1. **a** The DCF fluorescence intensity, corresponding to the level of ROS production, was detected. **b** Intracellular superoxide anion. The data shows the percentage and the fluorescence intensity of positive DHE staining cells from each group. Data represent mean ± SD. *$p < 0.05$, compared with the control group

purified mitochondrial fraction. MRCC I appeared to be the most affected one after Cr (VI) exposure. Although complex II was also altered to some extent, the change was not as significant as that of complex I. The activities of MRCC III and IV were not altered compared with control (Fig. 3a). The result suggested that MRCC I and II, especially the former may be the main target of Cr (VI) to induce mitochondrial ETC dysfunction and ROS accumulation. NDUFS3 encodes one of the iron-sulfur protein components of MRCC I. Mutations or inhibition of this gene are associated with MRCC I deficiency. The results shown in Fig. 3b revealed that Cr (VI) inhibited NDUFS3 at both mRNA and protein levels. GSH, SOD, and Trx are main antioxidative proteins that involved in

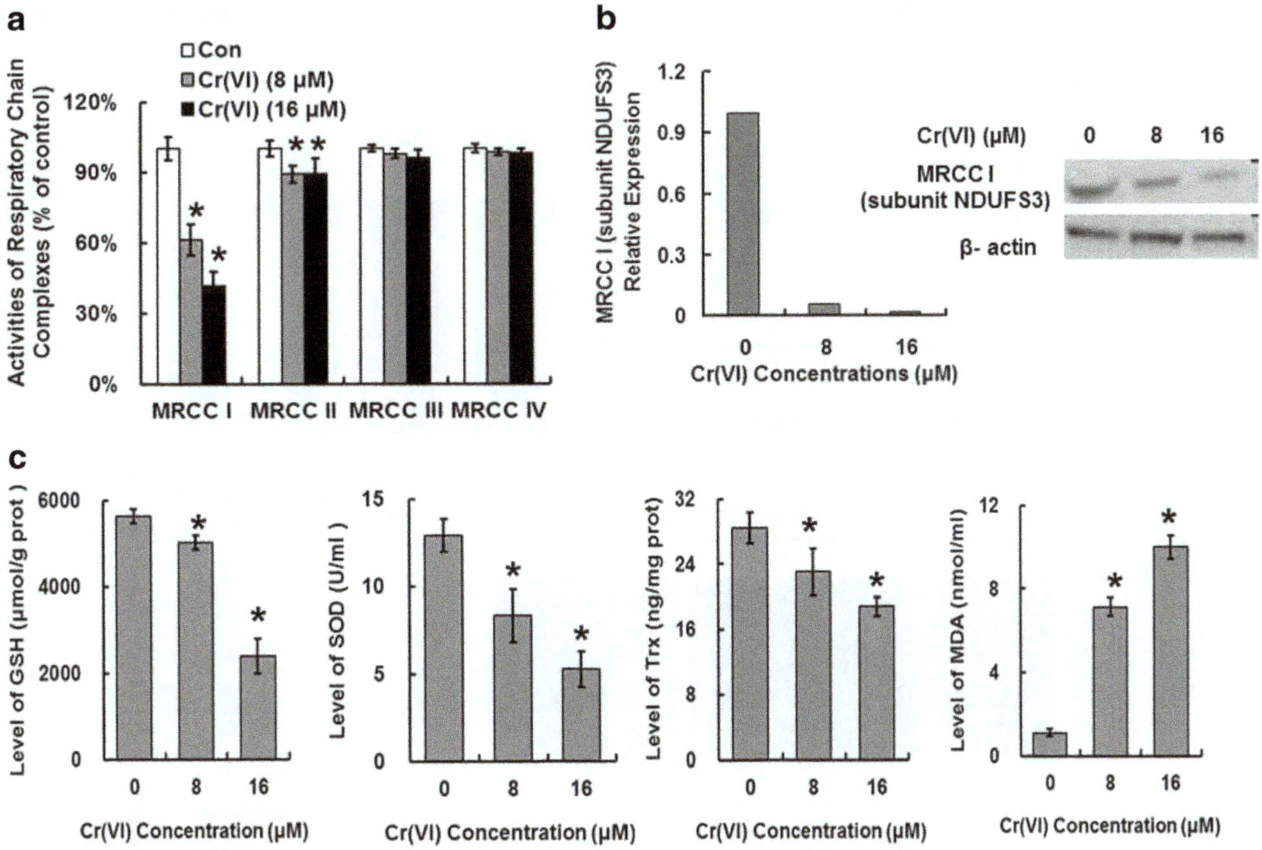

Fig. 3 The inhibition of ETC and antioxidant system were associated with Cr (VI)-induced ROS accumulation. The cells were treated as described in Fig. 1. **a** The activities of MRCC I-IV. **b** The mRNA and protein levels of MRCC I subunit NDUFS3. **c** GSH, SOD, Trx, and MDA levels. Data represent mean ± SD. *$p < 0.05$, compared with the control group

ROS clearance. It is reported that some chemotherapeutic agents cause ROS-dependent cytotoxicity by down-regulating the expression of the antioxidative proteins to facilitate ROS over-production, thus we tested these proteins expressions in Cr (VI)-treated hepatocytes to confirm the resource of ROS. As shown in Fig. 3c, Cr (VI) decreased GSH, SOD and Trx levels in the dose-dependent manner. Cr (VI) also increased MDA level which suggested the occurrence of lipid peroxidation.

Vit C inhibited ROS accumulation

The potential role of free radicals in hepatotoxicity associated with Cr (VI) exposure suggests that antioxidant supplementation may mitigate Cr (VI)-induced toxicity, thus we utilized Vit C in the present study to decrease intracellular ROS level. We analyzed the effect of Vit C (0–2430 μM) on cell survival rate and chose the concentration of 200 μM for the following studies according to the MTT result showed in Fig. 4a. To confirm the antagonistic effect of Vit C on Cr (VI)-induced free radical accumulation, L-02 hepatocytes were pretreated with Vit C (200 μM) for 2 h and then were exposed to Cr (VI) (8 and 16 μM) for 24 h. ROS assay was then performed as described before. As shown in Fig. 4b, Vit C decreased the fluorescence signal levels under microscope and the DCF fluorescence values by flow cytometry, suggesting the inhibition of Cr (VI)-induced ROS production. The DHE staining also showed that Vit C inhibited superoxide anion production by decreasing the percentage of positive staining cells (Fig. 4c).

Vit C protected against Cr (VI)-induced hepatotoxicity in vitro

The cells were exposed to Cr (VI) (0, 8 and 16 μM) with or without the pretreatment of 200 μM Vit C. Vit C significantly inhibited the increase of Cr (VI)-induced AST/ALT levels (Fig. 5a). We also examined effect of Vit C on other liver injury markers including IL-1β, TNF-α and LTB4 and obtained the similar results (Fig. 5b). Vit C also restrained Cr (VI)-induced antioxidant system dysfunction by inhibiting the decrease of GSH, SOD, and Trx levels (Fig. 5c). Fig. 5d showed the western blotting result. These results confirmed that Vit C exerted protective effect against Cr (VI)-induced hepatotoxicity in the L-02 hepatocytes.

Vit C protected against Cr (VI)-induced hepatotoxicity in vivo

All rats were given the drugs by gavage at a dose of 0.5 ml/100 g body weight daily for a week (seven consecutive

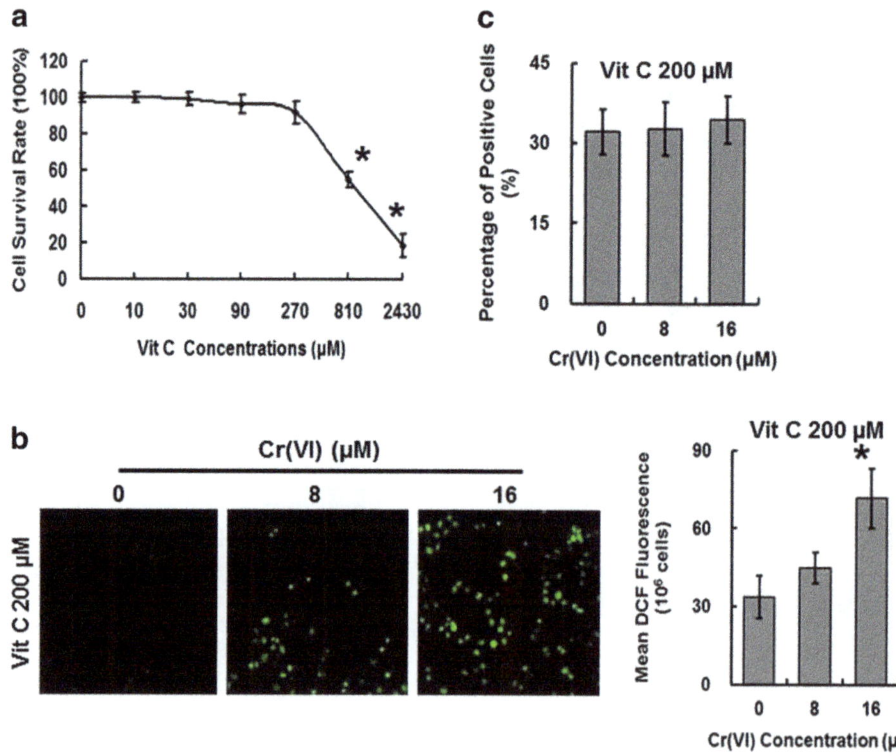

Fig. 4 Vit C inhibited ROS accumulation. **a** The hepatocytes were treated with different concentrations of Vit C (0–2430 μM) for 2 h and then analyzed for cell survival rate. (B-C) The L-02 hepatocytes were pretreated with Vit C (200 μM) for 2 h and then were exposed to Cr (VI) (8 and 16 μM) for 24 h. ROS production assay (**b**) and intracellular superoxide anion production assay (**c**) were conducted. Data represent mean ± SD. *$p < 0.05$, compared with the control group

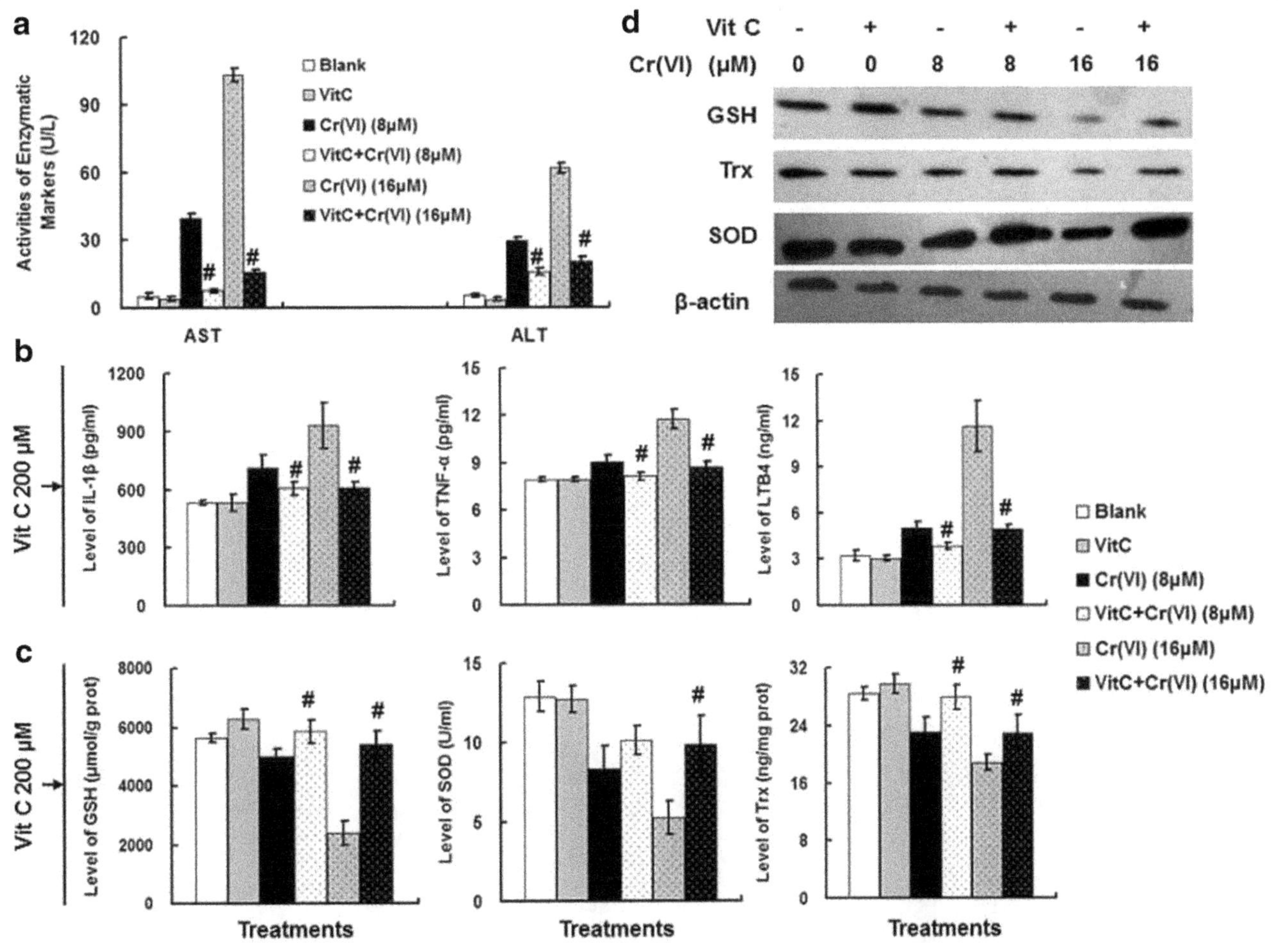

Fig. 5 Vit C protected against Cr (VI)-induced hepatotoxicity in vitro. The cells were exposed to Cr (VI) (0, 8 and 16 μM) with or without the combination of 200 μM Vit C. **a** The changes of activities of enzymatic markers AST and ALT. **b** The levels of IL-1β, TNF-α and LTB4. **c** The levels of GSH, SOD, and Trx. **d** The protein expression levels of GSH, SOD, and Trx. Data represent mean ± SD. $^{\#}p < 0.05$, compared with Cr (VI) alone treatment (8 or 16 μM) group

days). Groups are indicated by pretreatment + treatment as follows: Con, Vit C, Cr (VI) (8.84 mg/kg.bw), Vit C+ Cr (VI) (8.84 mg/kg.bw), Cr (VI) (17.68 mg/kg.bw), and Vit C + Cr (VI) (17.68 mg/kg.bw). As shown in Fig. 6a, a microscopic examination of the liver samples from all treatment groups revealed the typical histopathological features. Both the control and the Vit C (500 mg/kg.bw) group represented the normal rat liver showing normal hepatic architecture (H & E, ×200 magnification). The administration of Cr (VI) (8.84 mg/kg.bw) induced focal necrosis in the centrilobular region with infiltration of neutrophils and lymphocytes, while the hepatic lobules were clear and the hepatic cords were arranged in order. The histology of the livers from Vit C (500 mg/kg.bw) pretreatment plus Cr (VI) (8.84 mg/kg.bw) group showed slight inflammatory cell infiltration. And the Cr (VI) (17.68 mg/kg.bw) group revealed moderate to intense cytoplasmic vacuolization, central vein stenosis, and hepatocyte focal necrosis. Vit C (500 mg/kg.bw) pretreatment significantly alleviated Cr (VI) (17.68 mg/kg.bw)-induced pathological changes. We also examined the effect of Vit C on Cr excretion and Cr content in plasms and liver. Fig. 6b revealed that treatment of Cr (VI) significantly increased Cr content in stool, urine, liver and plasma in a dose-dependent manner. Vit C pretreatment plus Cr (VI) (17.68 mg/kg.bw) group showed higher fecal excretion and lower Cr content in liver and plasma compared with that of the Cr (VI) (17.68 mg/kg.bw) alone treatment group, indicating that Vit C treatment accelerated the fecal excretion of Cr in liver and plasma. High dose of Cr (VI) treatment increased AST activity, and Vit C pretreatment only alleviated high dose of Cr (VI)-induced AST activity elevation. Both low and high dose of Cr (VI) treatments increased ALT activity, and Vit C pretreatment showed obvious inhibitory effect on AST activity elevation (Fig. 6c). The examination of effect of Vit C on Cr (VI)-induced hepatic antioxidant system damage showed that Cr (VI) decreased GSH and SOD levels and increased MDA level, and Vit C

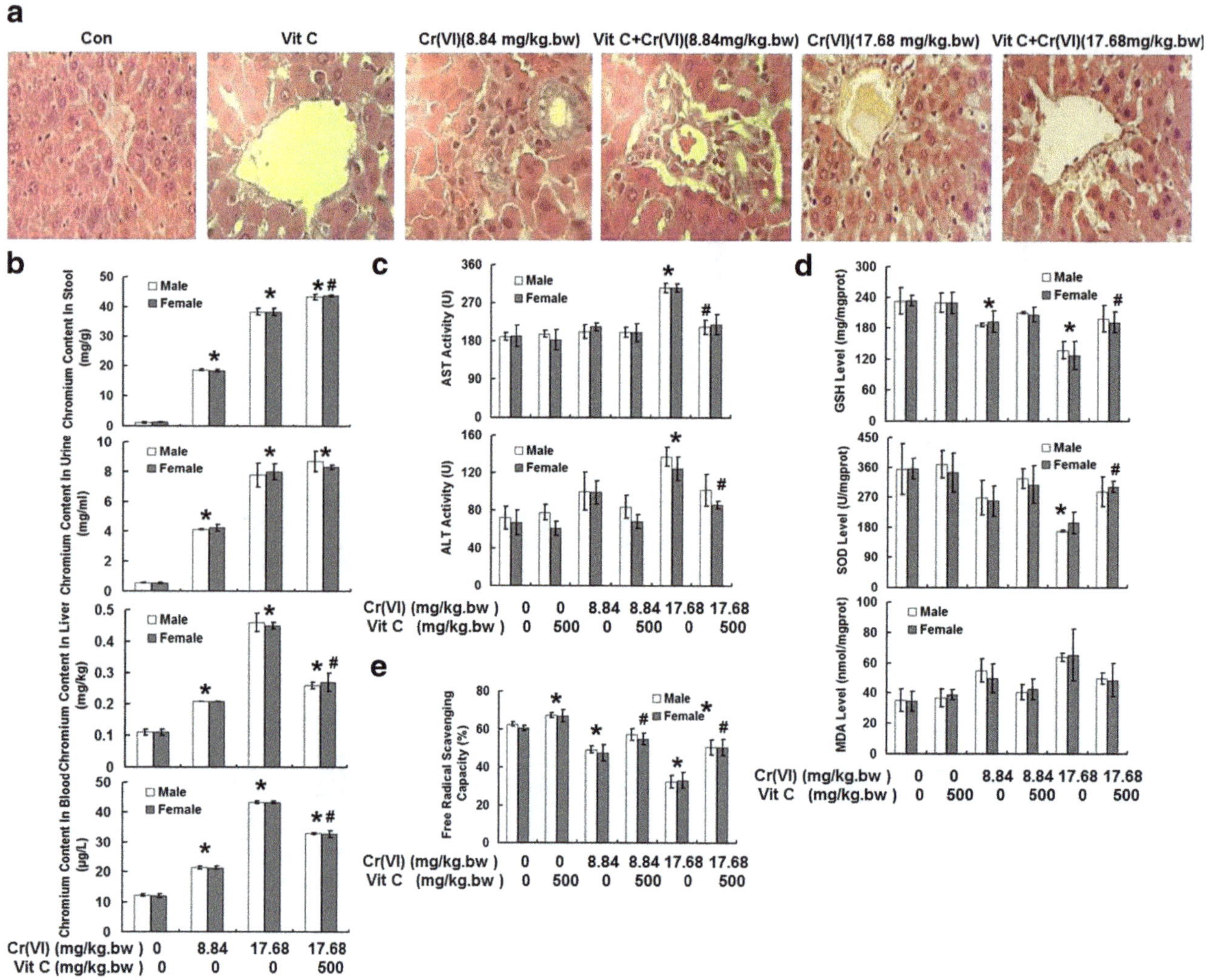

Fig. 6 Vit C protected against Cr (VI)-induced hepatotoxicity in vivo. All rats were given the drugs by gavage at a dose of 0.5 ml/100 g body weight daily for a week (seven consecutive days). Groups are indicated by pretreatment + treatment as follows: Con, Vit C, Cr (VI) (8.84 mg/kg.bw), Vit C+ Cr (VI) (8.84 mg/kg.bw), Cr (VI) (17.68 mg/kg.bw), and Vit C+ Cr (VI) (17.68 mg/kg.bw). **a** Effect of Vit C pretreatment on Cr (VI)-induced alterations in rat liver histology. **b** The chromium contents in stool, urine, liver and plasma. **c** AST and ALT activities. **d** GSH, SOD, and MDA levels. **e** Free radical scavenging capacity. Data represent mean ± SD. *$p < 0.05$, compared with control group. #$p < 0.05$, compared with the Cr (VI) alone treatment group

pretreatment reduced the antioxidant system damage (Fig. 6d). MDA quantification is known as the most widely used method to evaluate lipid peroxidation, the general mechanism accounts for cell injury and other cellular toxic ending. Cr (VI) inhibited free radical scavenging capacity, and Vit C pretreatment also showed the protective effect, suggesting that Vit C rescued the decrease of Cr (VI)-induced free radical scavenging capacity (Fig. 6e). Male and female rats showed similar results. Our present data revealed Vit C pretreatment effectively inhibited Cr (VI)-induced hepatotoxicity in the rat model, and the protective effect of Vit Cwas associated with the inhibition of various enzymatic markers and cytokines as well as the restoration of the antioxidant system function.

Discussion

It is known that heavy exposure to Cr (VI) is closely associated with the increased risk of liver primary cancers [13], thus study on the hepatotoxicity induced by Cr (VI) has become the hot spot in the research field of toxicology. Liver is particularly susceptible to injury for its involvement in xenobiotic metabolism. Under resting conditions the hepatocytes must maintain the critical balance between cellular oxidants and antioxidant defenses. The disruption of this balance may cause the entrance of the cells to an inflammatory state, resulting in the damage of both the cells involved and the surrounding tissues due to the induction of the inflammatory cytokines, the activation of various signaling pathways, and other molecular and cellular modifications. Inflammation is known as the protective mechanism to help the injured or infected organism to initiate cellular repair processes and to restore physiological functions. Liver inflammation has been shown to be associated with elevated production of various cytokines such as IL-1β, TNF-α and IFN-γ, which have been implicated in hepatocarcinogenesis [14, 15]. Although the activities of AST and ALT are the most commonly used and well-known enzymatic markers of liver injury, they only change in late stages and often lack sensitivity in early stages of various liver diseases [16]. IL-1β is known as an initiator cytokine that plays an important role in the regulation of the inflammatory responses [17]. As a major endogenous mediator of hepatotoxicity, TNF-α is a pro-inflammation cytokine that expresses in various liver injuries and plays an important role in tissue damage. Being another pro-inflammatory cytokine, IFN-γ is also a sensitive biomarker as well as a critical mediator of liver damage from several xenobiotic agents [18]. IL-10 is known to have anti-inflammatory effect for its ability to down-regulate the production of pro-inflammation cytokines such as IL-1β and IFN-γ from T cells and exerts its inhibitory effect on several model of liver injury [19]. We found IL-10 level was increased at low dose of Cr (VI) treatment but decreased at high dose of Cr (VI) treatment, indicating that IL-10 played a compensatory role at first, but then showed compensatory failure in severe liver injury. The data indicates that liver damage is likely occurring at the high dose of Cr (VI) treatment because we can speculate that the liver may be able to recover from the injury and regain its normal functions at low dose of Cr (VI) treatment. LTB4, which can be synthesized on activation of 5-lipoxygenase (5-LO), has also been confirmed to participate in different experimental models of liver injury [20].

Cr (VI) could enter the target cells and then undergoes metabolic reduction to Cr (III), causing the accumulation of ROS together with a cascade of various cellular toxic events. MRCC I is a large enzyme complex that embedded in the inner mitochondrial membrane and plays an important role in energy metabolism by proving proton-motive force required for ATP synthesis [21]. While other studies have confirmed that MRCC III is the important source of cellular ROS, in the present study we showed that MRCC I may be the precise site for ROS generation after Cr (VI) exposure. Complex I consists of at least 45 subunits of which 38 subunits are encoded by nuclear genome and 7 are encoded by the mitochondrial genome [22]. In order to investigate how Cr (VI) inhibits MRCC I, we checked the expression levels of all the subunits involved in MRCC I assembly by performing gene chip and RT-PCR. Data revealed that Cr (VI) significantly affected NDUFS3. The mechanisms involved in Cr (VI)-induced inhibition of MRCC I remain to be fully explored. There is evidence supporting that in hepatocytes, the pro-inflammatory cytokines such as TNF-α and IFN-γ can also induce ROS accumulation [23], but the related mechanism is not clear. ROS exhibit the dual role in biology. When produced by normal cellular metabolism and in limited quantities, ROS exert beneficial effects on mediating signaling pathways and contributing to cellular functions including proliferation and differentiation. However, the over-generation of ROS may act as key players in disease pathogenesis and induce cell and tissue damage by attacking vital cellular components such as DNA, lipids and proteins. OS is the state which can result from the increased formation of ROS and the unbalance between pro-oxidants and antioxidants [24]. Chaverrí et al. has reported that OS is associated with Cr (VI)-induced nephrotoxicity [25]. ROS scavenging enzymes, including SOD and GSH, are the members of antioxidants system whose function is to eliminate excess ROS. SOD is known to facilitate the conversion of superoxide to hydrogen peroxide. And GSH is a tripeptide responsible for protection against free radicals, and the depletion of GSH could decrease cellular antioxidant capacity and induce oxidative stress. It has been reported that infection with hepatitis C is accompanied with the accumulation of ROS and the inhibited antioxidant levels [26], thus we inferred that the decreased levels of antioxidant defenses, which were characterized by the inhibition of GSH, SOD and Trx levels, together with the augmented formation of ROS, appear to play an important part in Cr (VI)-induced liver injury. The role of free radicals in Cr (VI)-induced hepatotoxicity and the capacity of Cr (VI) to promote OS are important areas of research in toxicology, because such information may possess important therapeutic significance to prevent liver injury even cancer progression after Cr (VI) by antioxidants such as Vit C.

Previous reports suggest that Cr (VI) is a hepatotoxin and Cr (VI)-induced hepatotoxicity can be alleviated by several natural and synthetic compounds [27]. We think that free radical accumulation and the occurrence of OS is early event and the main mechanism of Cr (VI)-induced liver damage, thus the administration of antioxidant, especially in the early stage of Cr (VI) exposure, may significantly diminish liver injury and even inhibit hepatocarcinogenesis. The present research we conducted in vivo study. The purpose of utilization of experimental rat model of toxicant-induced hepatotoxicity is to evaluate the biochemical processes involved in various liver diseases and to explore the possible pharmacological effects of the liver protective agents such as Vit C. Based on our results, pretreatment with Vit C inhibited the above-mentioned hepatotoxicity-related alterations both in vitro and in vivo, and accelerated the fecal excretion of chromium in liver and plasma of the rates, indicating the hepatoprotective effect of Vit C against Cr (VI)-induced liver injury. Considering the difference between animals and humans and before we can provide valuable experimental evidence for the anti-oxidative therapy in clinic, we definitely need conduct further study because the effective dose and safe dose, during of treatment, and bio-availability of Vit C require thorough exploration.

The current federal maximum contaminant level for total Cr is 100 μg/l [28]. A 2-year cancer bioassay conducted by the National Toxicology Program (NTP) reported that administration of Cr (VI) in drinking water (in the form of sodium dichromate dihydrate [SDD]) induced tumors in the small intestines of rats at ≥172 mg/l SDD (≥60 mg/l Cr (VI)) [29]. The increasing evidence has suggested that both inflammation and ROS play important role in the induction of the carcinogenic phenotype. It is confirmed that inflammatory cell infiltration during cancer progression is accompanied with the generation of various cytokines, chemokines and growth factors, favoring increased cellular proliferation [30]. ROS generated from ETC and oxidation-reduction system after Cr (VI) exposure could cause oxidative damage to host DNA, resulting in activation of oncogenes and/or inactivation of tumor suppressor genes as well as various epigenetic modifications that favor tumor progression. Although we focused on liver injury and the protective effect of Vit C after Cr (VI) exposure in vitro and in vivo, the present study also provided important experimental evidence for the mechanism and treatment study of Cr (VI)-associated cancers. And in addition to the exploration of Cr (VI)-induced cytotoxicity and carcinogenicity, future attention should also be paid to the development of antioxidant-based strategies for primary prevention of liver injury even primary liver cancers in occupational Cr (VI) exposure individuals.

Conclusions

The present study confirmed that ROS played a role in Cr (VI)-induced hepatotoxicity and Vit C exhibited protective effect. Our current data provides important clues for studying the mechanisms involved in Cr (VI)-induced liver injury, and may be of great help to develop therapeutic strategies for prevention and treatment of liver diseases involving ROS accumulation for occupational exposure population.

Abbreviations

5-LO: 5-lipoxygenase; ALT: alanine aminotransferase; AST: aspartate aminotransferase; Cr (VI): hexavalent chromium; Cyt c: cytochrome c; ETC: electron transfer chain; GSH: glutathione; IFN-γ: interferon-γ; IL-10: interleukine-10; IL-1β: interleukine-1β; LTB4: leukotriene B4; MDA: malondialdehyde; MRCCs: mitochondrial respiratory chain complexes; NADH: Nicotinamide adenine dinucleotide; NADPH oxidase: nicotinamide adenine dinucleotide phosphate-oxidase; ROS: reactive oxygen species; SOD: superoxide dismutase; TNF-α: tumor necrosis factor-α; Trx: thioredoxin; Vit C: Vitamin C

Acknowledgements

Not applicable.

Funding

This research was financially supported by National Natural Science Foundation of China (NO. 81302456) and Natural Science Foundation of Hunan Province, China (NO. 2015JJ3135).

Authors' contributions

FX designed the experiments, supervised the project, and wrote the paper. XLZ, MZ and HFB performed the experiments. CGZ provided advice on technical development. XLZ analyzed the data. All authors read and approved the final manuscript.

Competing interests

The authors have no conflicts of interest to declare in relation to this article.

Author details

[1]Department of Health Toxicology, Xiangya School of Public Health, Central South University, NO. 238 Shangmayuanling Road, Kaifu District, Changsha 410078, Hunan, People's Republic of China. [2]Shajing Institution of Health Supervision of Baoan District, Shenzhen 518104, People's Republic of China.

References

1. Tchounwou PB, Yedjou CG, Patlolla AK, Sutton DJ. Heavy metal toxicity and the environment. EXS. 2012;101:133–64.
2. Sazakli E, Villanueva CM, Kogevinas M, Maltezis K, Mouzaki A, Leotsinidis M. Chromium in drinking water: association with biomarkers of exposure and effect. Int J Environ Res Public Health. 2014;11:10125–45.
3. Zhang X, Zhong T, Liu L, Ouyang X. Impact of soil heavy metal pollution on food safety in China. PLoS One. 2015;10:e0135182.
4. Xiao F, Feng X, Zeng M, Guan L, Hu Q, Zhong C. Hexavalent chromium induces energy metabolism disturbance and p53-dependent cell cycle arrest via reactive oxygen species in L-02 hepatocytes. Mol Cell Biochem. 2012;371:65–76.
5. Xie X, Zhao R, Shen GX. Impact of cyanidin-3-glucoside on glycated LDL-induced NADPH oxidase activation, mitochondrial dysfunction and cell viability in cultured vascular endothelial cells. Int J Mol Sci. 2012;13:15867–80.
6. Belyaeva EA, Sokolova TV, Emelyanova LV, Zakharova IO. Mitochondrial electron transport chain in heavy metal-induced neurotoxicity: effects of cadmium, mercury, and copper. Sci World J. 2012;2012:136063.
7. Chen Q, Vazquez EJ, Moghaddas S, Hoppel CL, Lesnefsky EJ. Production of reactive oxygen species by mitochondria: central role of complex III. J Biol Chem. 2003;278:36027.
8. Kim D, Kim GW, Lee SH, Han GD. Ligularia Fischeri extract attenuates liver damage induced by chronic alcohol intake. Pharm Biol. 2016;54:1–9.
9. Xiao F, Li Y, Luo L, Xie Y, Zeng M, Wang A, et al. Role of mitochondrial electron transport chain dysfunction in Cr (VI)-induced cytotoxicity in L-02 hepatocytes. Cell Physiol Biochem. 2014;33:1013–25.
10. Brustovetsky N, Brustovetsky T, Jemmerson R, Dubinsky JM. Calcium-induced cytochrome c release from CNS mitochondria is associated with the permeability transition and rupture of the outer membrane. J Neurochem. 2002;80:207–18.
11. Suliburska J, Krejpcio Z, Staniek H, Krol E, Bogdanski P, Kupsz J, et al. The effects of antihypertensive drugs on chromium status, glucose metabolism, and antioxidant and inflammatory indices in spontaneously hypertensive rats. Biol Trace Elem Res. 2014;157:60–6.
12. Bedard K, Krause KH. The NOX family of ROS-generating NADPH oxidases: physiology and pathophysiology. Physiol Rev. 2007;87:245–313.
13. Linos A, Petralias A, Christophi CA, Christoforidou E, Kouroutou P, Stoltidis M, et al. Oral ingestion of hexavalent chromium through drinking water and cancer mortality in an industrial area of Greece-an ecological study. Environ Health. 2011;10:50.

14. Sun B, Karin M. Obesity, inflammation, and liver cancer. J Hepatol. 2012;56:704–13.
15. Garcia-Nino WR, Tapia E, Zazueta C, Zatarain-Barron ZL, Hernandez-Pando R, Vega-Garcia CC, et al. Curcumin pretreatment prevents potassium dichromate-induced hepatotoxicity, oxidative stress, decreased respiratory complex I activity, and membrane permeability transition pore opening. Evid Based Complement Alternat Med. 2013;2013:424692.
16. Shih TY, Young TH, Lee HS, Hsieh CB, Hu YP. Protective effects of Kaempferol on Isoniazid- and Rifampicin-induced Hepatotoxicity. AAPS J. 2013;15:753–62.
17. Cover C, Liu J, Farhood A, Malle E, Waalkes MP, Bajt ML, et al. Pathophysiological role of the acute inflammatory response during acetaminophen hepatotoxicity. Toxicol Appl Pharmacol. 2006;216:98–107.
18. Küsters S, Gantner F, Künstle G, Tiegs G. Interferon gamma plays a critical role in T cell-dependent liver injury in mice initiated by concanavalin a. Gastroenterology. 1996;111:462–71.
19. Thompson K, Maltby J, Fallowfield J, Mcaulay M, Millwardsadler H, Sheron N. Interleukin-10 expression and function in experimental murine liver inflammation and fibrosis. Hepatology. 1998;28:1597.
20. Mei Chen BKL, Andrew D, Luster SZ, Murphy RC, Bair AM, Soberman RJ, et al. Joint tissues amplify inflammation and Alter their invasive behavior via Leukotriene B4 in experimental inflammatory arthritis. J Immunol. 2010;185:5503.
21. Efremov RG, Baradaran R, Sazanov LA. The architecture of respiratory complex I. Nature. 2010;465:441–5.
22. Rodenburg RJ. Mitochondrial complex I-linked disease. Biochim Biophys Acta. 1857;2016:938–45.
23. Adamson GM, Billings RE. Tumor necrosis factor induced oxidative stress in isolated mouse hepatocytes. Arch Biochem Biophys. 1992;294:223–9.
24. Halliwell B. Biochemistry of oxidative stress. Biochem Soc Trans. 2007;35:1147–50.
25. Pedraza-Chaverrí J, Barrera D, Medina-Campos ON, Carvajal RC, Hernández-Pando R, Macías-Ruvalcaba NA, et al. Time course study of oxidative and nitrosative stress and antioxidant enzymes in K2Cr2O7-induced nephrotoxicity. BMC Nephrol. 2005;6:4.
26. Lozano-Sepulveda SA, Bryan-Marrugo OL, Cordova-Fletes C, Gutierrez-Ruiz MC, Rivas-Estilla AM. Oxidative stress modulation in hepatitis C virus infected cells. World J Hepatol. 2015;7:2880–9.
27. Boşgelmez İİ, Söylemezoğlu T, Güvendik G. The protective and Antidotal effects of Taurine on Hexavalent chromium-induced oxidative stress in mice liver tissue. Biol Trace Elem Res. 2008;125:46.
28. Thompson CM, Kirman CR, Proctor DM, Haws LC, Suh M, Hays SM, et al. A chronic oral reference dose for hexavalent chromium-induced intestinal cancer. J Appl Toxicol. 2014;34:525–36.
29. Stout MD, Herbert RA, Kissling GE, Collins BJ, Travlos GS, Witt KL, et al. Hexavalent chromium is carcinogenic to F344/N rats and B6C3F1 mice after chronic oral exposure. Environ Health Perspect. 2009;117:716–22.
30. Coussens LM, Werb Z. Inflammation and cancer. Nature. 2002;420:860–7.

14

Hydrogen sulphide exposure in waste water treatment

Åse Dalseth Austigard[1], Kristin Svendsen[2*] and Kari K. Heldal[3]

Abstract

Background: The aims of this study was to assess exposure to hydrogen sulphide (H_2S) among waste water treatment workers (WWWs), and achieve a better measure of the risks of H_2S exposure than only using the eight-hour average value and the ceiling value because the exposure pattern of H_2S for WWWs is dominated by short-term peaks.

Methods: Ninety-three measurements of H_2S from 56 WWWs in three cities and three rural areas were collected. All exposure measurements were carried out from the start of the day until lunch time (sampling time 4–5 h) when most of the practical work was performed. The type of tasks and extent of flushing were registered. H_2S was measured using direct-reading instruments with logging: OdaLog L2/LL, Dräger X-am 5000 and Dräger Pac 7000 (0.1–200 ppm). Number and duration of peaks for different work tasks, seasons, places and extent of flushing were combined in an exposure index (IN), and evaluated in a mixed-model analysis, building a model aimed to predict exposure for different job tasks.

Results: Nine Percent (8 of 93) of all H_2S measurements have peaks above 10 ppm; in addition, 15% (14 of 93) have peaks of 5–10 ppm, 35% (33 of 93) have peaks of 1–5 ppm and 65% (62 of 93) have peaks of 0.1–1 ppm. 29% of the measurements of hydrogen sulphide showed no registered level > 0.1 ppm.
From the mixed-model analyses we see that exposure level, expressed as H_2S index IN, varied between places, work type, season and degree of flushing. For the work in a plant in the capital, the exposure index varied from 0.02 for working in spring doing some flushing, to 0.7 for working at the same plant in winter doing flushing more than three times or more than 10 min. Collecting sewage from cesspools in city 2 in winter doing a lot of flushing gave a hydrogen sulphide index of 230.

Conclusions: The use of a H_2S index, taking into consideration peak height, duration and number of peaks, could be a tool for exposure assessment for H_2S.

Keywords: Peak exposure, Waste water workers, Hydrogen sulphide, Exposure index

Background

As a part of a project aiming to elucidate the association between respiratory and neurological symptoms and exposure in waste water treatment workers (WWWs), results from the measurements of hydrogen sulphide (H_2S) when handling and transporting sewage in Norway are presented. To use the time weighted average (TWA) over one shift as a sole measure seemed inappropriate as one high peak could have health effects without being reflected by the TWA. However, no suggestions regarding what exposure measure having the most impact (peak level, peak frequency/number of peaks or peak duration) on health are reported in the literature.

WWWs commonly suffer from various health symptoms, including neurological and respiratory tract [1–5]. These effects have been ascribed to exposure to microorganisms and noxious gases such as H_2S or from exposure to low levels of different biological and chemical agents [1, 4, 6].

In particular H_2S exposure has been associated with cognitive impairment among WWWs [5] and neurological symptoms [2, 7].

H_2S is a gas that can be produced by bacterial processes during the decay of both plant and animal protein

* Correspondence: Kristin.svendsen@ntnu.no
[2]Institute of Industrial Economics and Technology Management, Norwegian University of Science and Technology, Alfred Getz vei 3, 7491 Trondheim, Norway
Full list of author information is available at the end of the article

or through the direct reduction of sulphate [8]. Therefore, it is a common pollutant in sewage plants and in agriculture as the process of cleaning the sewage needs the proteins to sediment from the water in which they are suspended. Further processing gives new possibilities for accumulation of H_2S until the processed sediments are spread in the fields.

H_2S can be extremely hazardous, being able to cause pulmonary oedema [9–11] sudden unconsciousness (> 500 ppm) or death by even a single exposure if the levels are over 1000 ppm [12, 13]. Repeated exposure to lower levels may result in more chronic respiratory symptoms [14] and symptoms from upper respiratory tract [15], the central nervous system, such as fatigue, headache, poor memory and dizziness [16]. As H_2S exposure is characterised by short peaks, often with high intensity, it represents an extremely hazardous risk for workers because of the toxicity in high concentration combined with the pattern of exposure [1, 17]. Exposure levels are unpredictable, but the occurrence is associated with disturbance of biological material sedimented under lack of oxygen. The disturbance might be due to flushing of pipelines, movement in sediment basins, lowering of pressure on sediments or tidal water lifting sediments in overflow pipes. These are pipelines draining the pumping stations and the treatment plants, so they are not flooded during maintenance or extensive rain. This is necessary, as much of the sewage pipelines in Norway also handle surface water.

Sewage is treated to reduce pollution of rivers, lakes and fjords. This pollution might lead to the extreme growth of algae, sedimentation that uses all the oxygen in the waters and thereby kills bottom life. Sewage treatment also prevents spreading of diseases and other kinds of pollution thrown in the sewage. Treatment is based on biological degradation, physical sedimentation and/or chemical treatment to enhance sedimentation.

Studies of WWWs' exposure to H_2S are sparse. TWA exposure levels over work shifts have been reported to be low [1, 18]. TWA measurements over 8 hours have shown mean levels < 1 ppm [1, 3, 18] regardless of jobs. Other reported measurement levels are either stationary or task based [1, 3, 6, 19]. All these results show that eight-hour TWA is < 1 ppm. However, peak exposure above 100 ppm from stationary measurements during handling of sewage has been reported [1, 19]. At these levels, H_2S does not smell, due to olfactory fatigue [20]. This means there is no smell to give exposure warning at levels of acute danger to life and health.

Several studies on exposure at low background levels of H_2S showed no adverse respiratory or neurological health effects, but studies from Iceland showed that exceeding 7.00 $\mu g/m^3$ (0.005 ppm) H_2S were associated with increase in emergency hospital visits due to heart disease in elderly population [21].

Studies from the geothermal areal Rotorura in New Zealand with long term exposure levels of H_2S at ~0.01–0.03 ppm provided no evidence of impairment of pulmonary function or with chronic obstructive pulmonary disease (COPD) [22].

The same authors studied H_2S and self reported asthma and asthma symptoms without finding any increased asthma risk [23].

A study on inhabitants in the same area of H_2S exposure and cognitive impairment found no association at these ambient levels [24].

Jäppinen [25] found that levels of 2 ppm H_2S might cause bronchial obstruction in asthmatic individuals. In non-asthmatic individuals they could not find noticeable respiratory effects at levels below 10 ppm.

A review of H_2S poisonings in the Alberta province of Canada over a 5 year period concluded that there were no long-term adverse effects apparent in the survivors. This conclusion was based on symptomatic description of the patients at their discharge from medical care as no follow-up tracings after discharge were available. Most of these incidences were related to the large Canadian oil industry [26].

As H_2S is an acutely toxic gas that could rapidly reach harmful or even lethal levels, a short term exposure level (STEL) or a ceiling value is established in several countries. In Norway, this ceiling value is 10 ppm [27]. The no observed effect level (NOEL) for lesions in the olfactory mucosa after short-term exposure has been reported to be 10 ppm [28].

The aim of the present study was to map the exposure to H_2S among sewer workers with regard to type of jobs, tasks, seasons and geographical place. In addition we wanted to suggest an index which may reflect another exposure measure than the TWA for H_2S.

Method

The study was conducted in two areas: around the capital and in five counties in the middle of Norway. Three big plants, all pump stations and the sewage network in the capital were included. In the middle of Norway, two cities and three rural counties were selected, with all their sewage work included. These counties were selected because of easy access and for their type of plants (the five biggest plants in Norway and one smaller, but still large plant) and because the plant sizes in the selected rural areas are found in smaller cities and all rural areas of Norway. All workers in the selected areas were invited to the study, and all participated, a total of 149 persons. H_2S measurements were performed for those available on the measurement days, which gave a total of 56 different workers.

All types of sewage work executed by four separate groups of workers were included:

i. Big plants:
daily inspection and cleaning activities. The inspection was mainly done from control rooms with automatic remote-control systems combined with visual control. The biggest city plant handled sewage from 600,000 person equivalents (PE) and the smallest city plant from 22,000 PE. The number of workers in each plant was from 4 to 20. The six plants were all located in rock halls and categorized as big plants.
ii. Pump stations and small plants:
maintenance and cleaning of the pump stations and plants. This work includes flushing with water under high pressure (100–200 bar) and emptying of sediments from pits or storage areas.
For rural workers, also working with the sewer network connected to the plant is included, as the work pattern is more complex and not easily separated during measurement.
The plants in the rural areas handled sewage from 2000 PE to 5000 PE and employed from one to three workers.
iii. Sewer network
This work includes flushing with water under high pressure (100–200 bar) and close contact with waste water.
iv. Collecting sewage from cesspools
The sewage was removed using a tanker lorry equipped with a pumping device and unloaded from the tanker lorry at the plants or into sewer tunnels leading to the plants. Cesspool dimensions vary from approximately 1 m^3 (one house) to over 20 m^3. One lorry load is normally 3.5 m^3. Intervals of emptying vary from 3 months (drinking water reservoir area) to 4 years (cottage, periodically habited). One and 2 years are the most common intervals. This work is not present in the capital.

Measurements of H_2S exposure were performed on 56 of the workers, at different seasons and always included at least two different seasons for each city or area.

During sampling, the number of flushings was registered. The job types were categorized. Table 1 gives an overview of places and job types.

Exposure measurements

Ninety three personal measurements have been collected among WWWs, focusing on distributing the measurements over seasons, work task, persons, areas and size of cleaning facilities, all in an effort to explore the exposure and to suggest an exposure index that is better than the time weighted average (TWA) to evaluate the connection between exposure and health effects.

Our initial thesis was that because of the nature of the toxicity and exposure pattern of H_2S, the levels could be expressed in an H_2S index combining the characteristics of peak height, number of peaks and duration of peaks during the whole shift. The index is intended to be used for the analysis of H_2S exposure and health effects in a coming study.

All exposure measurements were carried out from the start of the day until lunch time (sampling time 4–5 h) when most of the practical work was performed. Measurement time and time of active sewage work during measurement were registered. The workers carried a backpack, and the H_2S sensors were fastened on the carrying straps on the front of their chests. The inlets of the sensors were in the breathing zone of the worker. Sampling were performed during the whole year and therefore classified in four seasons, winter (26 measurements, 10 days), spring (14 measurements, 4 days), summer (25 measurements, 11 days) and autumn (28 measurements, 8 days) measurements. Fifty six workers

Table 1 The different cities and rural areas and the jobs and tasks measured.

Place	Type of plant and system	Type of jobs	Tasks
Capital	2 big plants, pump stations, sewer network	Working in big plant, Working with sewer network, Working at pump stations	Flushing and cleaning, maintenance, Inspection.
City 1	2 big plants, pump stations, sewer network, cesspools	Working in big plant, Working with sewer network, Working at pump stations, Collecting sewage from cesspools	Flushing and cleaning, maintenance, sucking sewage from cesspools
City 2	1 big plant, pump stations, 1 small plant, cesspools	Working in big plant, Collecting sewage from cesspools, Working in small rural plants including sewer network and pump stations	Inspection, flushing and cleaning, maintenance, sucking sewage from cesspools
Rural 1	1 small plant, pump stations, sewer network	Working in small rural plants including sewer network and pump stations	Flushing and cleaning, maintenance.
Rural 2	1 small plant, pump stations, sewer network	Working in small rural plants including sewer network and pump stations	Flushing and cleaning, maintenance.
Rural 3	1 small plant, pump station, sewer network, cesspools	Collecting sewage from cesspools, Working in small rural plants including sewer network and pump stations	Flushing and cleaning, maintenance, sucking sewage from cesspools

were measured, 30% more than once, and we obtained a total of 93 H_2S measurements over a total of 33 different days. Distribution of measurements per worker is illustrated in Fig. 1.

H_2S was measured with three different direct-reading logging instruments: OdaLog L2/LL, Dräger X-am 5000 and Dräger Pac 7000 (0.1–200 ppm; resolution 0.1 ppm). The instruments recorded 15 s concentration average, in a continuous log, four times per minute. H_2S exposure was registered by the number of peaks measured within these intervals: 0.1–1.0 ppm, 1.1–5.0 ppm, 5.1–10.0 ppm and above 10.0 ppm. The total duration of peaks were noted and given for two intervals: 0.1–5.0 ppm and above 5.0 ppm. Therefore, to handle these measurement results as one value, a H_2S index was suggested. We have thought of the index as dimensionless, even though it could be said to contain dimensions:

$$\begin{aligned} H_2S \text{ index} &= IN \\ &= H_2S_{01} \times 0.1 + H_2S_{duration01} \times 0.1 + H_2S_1 \\ &+ H_2S_5 \times H_2S_{duration5} \times 5 + H_2S_{10} \times 10 \\ &+ H_2S_{max}, \end{aligned}$$

where.

H_2S_{01}represents the number of peaks in the lowest interval (0.1–1.0 ppm).

$H_2S_{duration01}$represents the time with level between 0.1 to 5 ppm(counted as number of minutes).

H_2S_1represents the number of peaks between 1.1–5.0 ppm.

H_2S_5represents the number of peaks between 5.1–10.0 ppm.

$H_2S_{duration5}$represents the time with level above 5.0 ppm (counted as number of minutes).

H_2S_{10}represents the number of peaks higher than 10.0 ppm.

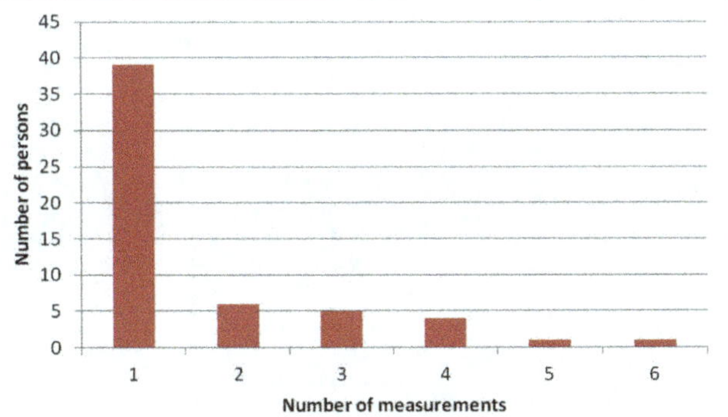

Fig. 1 Number of measurement per person. Bar graph illustrating the number of measurements per person and corresponding number of persons

H_2S_{max}represents the highest ppm level during measurement.

The values of number of peaks are multiplied with the set peak value: 0.1, 1, 5 or 10. This means that higher peaks are given more influence in the calculated index value when present.

Minutes is chosen as the time unit to be counted, as peak times are short. Most equipment can give values for such time, and it is easily counted from a graph or database.

This exposure index will be used as a determinant of exposure among others for different health effects in a later publication. The hypothesis is that not only average level but also the number of peaks and peak level are of relevance to health effects from the exposure. This is due to the behaviour of H_2S, with peaking exposure as normal events, but peak levels are camouflaged if only the average is given.

Statistical analysis

29% of the recordings gave H_2S index values of 0 (0 peaks above 0.1 ppm). No H_2S present is a rarity for this kind of work as long as active sewage work has been done, or deposits are present. Therefore $IN = 0$ was replaced with $0.04/\sqrt{2} = 0.028$, where 0.04 was 1/10 of the lowest calculated IN based on positive H_2S recordings as a substitute for the detection limit [29]. This is also necessary due to the analysis methods; otherwise the number of measurements counted in statistical processes will be lower. This would increase the calculated uncertainty and give a wrong impression of the accuracy of the method.

The index was log transformed before statistical analysis, as workplace measurements are supposed to be log normally distributed. Logarithmical transformations give the possibility to check whether the data are consistent over magnitudes, and ease the mathematical calculations.

To build our model for predicting exposure in Table 4, the exposure to H_2S, as H_2S index (IN), was modelled by linear mixed-effect regression to account for the correlation between repeated measurements on the same person. By linear mixed-effect regression we can evaluate multiple parameters occurring during measurements. Determinants of exposure (job type, season, place and degree of flushing) were treated as fixed effects and worker as a random effect. The models were built stepwise by forward/backward selection. Determinants that significantly improved the models, judged by a p-value < 0.05 of the likelihood ratio test, were kept in the model. The effect of determinants is shown as factors by back-transformation of the log transformed regression coefficients. From the final model, exposure levels of different combinations of job type, season, place and degree of flushing, can be calculated as follows:

$$E = e^{c+d1+d2...} = e^{c} \times \text{effect determinant } 1 \times \text{effect determinant } 2...,$$

where E is exposure as a calculated index for the specific set of determinants, c = intercept of the model and d1 and d2 are regression coefficients of determinants 1 and 2.

Arithmetic mean (AM) is a predictor of cumulative dose which is supposed to be the best exposure measure for long-term effects [30]. It can be calculated as

$$AM = GM \times e^{(0.5 \times \text{variance})}$$

where GM is the geometric mean, used for evaluating numbers that are log normally distributed, such as our H_2S data.

"Variance" in this formula is the total variance. In our model this equals the calculated within worker variance (variance(ww)), because the between worker variance (variance(bw)) is < 0.00. This means that the day to day variation of a worker is higher than the variance between workers.

Having both the AM and GM gives an even better understanding of the distribution of data and gives a measure for the dose relevant to long term effects, which might also be necessary to give good advice on exposure protection.

Differences in H_2S exposure as IN were analysed using one-way ANOVA with Bonferroni adjustments on the log transformed data, see Table 3.

All analyses were performed using IBM SPSS Statistics 20 (IBM, Armonk NY).

Results

As the H_2S peaks are normally steep, we have counted new peaks if the H_2S level fell under detection limit, or if it has fallen to a lower category and then risen again. The highest number of peaks was 58. This was over a period of 160 min, where 130 of them were active in sewage work, and with 115 min recorded levels above 0.1 ppm.

Median number of peaks during measurements were 2, average were 7. Median time above 0.1 ppm for the measurements were 4 min, average 12 min.

Counting the peaks was a time consuming task, especially on the measurements with complicated (many) peaks, but mostly the peaks were easily counted. Graphical presentation of the corresponding numbers for minutes above 0.1 ppm, number of peaks, highest peak value, measurement time and time with exposed work in the measurements are given in Figs. 2 and 3. Measurement numbers correspond in the two figures. The measurements are sorted by number of peaks.

Part of the graph from our highest exposed measurement (Fig. 4) illustrates the problem with using average, or count of peaks or duration of peaks as single measure of this exposure. All these three measures would give "Low risk" as a predicted result. The peak height would of course give "High risk" in this measurement. When the same pattern repeats at lower levels this is not necessarily the case. The measuring range was 0.1–200 ppm, so the peak level might have been higher than registered. Normally the work also would have lasted longer, but was this time interrupted.

9% (8 of 93) of all H_2S measurements have peaks above 10 ppm, in addition, 15% (14 of 93) have peaks of 5–10 ppm, 35% (33 of 93) have peaks of 1–5 ppm and 65% (62 of 93) have peaks of 0.1–1 ppm. 29% of the measurements of H_2S showed no registered sulphide level > 0.1 ppm. Pump stations and small plants, work in sewer networks and collecting sewage from cesspools all had shifts with peak H_2S above 10 ppm. The job with most excessive exposure to H_2S was collecting sewage from cesspools, with 16% of all shifts having peaks above 10 ppm.

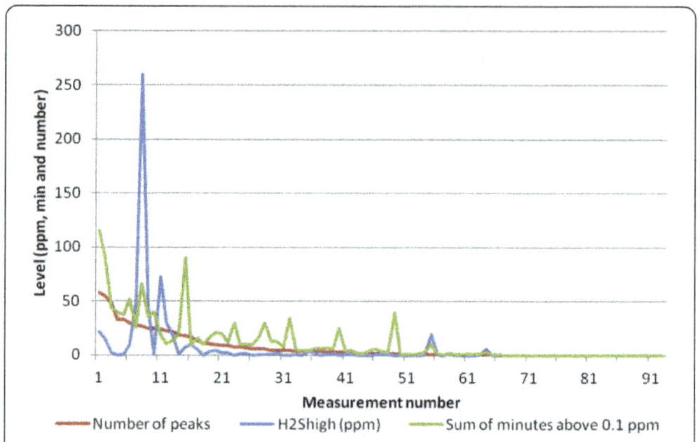

Fig. 2 Peaks, their duration and maximum level. Number of peaks and their corresponding time above 0.1 ppm and maximum level of H_2S

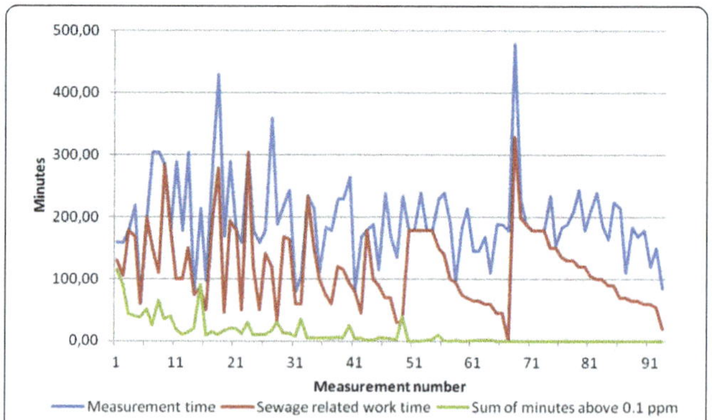

Fig. 3 Measurement time and exposed time. Corresponding values for measurement time and exposed time, where "exposed time" is time with active sewage work. The measurements are sorted by number of peaks

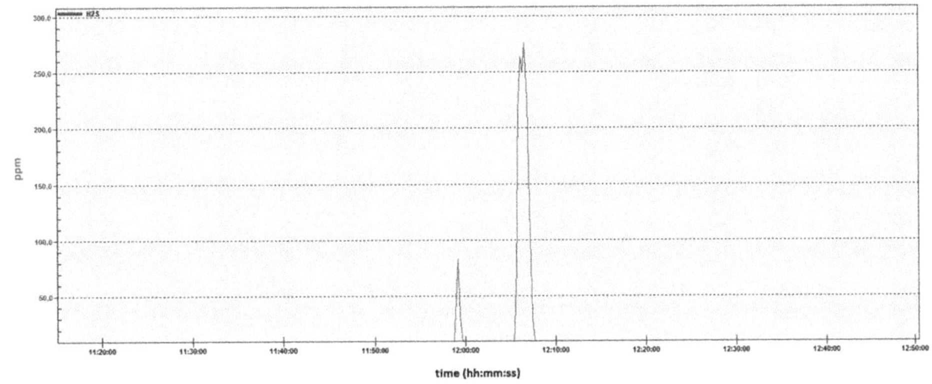

Fig. 4 Example of measurement. Part of the highest exposed measurement

During one shift, there could be as much as seven peaks above 10 ppm. The highest measured peak level (260 ppm) was also registered during this type of work. This was measured during collecting sewage that had been stored at a small plant for several months. The distribution of peaks for the different job types is given in Table 2.

The median, minimum and maximum H_2S index for the different type of jobs, places, seasons and degree of flushing are given in Table 3.

The one-way ANOVA showed the following results regarding statistically significant differences ($p < 0.05$) between the categories for the predictors.

Flushing: "More than 3 times or over 10 min" different from the two other categories
Time of year: "summer" different from the two other categories
Job type: "Inside big plants" different from "pump stations and small plants" and "collecting sewage from cesspools"
Place: Rural3 is different from Capital1, Capital2, Capital3 and City1.
City1 is different from Rural1, Rural2, Rural3.
City2 is different from Capital1 and City1.

From the mixed-model analyses, we see that exposure level, expressed as H_2S index, varied between places, work type, season and degree of flushing. For the work in a plant in the capital, the exposure index varied from 0.02 for working in spring doing some flushing, to 0.7 for working at the same plant in winter doing flushing more than three times or more than 10 min. Collecting sewage from cesspools in city 2 in winter doing a lot of flushing gave a H_2S index of 230.

Table 4 shows the model with determinants from the mixed-model analysis.

Example of calculation:

Geometric mean (GM) sulphide index of worker of pump stations and small plants in autumn, at place Rural 3 and some flushing then gives:

Table 2 Measurement findings per category of plant and system

	Number of measurements (shifts)	Number of measurements with peaks (percentage of measurements) [average number of peaks in measurements with peaks]					Median time in minutes for the peaks above level (min-max)		Highest measured peak level in ppm
		> 10 ppm	5 ppm–10 ppm	1 ppm–5 ppm	0.1 ppm–1 ppm	Zero peaks	0.1 ppm	5 ppm	
Big plants	31	0	1 (3%) [2.0]	4 (13%) [2.5]	20 (65%) [5.2]	11 (35%)	5.5 (1–40)	2 (2)	10
Pump stations and small plants	25	3 (12%) [4.0]	5 (20%) [5.6]	16 (64%) [7.6]	20 (80%) [8.9]	5 (20%)	11 (3–90)	3 (1–25)	30
Sewer network	12	1 (8%) [1.0]	0	1 (8%) [1.0]	4 (33%) [3.0]	8 (67%)	15 (1–40)	5 (5)	20
Collecting sewage from cesspools	25	4 (16%) [3.8]	8 (32%) [2.3]	12 (48%) [4.0]	18 (72%) [6.8]	7 (28%)	7 (1–80)	5 (1–11)	260

Table 3 Descriptives for the different determinants of exposure expressed as hydrogen sulphide index (IN)

Determinants	Number of measurements (shifts)	Median	(min-max)
Job type:			
Inside big plants	31	0.7	(0–36.7)
Pump stations and small plants	25	5.5	(0–281.0)
Sewer network	12	0.5	(0–55.5)
Collecting sewage from cesspools	25	3.0	(0–338.6)
Time of the year			
Winter	26	3.4	(0–281.0)
Spring	14	0.7	(0–5.30)
Summer	25	6.3	(0–338.6)
Autumn	28	0.3	(0–55.5)
Place:			
Capital 1	11	0.9	(0–5.0)
Capital 2	11	1.0	(0–7.4)
Capital 3	14	0.4	(0–75.1)
City 1	25	0.7	(0–25.8)
City 2	15	4.4	(0–338.6)
Rural 1	2	2.8	(0–5.5)
Rural 2	8	8.4	(0–177.5)
Rural 3	7	13.1	(3.7–281.0)
Flushing			
No	34	0.6	(0–55.5)
Some	31	1.2	(0–25.8)
More than 3 times or over 10 min	28	7.6	(0–338.6)

$$\text{IN} = \text{Intercept}^{*}\text{Job type}^{*}\text{Time of the year}^{*}\text{Place}^{*}\text{Flushing}$$
$$= 151.42 \times 0.18 \times 0.26 \times 1.77 \times 0.31 = 3.9$$

The arithmetic mean calculated for this work description is:

$$\text{Arithmetic mean (AM) sulphide index} = \text{GM} \times e^{(0.5\times\text{variations})} = 3.9 \times e^{0.92}$$
$$= 3.9 \times 2.51 = \underline{\underline{9.8}}$$

We have calculated overall data such as GM, AM, minimum and maximum for the measured situations both from our linear mixed model and from our proposed index. These values are presented in Table 5 for the four types of job.

In Fig. 5, IN values from measurements are plotted against the corresponding IN value calculated from the model. It also show the regression calculated by excel of IN below 10 from the index. Almost 80% of our measurements are in this category. At higher values of IN from the index, the model data underestimates IN. This can be seen by comparing max-data from Table 5.

The influence of the different factors in IN varies with the level of IN. For levels below 10, obviously, the duration of peaks 0.1 ppm and the maximum level dominates. The dominating elements shift as the value of IN increases, and for values of IN> 100 number of and duration of the lowest peaks are negligible. The average percentage contributions for the different factors in different intervals of IN are shown in Fig. 6.

Table 4 Linear mixed effect model of exposure determinants for hydrogen sulphide index (IN) in sewage workers

Factor	B	SE	e^B
Intercept	5.02*	1.35	151.42
Job type:			
Inside big plants	−2.55	1.52	0.08
Pump stations and small plants	−1.73	1.51	0.18
Working on sewer network	0	0	1.00
Collecting sewage from cesspools	0.42	1.46	1.52
Time of the year:			
Winter	0	0	1.00
Spring	−2.49*	0.88	0.08
Summer	−1.10	0.82	0.33
Autumn	−1.36*	0.65	0.26
Place:			
Capital 1	−1.14	1.10	0.32
Capital 2	0.07	1.22	1.07
Capital 3	−2.80*	1.09	0.06
City 1	−2.07*	1.00	0.13
City 2	0	0	1.00
Rural 1	−1.90	1.33	0.15
Rural 2	−0.38	0.69	0.68
Rural 3	0.57	0.90	1.77
Flushing			
No	−1.10*	0.47	0.33
Some	−1.16*	0.45	0.31
More than 3 timers or over 10 min	0	0	1.00
Random effects	Variance		
Within worker	1.83		
Between worker	< 0.000		

B regression coefficient, *SE* Standard error, e^B Determinants for calculating GM for different operations of work
*$p < 0.05$

Discussion

It was not surprising that collecting sewage from cesspools gave the highest IN (339), as most risks were present there: storage for several months (might be

Table 5 Comparable calculations of IN from model and proposed index, based on measurement data and situations

Calculations of index IN	From Mixed model data				From Measurement data			
	GM	AM	Max	Min	GM	AM	Max	Min
Inside big plant	1.0	1.3	4.0	0.3	0,4	2.6	36.7	0.028
Pump stations and small plants	5.6	11.2	48.2	1.3	3,8	32.0	281.0	0.028
Sewer network	1.1	1.3	3.0	0.8	0.3	5.9	55.5	0.028
Collecting sewage from cesspools	3.8	19.6	76.0	0.7	2.2	41.4	338.6	0.028

years) and often extensive flushing with high-pressure water to break the compact layer that covered the sewage. When breaking this layer, H_2S was released from the sewer. The intensity of the H_2S exposure was, however dependent on the time between emptying the cesspools. The measurement data from areas with frequent emptying (maximum one-year periods) did not have these peaks. The workers that collected sewage from frequently emptied cesspools did not need to use high-pressure water, but was able to suck up the sewage directly. There were no other noticeable differences between the cesspools. Frequent emptying of cesspools therefore seems important to avoid the use of high-pressure water (flushing), which easily releases H_2S. This is shown in Table 4 of the mixed model as a factor 0.33 for no flushing and 1.00 for flushing more than 3 times per shift.

Another type of work that resulted in high peaks of H_2S on a regular basis was maintenance on pump stations and small plants. The highest measured peak was 30 ppm and the highest number of peaks above 10 ppm in one shift was four (IN_{max} 281). They had more of the lower peaks and the lower peaks lasted for a longer time than cesspool emptying.

Other types of sewage work showed less frequent peaks above 10 ppm, but all types of jobs resulted in some H_2S exposure. This H_2S index also demonstrates that the degree of flushing has a great impact on the H_2S exposure.

The different places of work give different exposure to H_2S. This is partly because the different places had different work types. Some of the urban plants did not collect sewage from cesspools, nor did they have small plants to deal with. The work in rural areas, on the other hand, consisted of the two most exposed work types. This might have more to do with the technical standard than to size. As an example, all the big plants had ventilation from beneath covered sewage areas.

Our H_2S index was constructed with weight on both low levels, duration and peak height because studies have indicated health effects from ambient air levels of H_2S as low as 0.03 ppm [31] and at 0.3 ppm [16]. It seems, therefore, relevant to test a model that also emphasizes the lower exposure levels at 0.1 ppm. At this low level, the duration of exposure might have the same or higher significance than the level, as the documentation of health effects from these low levels originate from studies of ambient air concentrations measured over hours and days [16, 32–34]. However, in our IN model, these low levels of exposure were weighted less than higher levels.

As another set point for the duration, the Norwegian threshold limit value (TLV) at 5 ppm was chosen as this is the normal low alarm level for warning in personal alarm sensors worn by the WWWs. The weighting of our model was chosen in accordance with our equipment and the TLV and the STEL. The weighting of the different peaks and durations could, however, be changed. This index is no exact measure of the H_2S level, but a relative estimate of exposure. By building an exposure

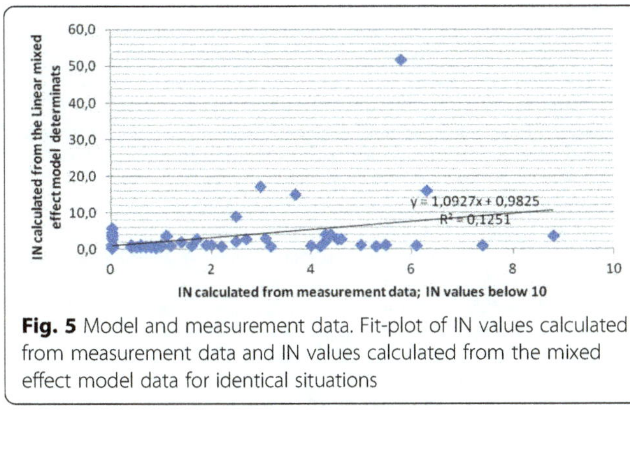

Fig. 5 Model and measurement data. Fit-plot of IN values calculated from measurement data and IN values calculated from the mixed effect model data for identical situations

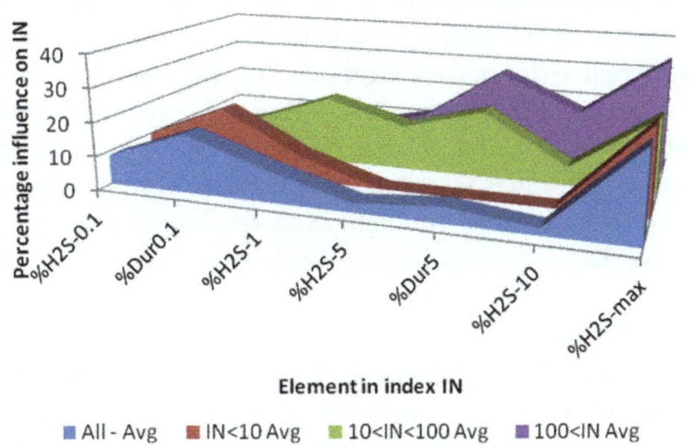

Fig. 6 Contribution to IN. Distribution of percentage average contribution to IN for different intervals of IN

model based on the index values of our measurements, we try to give a tool to estimate H_2S exposure by task, place, season and extent of flushing.

When we treat the index as dimensionless, this is to simplify the use of the index and avoid misunderstandings with ppm values.

We chose to count number of minutes as our measure for time. It could be argued that we should have used 15 s periods, as this was our time resolution. One minute periods was chosen to ease the counting of our peaks. Improvement of the accuracy of the time could be done by counting number of resolution periods instead. If we then divide that number of periods by the number of periods in 1 minute, the values are still comparable to our index.

When using our H_2S index for modelling exposure, we see that the exposure may vary with place. For city 2, where several work types were performed, the H_2S index (geometric mean) varied between 0.3 for the workers that were inside the big plant when working in spring and doing no flushing, to 230 for those that collected sewage from cesspools in winter and doing flushing more than three times on the shift. The workers from city 1, also collecting sewage from cesspools, but without flushing with water (just sucking the sewage), had H_2S index for winter of 30. This reflects the real difference between these two places. They performed a work operation that seemed to be the same, but the work was performed in two distinctly different ways, resulting in different exposure to H_2S.

The detection limits in our measurements were 0.1 ppm. Our index may therefore not be valid for lower concentrations, and to use this index at lower values it must be given additional elements according to exposure profile.

Most of our measurements gave IN< 10, and all these measurements are below the Norwegian TLV and ceiling value. This is the normal exposure situation for WWWs in Norway. Almost 80% of our measurements are in this category. As shown in Fig. 5, there is a very good consistency between model values and index values of IN at values of IN below 10. Using the proposed index we can predict the normal exposure for WWWs quite well, but as the measurements show, there are regularly peaks and exposure duration that challenge the acceptable exposure. All values in our data set with IN> 100 have peaks above ceiling value. At such levels the model gives lower values than IN values from real measurements.

Conclusion

This study shows that working with sewage often brings exposure to H_2S. The exposure could have different patterns, and finding one measure for comparison between different tasks or workers could be challenging. The use of a H_2S index, taking into consideration peak height, duration and number of peaks, could be a tool for exposure assessment for H_2S. By using the model in sewage work in other places, IN can be predicted as an estimate.

Abbreviations

AM: Arithmetic mean; COPD: Chronic obstructive pulmonary disease; GM: Geometric mean; H_2S: Hydrogen sulphide; IN: Exposure index for H_2S; m^3: Cubic metres; NOEL: No observed effect level; PE: Eerson equivalents; ppm: Parts per million; s: Seconds; STEL: Short term exposure level. Normally 15 min average level; TLV: Threshold limit value. Normally 8 h average level; TWA: Time weighted average; WWWs: Waste water workers

Acknowledgements

No

Funding

The project was funded by Norwegian Water, The Labour Inspectorate and The Norwegian Labour Organization.

Authors' contributions

All authors contributed with data collection, data handling and manuscript preparation.

Competing interests

The authors declare that they have no competing interests.

Author details

[1]Municipality of Trondheim, Working Environment Office, Trondheim, Norway. [2]Institute of Industrial Economics and Technology Management, Norwegian University of Science and Technology, Alfred Getz vei 3, 7491 Trondheim, Norway. [3]The National Institute of Occupational Health, Oslo, Norway.

References

1. Lee JA, Thorne PS, Reynolds SJ, O'Shaughnessy PT. Monitoring risks in association with exposure levels among wastewater treatment plant workers. J Occup Environ Med. 2007;49(11):1235–48. https://doi.org/10.1097/JOM.0b013e3181568b40.
2. Douwes J, Mannetje A, Heederik D. Work-related symptoms in sewage treatment workers. Ann Agric Environ Med. 2001;8(1):39–45.
3. Thorn J, Beijer L. Work-related symptoms and inflammation among sewage plant operatives. Int J Occup Environ Health. 2004;10(1):84–9. https://doi.org/10.1179/oeh.2004.10.1.84.
4. Heldal KK, Madso L, Huser PO, Eduard W. Exposure, symptoms and airway inflammation among sewage workers. Ann Agric Environ Med. 2010;17(2):263–8.
5. Farahat SA, Kishk NA. Cognitive functions changes among Egyptian sewage network workers. Toxicol Ind Health. 2010;26(4):229–38. https://doi.org/10.1177/0748233710364966.
6. Teixeira JV, Miranda S, Monteiro RA, Lopes FV, Madureira J, Silva GV, et al. Assessment of indoor airborne contamination in a wastewater treatment plant. Environ Monit Assess. 2013;185(1):59–72. https://doi.org/10.1007/s10661-012-2533-0.
7. Watt MM, Watt SJ, Seaton A. Episode of toxic gas exposure in sewer workers. Occup Environ Med. 1997;54(4):277–80.
8. IPCS. In: Hydrogen sulfide, WH Organization, editors. Environmental health criteria 19. Geneva: World Health Organization; 1981.
9. Beliles RP, Beliles EM. Phosphorus, selenium, tellurium, and sulfur. In: Clayton FE, editor. Patty's industrial hygiene and toxicology. New york: John Wiley; 1993. p. 811–8.
10. Schneider JS, Tobe EH, Mozley PD Jr, Barniskis L, Lidsky TI. Persistent cognitive and motor deficits following acute hydrogen sulphide poisoning. Occup Med (Lond). 1998;48(4):255–60.

11. Tvedt B, Skyberg K, Aaserud O, Hobbesland A, Mathiesen T. Brain damage caused by hydrogen sulfide: a follow-up study of six patients. Am J Ind Med. 1991;20(1):91–101.
12. Guidotti TL. Hydrogen sulphide. Occup Med (Lond). 1996;46(5):367–71.
13. Hessel PA, Herbert FA, Melenka LS, Yoshida K, Nakaza M. Lung health in relation to hydrogen sulfide exposure in oil and gas workers in Alberta, Canada. Am J Ind Med. 1997;31(5):554–7.
14. Richardson DB. Respiratory effects of chronic hydrogen sulfide exposure. Am J Ind Med. 1995;28(1):99–108.
15. Mousa HA. Short-term effects of subchronic low-level hydrogen sulfide exposure on oil field workers. Environ Health Prev Med. 2015;20(1):12–7. https://doi.org/10.1007/s12199-014-0415-5.
16. Legator MS, Singleton CR, Morris DL, Philips DL. Health effects from chronic low-level exposure to hydrogen sulfide. Arch Environ Health. 2001;56(2): 123–31. https://doi.org/10.1080/00039890109604063.
17. NEG, Hydrogen Sulphide, in Arbete och Hälsa, TNEGfCDoHRf Chemicals, Editor. 2001, National Institute for Working Life: Stockholm.
18. Melbostad E, Eduard W, Skogstad A, Sandven P, Lassen J, Sostrand P, et al. Exposure to bacterial aerosols and work-related symptoms in sewage workers. Am J Ind Med. 1994;25(1):59–63.
19. Sostrand P, Tvedt B, Eduard W, Bye E, Heldal K. Hazardous peak concentrations of hydrogen sulfide gas related to the sewage purification process. AIHAJ. 2000;61(1):107–10.
20. Glass DC. A review of the health effects of hydrogen sulphide exposure. Ann Occup Hyg. 1990;34(3):323–7.
21. Finnbjornsdottir RG, Carlsen HK, Thorsteinsson T, Oudin A, Lund SH, Gislason T, et al. Association between daily hydrogen sulfide exposure and incidence of emergency hospital visits: a population-based study. PLoS One. 2016; 11(5):e0154946. https://doi.org/10.1371/journal.pone.0154946.
22. Bates MN, Crane J, Balmes JR, Garrett N. Investigation of hydrogen sulfide exposure and lung function, asthma and chronic obstructive pulmonary disease in a geothermal area of New Zealand. PLoS One. 2015;10(3): e0122062. https://doi.org/10.1371/journal.pone.0122062.
23. Bates MN, Garrett N, Crane J, Balmes J. Associations of ambient hydrogen sulfide exposure with self-reported asthma and asthma symptoms. Environ Res. 2013;122:81–7. https://doi.org/10.1016/j.envres.2013.02.002.
24. Reed BR, Crane J, Garrett N, Woods DL, Bates MN. Chronic ambient hydrogen sulfide exposure and cognitive function. Neurotoxicol Teratol. 2014;42:68–76. https://doi.org/10.1016/j.ntt.2014.02.002.
25. Jappinen P, Vilkka V, Marttila O, Haahtela T. Exposure to hydrogen sulphide and respiratory function. Br J Ind Med. 1990;47(12):824–8.
26. Burnett WW, King EG, Grace M, Hall WF. Hydrogen sulfide poisoning: review of 5 years' experience. Can Med Assoc J. 1977;117(11):1277–80.
27. Arbeidstilsynet, Forskrift om tiltaks og grenseverdier, Df Arbeidstilsynet, Editor. 2015, Gyldendal Akademiske: Trondheim.
28. Brenneman KA, James RA, Gross EA, Dorman DC. Olfactory neuron loss in adult male CD rats following subchronic inhalation exposure to hydrogen sulfide. Toxicol Pathol. 2000;28(2):326–33.
29. Hornung R, Reed L. Estimation of average concentration in the presence of nondetectable values. Appl Occup Hyg. 1990;5(1):6.
30. Rappaport SM. Assessment of long-term exposures to toxic substances in air. Ann Occup Hyg. 1991;35(1):61–121.
31. Carlsen HK, Zoega H, Valdimarsdottir U, Gislason T, Hrafnkelsson B. Hydrogen sulfide and particle matter levels associated with increased dispensing of anti-asthma drugs in Iceland's capital. Environ Res. 2012;113: 33–9. https://doi.org/10.1016/j.envres.2011.10.010.
32. Kilburn KH, Thrasher JD, Gray MR. Low-level hydrogen sulfide and central nervous system dysfunction. Toxicol Ind Health. 2010;26(7):387–405. https://doi.org/10.1177/0748233710369126.
33. Fiedler N, Kipen H, Ohman-Strickland P, Zhang J, Weisel C, Laumbach R, et al. Sensory and cognitive effects of acute exposure to hydrogen sulfide. Environ Health Perspect. 2008;116(1):78–85. https://doi.org/10.1289/ehp.10531.
34. Heaney CD, Wing S, Campbell RL, Caldwell D, Hopkins B, Richardson D, et al. Relation between malodor, ambient hydrogen sulfide, and health in a community bordering a landfill. Environ Res. 2011;111(6):847–52. https://doi.org/10.1016/j.envres.2011.05.021.

15

Evaluating a framework for tuberculosis screening among healthcare workers in clinical settings, Inner Mongolia, China

Shiming Cheng[1†], Deanna Tollefson[2†], Guangxue He[1†], Yuan Li[3†], Hui Guo[1], Shua Chai[2,3], Fangfang Gao[4], Fei Gao[4], Guoxin Han[4], Liping Ren[4], Yulin Ren[4], Jianbo Li[5], Lixia Wang[1], Jay K. Varma[2,3], Dongmei Hu[1], Haiying Fan[1], Fei Zhao[1], Emily Bloss[2], Yu Wang[1*] and Carol Y. Rao[2,3*]

Abstract

Background: Health care workers are at high risk for tuberculosis (TB). China, a high burden TB country, has no policy on medical surveillance for TB among healthcare workers. In this paper, we evaluate whether China's national TB diagnostic guidelines could be used as a framework to screen healthcare workers for pulmonary TB disease in a clinical setting in China.

Methods: Between April–August 2010, healthcare workers from 28 facilities in Inner Mongolia Autonomous Region, China were eligible for TB screening, comprised of symptom check, chest X-ray and tuberculin skin testing. Healthcare workers were categorized as having presumptive, confirmed, or clinically-diagnosed pulmonary TB, using Chinese national guidelines.

Results: All healthcare workers (N=4347) were eligible for TB screening, of which 4285 (99%) participated in at least one TB screening test. Of the healthcare workers screened, 2% had cough for ≥ 14 days, 3% had a chest X-ray consistent with TB, and 10% had a tuberculin skin test induration ≥ 20 mm. Of these, 124 healthcare workers were identified with presumptive TB (i.e., cough for ≥ 14 days in the past 4 weeks or x-ray consistent with TB). Twelve healthcare workers met the case definition for clinically-diagnosed pulmonary TB, but none were diagnosed with TB during the study period.

Conclusion: A substantial proportion of healthcare workers in Inner Mongolia had signs, symptoms, or test results suggestive of TB disease that could have been identified using national TB diagnostic guidelines as a screening framework. However, achieving medical surveillance in China will require a framework that increases the ease, accuracy, and acceptance of TB screening in the medical community. Routine screening with improved diagnostics should be considered to detect tuberculosis disease among healthcare workers and reduce transmission in health care settings in China.

Keywords: Case detection, Medical surveillance, Clinically diagnosed cases, Active case finding, Healthcare workers, X-ray, Tuberculosis, Tuberculin skin test

* Correspondence: wangyu@chinacdc.cn; crao@cdc.gov
†Equal contributors
[1]China Center for Disease Control and Prevention, 155 Changbai Road Changping District, Beijing 102206, People's Republic of China
[2]U.S. Centers for Disease Control and Prevention (CDC), 1600 Clifton Road NE, MS-93, Atlanta, GA 30329, USA
Full list of author information is available at the end of the article

Background

Since 1990, China has experienced substantial declines in the burden of tuberculosis (TB) nationally [1], yet the country continues to have the third largest number of incident TB cases and the highest number of multi-drug resistant (MDR) TB cases in the world [2]. Healthcare workers (HCWs) are a high risk group for TB infection in China [3–8], possibly due to inadequate infection control practices in healthcare settings [3]. However, medical surveillance of HCWs for TB disease is not routine, and there are no guidelines to screen HCWs for TB disease in China [9]. As such, HCWs may develop TB disease, not be diagnosed in a timely manner and thus contribute to ongoing TB transmission. Accurate and timely diagnosis of TB disease is essential to ensure proper patient care and appropriate public health response.

Guidelines for routine TB screening among HCWs can help reduce ongoing transmission of TB and be used to monitor and evaluate existing nosocomial TB infection control policies [9]. In lieu of these, China's national TB diagnostic guidelines can serve as a framework for routine screening of HCWs for TB disease [10, 11], but the application of the diagnostic guidelines in this context has not been evaluated. To address this gap, we evaluated using China's national TB diagnostic guidelines to screen HCWs for pulmonary TB disease in a clinical setting in Inner Mongolia. Inner Mongolia is an Autonomous Region in northern China, with a population of approximately 24 million people in the 2010 census. In 2010, the notification rate of active TB in China's Inner Mongolia Autonomous Region was 74.1 per 100,000 and the notification rate for smear positive TB was 35.4 per 100,000 [12].

Methods

Study population

Facilities that diagnosed TB cases were selected based on their capability to conduct chest X-rays and their willingness to participate. All HCWs in the 28 selected healthcare facilities were eligible to participate. A HCW was defined as any person who received payment for working in the facility, regardless of the type of employment (e.g., clinicians, nurses, laboratorians, and administrative, janitorial, and cafeteria staff). The number of eligible HCWs at a facility ranged from 9 to 1000. HCWs undergoing TB treatment were excluded.

Definitions

We used 2008 Chinese national diagnostic guidelines to define a TB case. Chinese national guidelines rely on clinical judgement based on symptoms, chest radiography, tuberculin skin test (TST), and smear microscopy to diagnose TB; the national guidelines do not include use of culture for TB diagnosis. Per these guidelines, a confirmed pulmonary TB case was defined as a person with sputum smear positive acid-fast bacilli (AFB) results; a clinically-diagnosed TB case was defined as a person with a chest X-ray consistent with TB and either a cough for more than 14 days in the past 4 weeks or a tuberculin skin test reading ≥20 mm [10, 11]. We defined a presumptive TB case as a person who, per Chinese national guidelines, was eligible for smear microscopy testing: i.e., one who had a chest X-ray consistent with TB or one who had cough for more than 14 days in the past 4 weeks.

Screening for TB

Between April and August 2010, HCWs were screened for active pulmonary TB disease following Chinese national guidelines, the first step of which included offering all HCWs a symptom screen, a chest x-ray, and TST. Project personnel administered a standardized questionnaire that included a TB symptom screen, such as cough for more than 14 days, and collected information on HCW demographics and risk factors for TB disease. A sub-set of participating health care workers were offered chest X-rays and TSTs; these HCWs were conveniently sampled by facility staff. Radiologists from each participating clinic independently reviewed chest X-rays for participating HCWs from their own facilities; no additional training was provided on taking and reading chest X-rays. Study staff were trained by China CDC to place TSTs and read and interpret the results, since TSTs were not routinely administered. Study staff performed a single-step TST using 5 IU (0.1 ml) of domestically-produced tuberculin derived from *M. bovis* BCG (Chengdu Institute of Biological Products, Chengdu, China).

Per national guidelines, facility staff were to refer an HCW for sputum smear microscopy if he/she had a chest X-ray suggestive of TB or symptoms of cough greater than 2 weeks, and were to follow routine facility procedures to record and report diagnosed cases. Presumptive TB cases should provide spot, morning and night sputum specimens. To identify TB cases, we searched the national electronic TB surveillance system for HCWs who were eligible for sputum smear evaluation (matching by name, age, gender and current address) to ascertain if they were diagnosed with active TB within 5 years of the project (from July 2010–July 2015).

Data analysis

All data were collected on paper forms and double-entered into Microsoft Excel (Redmond, WA, USA). Project staff conducted periodic site visits to monitor data quality and to provide ongoing training, as necessary. Frequencies and proportions were calculated and compared for all HCWs at each stage of the TB screening process. Data were analyzed using SAS 9.3 (SAS Institute, Cary, NC, USA).

Ethical considerations

HCWs provided written informed consent. The Chinese Ethical Committee for Tuberculosis Operational Research and the Chinese Center for Disease Control and Prevention approved this project.

Results

Within the 28 facilities, 4347 HCWs were eligible to participate in the study. Of these, 3011 (69.3%) underwent symptom screening, 2311 (53%) received a chest x-ray, and 2568 (59%) received a TST (Fig. 1); 4285 HCWs participated in at least one of these screenings. There were no significant differences in the demographic characteristics between HCWs participating in each of the screening methods (data not shown). Among HCWs screened for symptoms, most were primarily medical doctors or nurses (47%), females (66%), never smokers (77%), and at least 40 years old (53%); half of participants had spent more than 15 years working in health care settings (52%) (Table 1). Most HCWs had never had a TST (80%) and, of the 591 HCWs who ever had a TST, 217 (37%) had a skin test within the last 5 years.

Among HCWs screened for symptoms, the majority of HCWs reported no TB symptoms (2714, 90%) (Table 1). Among HCWs receiving TST, 251 (10%) had a TST ≥20 mm. Among HCWs receiving chest X-rays, 125 (5%) had an abnormal result; this included 59 (47%) chest X-rays that were consistent with TB.

X-ray and symptom screening identified 124 HCWs with presumptive TB, who were thus eligible for sputum smear evaluation: 59 who had X-rays consistent with TB and 65 who reported cough for more than 14 days in the past 4 weeks (Fig. 1). There were no cases with both X-ray consistent with TB and cough for more than 14 days in the past 4 weeks. An unknown number of HCWs who should have been referred for sputum smear microscopy completed the test during the study period (i.e., April–August 2010) as facility staff only reported positive smear tests for HCWs and no smear results were reported. Between July 2010 and July 2015, however, 1 out of the 124 HCW eligible for sputum smear was reported in the

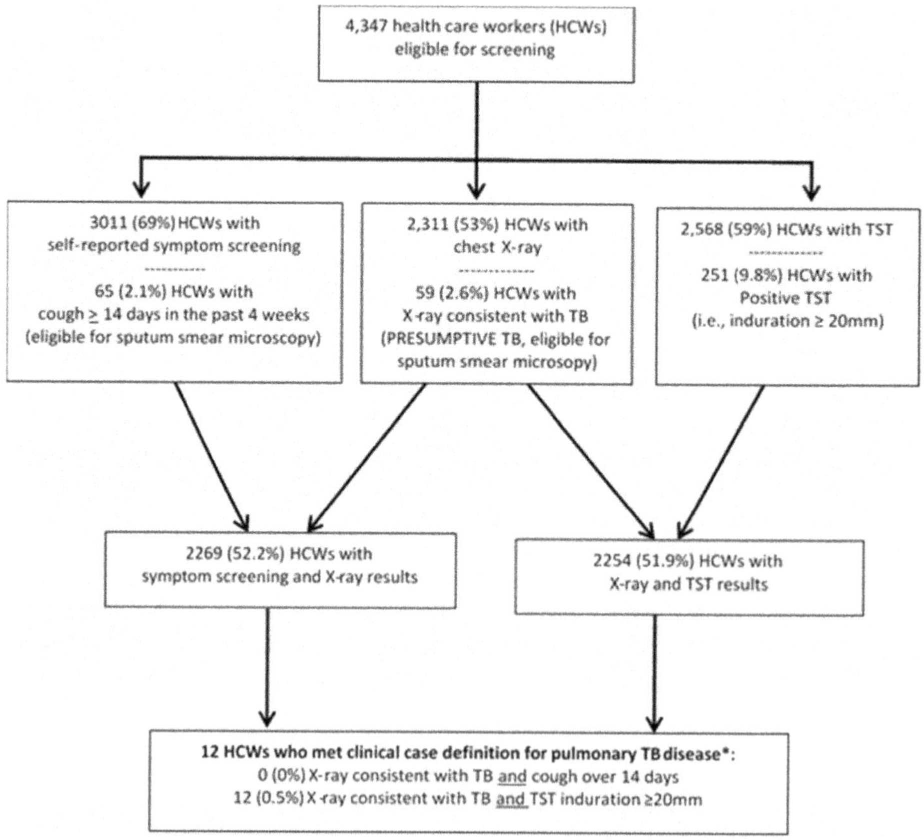

Fig. 1 TB screening and diagnostic algorithm as used among health care workers (HCWs) in Inner Mongolia. *No HCWs were actually diagnosed with active pulmonary TB during the course of the evaluation.

Table 1 Characteristics of health care workers (HCWs) screened for symptoms or sputum testing or clinically-diagnosed TB

Characteristic	HCWs with symptom screening (n = 3011[a])	HCWs eligible for sputum testing[b] (n = 124[a])	Met case definition for clinically-diagnosed TB[c] (n = 12)
	n (%)	n (%)	n (%)
DEMOGRAPHICS			
Sex			
Female	1997 (66%)	67 (54%)	9 (75%)
Male	1014 (34%)	57 (46%)	3 (25%)
Age, years			
18–29	598 (20%)	14 (11%)	1 (8%)
30–39	824 (27%)	32 (26%)	4 (33%)
40–49	1029 (34%)	40 (33%)	4 (33%)
≥ 50	558 (19%)	36 (30%)	3 (25%)
Education			
College or above	852 (28%)	52 (43%)	6 (50%)
Some college or tech school	1480 (49%)	48 (39%)	4 (33%)
High school or below	674 (22%)	22 (18%)	2 (17%)
Self-reported BCG			
Did not have BCG	1521 (51%)	55 (45%)	2 (17%)
Had BCG	1468 (49%)	66 (55%)	10 (83%)
Smoking status			
Never smoker	2319 (77%)	80 (66%)	10 (83%)
Former/current smoker	681 (23%)	41 (34%)	2 (17%)
TB infection and disease history			
Previous diagnosis of TB	147 (5%)	27 (22%)	4 (33%)
Previous TST	591 (20%)	37 (30%)	7 (58%)
Tested within last 5 years	217 (37%)	10 (27%)	2 (29%)
Previously positive TST[d]	239 (41%)	24 (67%)	4 (57%)
WORK-RELATED TB RISK FACTORS			
Work type			
Clinician or nurse	1420 (47%)	62 (51%)	7 (58%)
Clinical support[f]	713 (24%)	25 (20%)	1 (8%)
Administrative	411 (14%)	21 (17%)	2 (17%)
Other (e.g., cleaner, cook)	462 (15%)	14 (11%)	2 (17%)
Working time in health care			
≤ 5 years	746 (25%)	23 (19%)	2 (18%)
6–15 years	679 (23%)	19 (16%)	4 (36%)
> 15 years	1530 (52%)	78 (65%)	5 (45%)
Direct contact with TB cases			
TB patients	1295 (43%)	83 (68%)	10 (83%)
Coworkers with history of TB	254 (8%)	19 (16%)	4 (33%)
Household member with TB	230 (8%)	10 (8%)	1 (8%)
Average daily time with patients			
0 h	803 (27%)	23 (19%)	1 (8%)
< 1 h	458 (15%)	21 (17%)	4 (33%)
1–4 h	506 (17%)	22 (18%)	3 (25%)
> 4 h	1234 (41%)	55 (45%)	4 (33%)

Table 1 Characteristics of health care workers (HCWs) screened for symptoms or sputum testing or clinically-diagnosed TB *(Continued)*

Characteristic	HCWs with symptom screening (n = 3011[a]) n (%)	HCWs eligible for sputum testing[b] (n = 124[a]) n (%)	Met case definition for clinically-diagnosed TB[c] (n = 12) n (%)
OTHER SCREENING RESULTS			
Symptoms in the last 4 weeks			
None	2714 (90%)	49 (40%)	7 (58%)
Cough only	191 (6%)	53 (43%)	3 (25%)
Fever or night sweats, no cough	35 (1%)	1 (0.8%)	1 (8%)
Fever or night sweats, any cough	31 (1%)	13 (10%)	0
TST (mm)	n=2568[e]		
< 5	714 (28%)	20 (18%)	0
5–14	1232 (48%)	49 (45%)	0
15–19	356 (14%)	24 (22%)	0
≥ 20	251 (10%)	15 (15%)	12 (100%)
X-ray results	n=2269[e]	n=103[e]	
Consistent with TB	57 (2%)	59 (57%)	12 (100%)
Abnormal, not consistent with TB	65 (3%)	1 (1%)	0
Normal	2147 (95%)	43 (42%)	0

Footnotes:
[a]Categories may not total n due to missing data
[b] Defined as HCWs who had a chest X-ray consistent with TB OR a cough lasting ≥ 14 days in the past 4 weeks
[c] Defined as HCWs who had a chest X-ray consistent with TB AND a TST induration ≥ 20 mm
[d] HCW self-report of TST positivity. We did not ask what induration size was considered positive. Chinese guidelines categorize 5–9 mm as general positive, 10–19 mm as medium positive and ≥ 20 mm as very positive (See: *Ministry of Health People's Republic of China. Diagnostic criteria for pulmonary tuberculosis. 2008.* [11])
[e] The denominators in these sub-sections are a subset of the HCWs within the column. The denominators are: a subset of HCWs with symptom screening who received TST, a subset of HCWs with symptom screening who received chest x-ray, and a subset of HCWs eligible for sputum testing who received chest x-ray
[f] Clinical support jobs were radiographer/X-ray technician, laboratorian, public health/preventive medicine, and pharmacists

national electronic TB surveillance system as having active TB disease.

Of the 2269 participants who completed both the symptom screening and a chest x-ray, 12 HCWs (0.53% or 529 per 100,000; 95% confidence interval [208, 849]) met the case definition for clinically-diagnosed, active pulmonary TB (i.e., X-ray consistent with TB and TST induration of at least 20 mm). However, despite meeting the case definition for active pulmonary TB disease, these 12 cases were not diagnosed with TB by their healthcare facilities. The majority of HCWs meeting the case definition for clinically-diagnosed TB were clinical staff (i.e., medical doctors or nurses) (7/12), had direct contact with TB patients (10/12) and had been working in healthcare settings for at least 6 years (9/12) (Table 1). Two-thirds of the HCWs who met the case definition for clinically diagnosed pulmonary TB were asymptomatic (i.e. reported no fever, night sweats, or cough in the last 4 weeks) (7/11) while nearly three quarters of HCWs with X-rays consistent with TB were asymptomatic (43/59).

Discussion

TB is an under-recognized disease among healthcare workers in China. This study found that in Inner Mongolia, using China's national TB diagnostic guidelines as a framework to screen HCWs for TB could have identified 12 HCWs with TB. Twelve HCWs met national guideline definitions for clinically diagnosed TB, which is equivalent to a prevalence of 529 (95% CI 208, 849) TB cases per 100,000, a number higher than the national TB prevalence (108 per 100,000) [13] and the provincial TB prevalence for Inner Mongolia (74 per 100,000) [12]. However, during the study period, none of the HCWs meeting the criteria for clinically diagnosed TB were confirmed microbiologically, formally diagnosed with TB disease, or treated with anti-TB medications, and thus were not reported as TB cases. This suggests that while screening for TB among HCWs in China is urgently needed, using the national TB diagnostic algorithm as a framework for medical surveillance in itself may be insufficient. Effectiveness of screening programs may be hampered by lack of recognition of TB disease among HCWs, poor understanding or acceptance of diagnostic guidelines, and poor quality of tests used to diagnose TB, which would need to be addressed to achieve optimal medical TB surveillance in China.

Medical surveillance for occupationally-acquired diseases among HCWs is not routine in China [9] despite global recommendations to conduct on-site surveillance of TB among HCWs [14]. We found 20 % of participating HCWs reported ever having a TST and fewer than half of those had the test within the last 5 years. If an HCW is diagnosed with TB in China, it is not generally acknowledged as an occupationally-acquired infection [9], even though our study found a high proportion of HCWs who met the case definition for sputum referral or for clinically-diagnosed TB had work related exposures (i.e., contact with TB patients or with coworkers with TB). The participation rate for the initial screening was high, with 98.5% participating in at least one screening method, indicating that there is capacity to conduct medical surveillance if prioritized by hospital management. Regular TB screening of HCWs would facilitate early identification of TB in this vulnerable population and reduce risk of TB transmission in healthcare settings.

This evaluation identified challenges in uptake of the current national TB diagnostic algorithm as a framework to screen HCWs for TB. Namely, the study found it difficult to achieve HCW participation in the full screening process, especially with smear microscopy. The low yield of smear positive TB cases identified in this study suggests that HCWs who should have been referred for sputum smear testing may not have completed testing. Previous studies in China have found that persons eligible for sputum smears are frequently not offered the test, and the number of individuals who complete a sputum exam among those offered a test is even lower [15, 16]. Most of the presumptive TB cases and participants who met the case definition of clinically-diagnosed pulmonary TB in this evaluation were asymptomatic which could have affected the perceived urgency for sputum testing. However, other barriers to being offered and completing sputum exams in China have been found to include economic constraints and innate beliefs held by both doctors and presumptive TB cases that sputum tests are unimportant [15, 16]. In addition, China does not have established protocols for referral and follow-up of asymptomatic HCWs with suspected TB. For routine TB screening to be effective among HCWs in China, additional research is needed to better understand the low uptake of sputum screening. Alternative laboratory-based screening methods that are more acceptable to HCWs may need to be considered, along with active follow up of presumptive TB cases to ensure they undergo appropriate laboratory-based TB testing.

The study also found that imperfections of the diagnostic tests used in the national TB diagnostic algorithm could hinder its use to conduct successful medical TB surveillance in HCWs. For example, identification of no smear positives in this study may have been partly due to challenges with the AFB sputum test as sensitivity for smear microscopy can range between 20 and 80% based on how samples are collected, stored, transported, and analyzed [17–19]. In contrast, radiography is non-specific for TB diagnosis, which makes diagnosis based on x-ray challenging [20–23]. Similarly, the utility of TST is also debatable, not only for active TB but for latent TB. The validity of TST results using Chinese domestically produced tuberculin have been questioned due to concerns about cross-reactivity with BCG vaccination [4, 7], which is provided to everyone at birth in China. Furthermore, healthcare facilities in China do not routinely perform TST on HCWs because of poor infrastructure for performing TST, high endemic rates of TB transmission, lack of policy on prophylaxis for TB infection, and limited recognition of the contribution of healthcare worker TB surveillance to TB control [7, 9]. A screening algorithm with more accurate testing methods could be needed to make routine medical surveillance for TB worthwhile in China.

The high number of HCWs who met the case definition for clinically-diagnosed pulmonary TB in this study but lacked microbiological testing suggests routine screening for active TB disease among healthcare workers in China could benefit by inclusion of more accurate and better accepted diagnostic tests, like WHO-approved rapid tests (e.g., Xpert® MTB/RIF [Xpert]). Due to their ease of use and rapid turn-around of results, these tests could be more appealing to healthcare workers; expanding use of these WHO-approved rapid tests could thus improve uptake of bacteriological testing. China's Food and Drug Administration has approved use of Xpert for drug resistance testing among smear positive TB cases [24], but expanding the use of Xpert for TB diagnosis of smear negative TB cases has improved accuracy of TB diagnosis in other high-burden TB settings [25–27]. Although Xpert tests are expensive, modeling suggests that coupling same-day sputum microscopy with Xpert testing could reduce TB incidence and mortality in high-burden settings [28]. Considering the high rate of MDR TB in China, incorporating drug resistance testing into routine medical surveillance for all HCWs would also be beneficial [29].

This evaluation has several limitations. This project was conducted in one autonomous region in China and may not be representative of China as a whole. We relied upon routine diagnostic practices and technologies used at the facility level, so we could not control for the quality of X-rays, sputum collection, or microscopy reading. As a result, quality may have varied substantially between the 28 facilities, which had a wide range of capacity for TB screening and referral. The lack of culture, or other confirmatory tests, within the screening algorithm also made it impossible to assess diagnostic accuracy. In addition, single-step TST tests were conducted which could have led to under-identification of TST positive participants due to the booster effect, thus under-diagnosing participants who met the case definition of clinically-diagnosed pulmonary TB. Conversely, the high prevalence of BCG vaccination in China and the local TST's potential to cross-react with BCG vaccination could have resulted in an artificially high number of HCWs developing positive TSTs, thus overestimating number of participants who med the case definition of clinically-diagnosed pulmonary TB. Furthermore, as this study relied on the national TB policies and practices already in place for testing presumptive TB patients, facilities only reported on positive smear results, so the number of HCWs who completed AFB sputum testing was unknown; this could have led to underestimation of sputum smear positive TB cases. Similarly, we had to rely on the routine national electronic reporting system to know whether presumptive TB patients were diagnosed with TB after the study period because it was outside the scope of the study to follow HCWs after TB screening. Finally, no information was available on HCWs who chose not to participate in, or were not offered, TB screening, so intrinsic differences between participating and non-participating HCWs are unknown. Additional research is needed to elucidate reasons for HCW participation, or lack of participation, in the TB screening process.

Conclusions

Although the burden of TB in China has declined substantially since 1990, the country continues to bear a large portion of the world's incident TB cases, with healthcare workers being at high risk for TB. China currently has no policy on medical surveillance for TB among HCWs. This study suggests that while using the current national TB diagnostic algorithm to screen HCWs for TB in China could be a start to actively find TB in this at-risk population, this framework would require adjustments to increase the ease, accuracy, and acceptance of TB screening in order to achieve optimal medical surveillance for TB in China. To do this, there is a need for stronger approaches to obtain microbiological evaluation on presumptive TB cases, which could include expanded use of Xpert or other WHO-approved rapid tests. Operational research would be necessary to fully elucidate the feasibility, costs, and benefits of adapting a revised TB screening algorithm for routine medical TB surveillance in China.

Abbreviations

AFB: Acid-fast bacilli; BCG: Bacillus Calmette-Guérin; China CDC: China Center for Disease Control and Prevention; HCWs: Healthcare workers; MDR: Multidrug resistant; TB: Tuberculosis; TST: Tuberculin skin test; US CDC: United States Centers for Disease Control and Prevention; Xpert: Xpert® MTB/RIF

Acknowledgements

We thank X. Nie, Q. Zhang, and N. Ta for their help in project management. We thank the staff at the participating facilities in Inner Mongolia for project organization and coordination, and administering the surveys and x-rays. We also thank the national radiologists in Beijing for their expert review of the x-ray films.

Funding

This publication was supported by the Cooperative Agreement Number 5U2GGH000018 from the U.S. Centers for Disease Control and Prevention. The findings and conclusions in this report are those of the authors and do not necessarily represent the official position of US CDC.

Authors' contributions

SMC, GXH, LXW, SC, JKV, YW and CYR designed the study and oversaw implementation. Colleagues from Inner Mongolia (FFG, FG, GXH, LPR, YLR, and JBL) implemented the study and collected data. Colleagues from the China CDC (GXH, HG, HYF, and DMH) monitored study implementation and data collection. CYR initiated the manuscript. YL analyzed the data and DT wrote the manuscript, under direction from CYR and EB. CYR and EB edited the manuscript. All authors read and approved the final manuscript.

Competing interests

None of the authors have a commercial or other financial interest associated with the information presented.

Author details

[1]China Center for Disease Control and Prevention, 155 Changbai Road Changping District, Beijing 102206, People's Republic of China. [2]U.S. Centers for Disease Control and Prevention (CDC), 1600 Clifton Road NE, MS-93, Atlanta, GA 30329, USA. [3]U.S. Centers for Disease Control and Prevention (CDC), Beijing, China. [4]Inner Mongolia Center for Tuberculosis Control and Prevention, Middle Hugao Rd, New District, Hohhot, Inner Mongolia 010080, People's Republic of China. [5]Ulanqab General Hospital, No.157, Jiefang Road, Jining District, Ulanqab, Inner Mongolia 012000, People's Republic of China.

References

1. Wang L, Zhang H, Ruan Y, Chin DP, Xia Y, Cheng S, et al. Tuberculosis prevalence in China, 1990-2010; a longitudinal analysis of national survey data. Lancet. 2014;383(9934):2057–64.
2. World Health Organization. Global Tuberculosis Report 2017. 2017. http://www.who.int/tb/publications/global_report/en/ . Accessed 13 Mar 2018.
3. He GX, van den Hof S, van der Werf MJ, Wang GJ, Ma SW, Zhao DY, et al. Infection control and the burden of tuberculosis infection and disease in health care workers in China: a cross-sectional study. BMC Infect Dis. 2010;10:313.
4. He GX, Wang LX, Chai SJ, Klena JD, Cheng SM, Ren YL, et al. Risk factors associated with tuberculosis infection among health care workers in Inner Mongolia, China. Int J Tuberc Lung Dis. 2012;16(11):1485–91.
5. Wei Z, Yang M, Quan B, Wang Y, Wu Y, Ji B. Prevalence of latent

tuberculosis infection among healthcare workers in China as detected by two interferon-gamma release assays. J Hosp Infect. 2013;84(4):323–5.
6. Zhang X, Jia H, Liu F, Pan L, Xing A, Gu S, et al. Prevalence and Risk Factors for Latent Tuberculosis Infection among Health Care Workers in China: A Cross-Sectional Study. PLoS One. 2013;8(6):e66412.
7. Zhou F, Zhang L, Gao L, Hao Y, Zhao X, Liu J, et al. Latent tuberculosis infection and occupational protection among health care workers in two types of public hospitals in China. PLoS One. 2014;9(8):e104673.
8. He G, Li Y, Zhao F, Wang L, Cheng S, Guo H, et al. The prevalence and incidence of latent tuberculosis infection and its associated factors among village doctors in China. PLoS One. 2015;10(5):e0124097.
9. Chai SJ, Mattingly DC, Varma JK. Protecting health care workers from tuberculosis in China: a review of policy and practice in China and the United States. Health Policy Plan. 2013;28(1):100–9.
10. Ministry of Health People's Republic of China. Guidelines for implementing the National Tuberculosis Control Program in China. Beijing: Peking Union Medical College Publishing House; 2008 (in Chinese).
11. Ministry of Health People's Republic of China. Diagnostic criteria for pulmonary tuberculosis (WS 288–2008). Beijing: People's Medical Publishing House Press; 2008 (in Chinese).
12. Chin J. The prevalence of pulmonary tuberculosis in a national survey across China in 2010. Tubere Respir Dis. 2012;35(09):665–8 (in Chinese).
13. World Health Organization. Global tuberculosis control: WHO report 2011. http://apps.who.int/iris/bitstream/10665/44728/1/9789241564380_eng.pdf?ua=1. Accessed 13 Mar 2018.
14. World Health Organization. WHO policy on TB infection control in health-care facilities, Congregate settings and households. 2009. http://www.who.int/tb/publications/tb-facilities-policy/en/. Accessed 13 Mar 2018.
15. Long Q, Li Y, Wang Y, Yue Y, Tang C, Tang S, et al. Barriers to accessing TB diagnosis for rural-to-urban migrants with chronic cough in Chongqing, China: a mixed methods study. BMC Health Serv Res. 2008;8:202.
16. Li Y, Ehiri J, Tang SL, Li DK, Bian YQ, Lin H, et al. Factors associated with patient, and diagnostic delays in Chinese TB patients: a systematic review and meta-analysis. BMC Med. 2013;11:156.
17. Steingart KR, Ramsay A, Pai M. Optimizing sputum smear microscopy for the diagnosis of pulmonary tuberculosis. Expert Rev Anti-Infect Ther. 2007; 5(3):327–31.
18. Parsons LM, Somoskovi A, Gutierrez C, Lee E, Paramasivan CN, Abimiku A, et al. Laboratory diagnosis of tuberculosis in resource-poor countries: challenges and opportunities. Clin Microbiol Rev. 2011;24(2):314–50.
19. Ho J, Marks GB, Fox GJ. The impact of sputum quality on tuberculosis diagnosis: a systematic review. Int J Tuberc Lung Dis. 2015;19(5):537–44.
20. Jaeger S, Karargyris A, Candemir S, Siegelman J, Folio L, Antani S, et al. Automatic screening for tuberculosis in chest radiographs: a survey. Quant Imaging Med Surg. 2013;3(2):89–99.
21. Davies PD, Pai M. The diagnosis and misdiagnosis of tuberculosis. Int J Tuberc Lung Dis. 2008;12(11):1226–34.
22. Piccazzo R, Paparo F, Garlaschi G. Diagnostic accuracy of chest radiography for the diagnosis of tuberculosis (TB) and its role in the detection of latent TB infection: a systematic review. J Rheumatol Suppl. 2014;91:32–40.
23. Herath S, Lewis C. Pulmonary involvement in patients presenting with extra-pulmonary tuberculosis: thinking beyond a normal chest x-ray. J Prim Health Care. 2014;6(1):64–8.
24. China Food and Drug Administration (FDA). Mycobacterium tuberculosis rpoB gene and mutation detection kit (real-time PCR method) (trade name: Xpert (R) MTB / RIF) 2014.02.26. http://app2.sfda.gov.cn/datasearchp/index1.do?tableId=27&tableName=TABLE27&tableView=进口器械&Id=28263. Accessed 13 Mar 2018 (in Chinese).
25. Creswell J, Rai B, Wali R, Sudrungrot S, Adhikari LM, Pant R, et al. Introducing new tuberculosis diagnostics: the impact of Xpert((R)) MTB/RIF testing on case notifications in Nepal. Int J Tuberc Lung Dis. 2015;19(5):545–51.
26. Theron G, Pooran A, Peter J, van Zyl-Smit R, Kumar Mishra H, Meldau R, et al. Do adjunct tuberculosis tests, when combined with Xpert MTB/RIF, improve accuracy and the cost of diagnosis in a resource-poor setting? Eur Respir J. 2012;40(1):161–8.
27. Hu P, Bai L, Liu F, Ou X, Zhang Z, Yi S, et al. Evaluation of the Xpert MTB/RIF assay for diagnosis of tuberculosis and rifampin resistance in county-level laboratories in Hunan province, China. Chin Med J. 2014;127(21):3744–50.
28. Dowdy DW, Davis JL, den Boon S, Walter ND, Katamba A, Cattamanchi A. Population-level impact of same-day microscopy and Xpert MTB/RIF for tuberculosis diagnosis in Africa. PLoS One. 2013;8(8):e70485.
29. Zhao Y, Xu S, Wang L, Chin DP, Wang S, Jiang G, et al. National survey of drug-resistant tuberculosis in China. N Engl J Med 2012;366(23):2161–2170.

Respiratory symptoms, fractional exhaled nitric oxide & endotoxin exposure among female flower farm workers in Ethiopia

Amare W Nigatu[1*], Magne Bråtveit[1], Wakgari Deressa[2] and Bente E Moen[1]

Abstract

Background: Greenhouse workers are exposed to organic dusts, and they are thereby at risk of developing airway disorders. This study aims to measure personal endotoxin exposure, assess respiratory symptoms and measure fractional exhaled nitric oxide (FeNO) among female flower farm workers in Ethiopia.

Methods: A cross-sectional study involving female workers (n = 248) from four flower farms was conducted. The workers were interviewed for respiratory symptoms using a standard questionnaire. Workers from two of these farms also participated in personal endotoxin sampling (46 workers, 75 measurements) on glass fiber filters (0.2 μm pore size) inside conductive 25 mm Millipore cassettes for sampling of the "total dust" fraction. They also participated in FeNO (n = 114) measurements with a portable electrochemistry-based sensor. Chi-square and independent t-tests were used to compare categorical and continuous variables respectively. A mixed-effects model was used to analyze exposure determinants.

Results: Endotoxin exposure had a geometric mean (GM) of 22.8 endotoxin units (EU)/m^3 with a maximum of 180 EU/m^3. Greenhouse workers had significantly higher endotoxin exposure than workers outside the greenhouses (GM = 26.7 vs. 19.3 EU/m^3 respectively; $p < 0.05$). The mean age of the workers was 24 years, and their mean working time in the flower farm was 21 months. Greenhouse workers had higher prevalence of self-reported respiratory symptoms than those outside greenhouses. However, after adjusting for education only blocked nose remained significant. The FeNO concentration ranged 5–166 ppb (GM = 14 ppb). Two workers had FeNO concentration above 50 ppb. FeNO levels differs significantly between the farms but there was no difference between workers inside and outside greenhouses.

Conclusion: Greenhouse workers at flower farms had higher prevalence of blocked nose than workers outside, which may indicate the presence of rhinitis. Endotoxin exposure was low. There were few workers with objective signs of airway inflammation; this might be because the mean working time in the greenhouses was only two years. We suggest further studies to evaluate the effect of longer employment and exposure time as well as to investigate possible exposure to pesticides and other components in the bio-aerosols.

Keywords: Endotoxin exposure, Respiratory symptoms, Fractional exhaled nitric oxide, Greenhouse, Flower farm

Background

The cultivation of roses inside greenhouses is a rapidly growing economic activity in Ethiopia, and covers 120 hectares of land with over 50,000 workers [1]. The greenhouses are characterized by elevated temprature, humidity and poor ventilation [2-4]. Pesticides of different types, chemical fertilizers and to some extent biological agents are widely used to enhance the growth of flowers [5].

It is likely that people in the agriculture sector are exposed to organic dusts during their daily routines [6-8]. Part of the agriculture process involves work in greenhouses, including cultivation of flowers and vegetables. Because of the enclosed space and poor ventilation, greenhouse work might also be associated with high exposure levels to organic dust [9]. Several studies among greenhouse workers have shown high prevalence of respiratory symptoms such as chronic cough, dyspnea,

* Correspondence: Amare.Nigatu@igs.uib.no
[1]Department of Global Public Health and Primary Care, University of Bergen, Bergen, Norway
Full list of author information is available at the end of the article

chest tightness and rhinitis, as compared to controls [2,10-12]. In 2012 we conducted a study among flower farm workers in Ethiopia and found that workers inside the greenhouse had significantly higher self-reported prevalence of chronic respiratory symptoms compared to workers outside the greenhouse as well as compared to a control group of supermarket workers [13]. No objective measurements of occupational exposure or respiratory health were performed in that study.

The organic dust in greenhouses has many components such as fungal spores, bacteria, and endotoxins [4,14,15]. Endotoxins are a cell-wall component of gram-negative bacteria, and can be inhaled by workers [16,17]. It is suggested that they are involved in the development of respiratory disorders such as obstructive lung disease [17]. As many of the Ethiopian farm workers had respiratory symptoms, which can be considered typical for airway obstruction [9,13], we decided to measure endotoxin exposure levels in their work environment.

Adverse respiratory effects due to organic dust exposure might be associated with eosinophilic inflammation and increased fractional exhaled nitric oxide (FeNO) among workers [18]. The measurement of FeNO involves a simple and non-invasive method. The technique uses a portable device. This gives fast and reliable results in the field [19]. Occupational exposure to organic dust and measurement of FeNO in the agricultural sector has been used in the Western countries to study several work settings [20]. However, few of these studies are conducted among greenhouse workers [4,11]. Moreover, there is no information about endotoxin exposure and FeNO among flower farm workers in Ethiopia.

The objective of the present study was to evaluate the exposure to endotoxins; to assess the prevalence of respiratory symptoms and to measure FeNO among female workers inside and outside greenhouses in flower farms in Ethiopia.

Methods and materials

Study design and study settings

A cross-sectional study was conducted from July to October 2013 in four flower farms in the three main geographical areas for cultivation of roses in Ethiopia (Hollota/Addis-Alem, Debrezeit and Ziway areas). Due to practical reasons such as location and accessibility, we used convenient sampling to select the farms. The workers in each of the farms were divided into two observational groups based on their workstation (inside vs. outside greenhouses) for an interview, FeNO measurement and endotoxin sampling under their normal working conditions. All the four farms were included in the assessment of respiratory symptoms, but due to limited resources only two farms were included in the measurements of endotoxin and FeNO. The farms were visited before the actual data collection and the farm managements were informed about the purpose of the study.

The farms only grow roses, and vary in size from 5–51 hectares, while the total number of workers ranged from 350 to 1,300 (Table 1). The production rate is relatively constant, but at times there is peak production to meet increased demands. All the farms use chemical fertilizers and pesticides to enhance the growth of flowers and to control pests. In addition, Farm I also uses mites as biological control, however, we did not collected information on the types of mites used. The pesticides are manually mixed at a central location inside greenhouses and distributed through pipelines. The sprayers use a nozzle or sprayer gun to spray the pesticide. In all the farms, except Farm IV, spraying takes place in the morning during which time the other greenhouse workers are relocated to other greenhouses until the spraying is completed. In Farm IV spraying is done late in the afternoon after all greenhouse workers have completed their work and left the farm.

The great majority of the workers are females, who either harvest and weed flowers inside greenhouses or trim and pack roses in a pack-house before storage in a cold room until transporting them to Addis Ababa for export. The few men work as pesticide sprayers and also perform other activities including repairing the greenhouses, collecting and disposing of wastes as well as transporting harvested flowers.

Study participants

Female workers from the selected farms participated in the study. Based on the prevalence of shortness of breath (70%) among Ethiopian flower farm workers [13], a total of 248 participants (divided in two groups, i.e., inside vs. outside greenhouse) were needed to achieve 80% statistical power with significance level set to $P < 0.05$. The plan was to have equal number of workers from each of the four farms as well as from inside and outside greenhouses, and overall 122 and 126 workers participated from inside and outside greenhouses, respectively. The same participants from Farm I & II ($n = 114$) were also invited to participate in the FeNO measurements. Participants were randomly selected by the researcher from the personnel registration book in Farm II & III, while in Farm I & IV, the selection was done together with the farm administration. The principal investigator did all the interviews and the FeNO measurements in a separate room inside the farm compound. The FeNO instruction was sometimes done in groups of 2–4 workers.

Interview

A part of the standardized questionnaire from the British Medical Research Council (BMRC) on respiratory health was used to assess chronic respiratory symptoms. The

Table 1 Description of the flower farms and workers participated in the study

Farm characteristics	Farm ID			
	I	II	III	IV
Farm size (hectares)	51	12	5	41
Number of greenhouses	21	7	3	5
Number of pack-houses	2	1	1	2
Number of workers	1,300	700	350	1295
Sample Size				
Interview	67	47	41	93
FeNO measurement	67	47	NA	NA
Endotoxin measurement	25	21	NA	NA
Pest control methods	CP, BA	CP	CP	CP
Pesticide spraying time	6:00–10:00 AM	6:00–10:00 AM	6:00–10:00 AM	3:00–6:00 PM
Flower cultivated	Roses	Roses	Roses	Roses

NA: Not Applicable; CP: Chemical Pesticides; BA: Biological Agents.

questionnaire was adapted to the Ethiopian context, and translated from English to the local language; the symptoms included cough first thing in the morning, day/night time cough, shortness of breath, chest tightness and wheezing as well as previous diseases such as bronchitis, pulmonary TB, asthma and chest injury (yes/no). In addition, questions about upper airway symptoms (runny nose, sneezing and blocked nose) were also included [21]. Moreover, previous flower farm experience (months), socio-demographic characteristics such as age, education (years in school), types of job (cutter & weeder, packing, deleafing, grading, quality control), present and previous smoking habits (yes/no) and the use of Personal Protective Equipment: gloves and respiratory protective device (yes/no) were also asked.

FeNO measurement

FeNO measurements were taken for each person in a sitting position during the working day between 10:00 and 15:00 hours, using a portable electrochemistry-based sensor (NIOX MINO; Aerocrine AB, Solana, Sweden) in accordance with the American Thoracic Society & European Respiratory Society recommendations for online measurement of FeNO [22,23]. The mean ambient NO, room temperature and relative humidity of the room where FeNO measurement performed were registered daily; below 5 ppb, 22°C (18 – 28°C) and 70%, respectively.

Endotoxin sampling and analysis

Full-shift personal endotoxin air samples were collected in the two selected farms (inside vs. outside greenhouses). The number of endotoxin samples was based on the Rappaport and Kupper's recommendations for exposure studies; 10–20 measurements per observational group, two measurements of 5–10 randomly selected individuals per group [24]. Totally 46 female workers were invited for sampling; 25 from Farm I, and 21 from Farm II. Among these, 31 workers had repeated samples.

Sampling was performed from the workers' breathing zone during the summer months, which is a rainy season in Ethiopia. Side Kick Casella Pump at a flow rate of 2 L/minute connected to 25 mm closed-face conductive Millipore cassettes containing a glass fiber filter with 0.2 μm pore size was mounted onto each worker for sampling of the "total dust" fraction. The mean sampling times were 350 (275 – 425) minutes and 358 (240 – 405) minutes for Farm I and II, respectively. The pumps were calibrated using a Rotameter every day before starting the measurement, and the air flow rate was also measured at the end of the measurements. Two samples were excluded due to a reduction in air flow of more than 10% during the sampling day. Filters were kept cold at about 4°C inside a box filled with ice bags until the samples were transported to Norway and then to Sweden for analysis at Lund University Medical Laboratory. The samples were transported as hand luggage on the flights, and were outside the cold box for a total of about 15 hours. The glass fiber filters were immersed into 0.05% Tween-20 pyrogenic free water and shaken on a rotary shaker for 1 h. Endotoxin extracts were analyzed using kinetic chromogenic Limulus amebocyte Lysate (LAL) Assay. The results were expressed as Endotoxin Unit (EU) per filter. A total of 27 samples had endotoxin values below the Limit of Quantification (LOQ), which was set to 10 EU per filter by the laboratory. In calculations of exposure levels (EU/m^3), the amount of endotoxins on the respective filters were divided by the air volume that had passed through that filter. The measurements below LOQ were set as LOQ/2$^{1/2}$ in further data handling. This cut-off level has been suggested when less than 50% of the data are nondetectable, and the geometric standard deviation is below 3.0 [25]. The resulting limit of detection (LOD) for the endotoxin exposure corresponding to the 27 samples < LOQ varied from 8.7 to 14.7 EU/m^3 due to different air volumes.

Ethics

The research proposal was submitted and approved by the Ethical committees both in Norway and Oromia Regional State Health Bureau, Ethiopia. All the participants were informed about the purpose of the study and written consent was obtained.

Statistical analysis

The data was plotted into SPSS version 21 and analyzed using descriptive statistics. The distribution of endotoxin and FeNO data were skewed, and were therefore log-transformed in order to compare the levels between the groups. Chi-square test for categorical variables, and independent t-tests for continuous variables were used to test differences between the groups. The significance level was set to 0.05. A linear mixed-effects model was used to analyze the determinants of endotoxin exposure among the female workers, since we had repeated measurements of endotoxins on several of the workers. The individual female participants were included in the model as random effects. The farms (Farm I vs. Farm II) and workstation (inside vs. outside greenhouses) were set as fixed effects. Logistic regression was used to test differences in symptoms between groups by adjusting for education. Education was the only potential confounder among those tested that was significantly different between workers inside vs. outside greenhouses.

Results

Characteristics of the study participants

The workers were categorized by workstation based on whether they work inside the greenhouse or not. The response rate for the interview was 100%. The mean age of all female workers was 24 years (range 14 – 60 years). There were no differences in age, previous respiratory diseases and duration of work experience between inside and outside greenhouse workers (Table 2). Workers outside the greenhouse had significantly higher education than those working inside (Table 2). None of the female workers were current smokers or had any previous history of smoking. The majority of the workers (97%) used biofuel (wood, cow dung & charcoal) as energy source for cooking and other domestic purposes. A quarter of the participants had domestic animals, and 7% shared their living space with the animals.

Table 2 Characteristics of the female flower farm workers by workstation (inside vs. outside greenhouse)

N	IGH	OGH
	122	126
Years of age		
Mean (Range)	24 (14 – 48)	23 (16 – 60)
Cooking energy N (%)		
Biofuel-wood-dung-wood-charcoal	119 (98)	122 (97)
Kerosin	2 (1.6)	4 (3)
Both	1 (0.8)	0
Educational level N (%)		
No Education (0–4 school years)	55 (45)	25 (20)*
Education (>5 school years)	67 (55)	101 (80)
Work experience in Months		
Mean (range)	21 (1–96)	22 (1–96)
Previous Agricultural experience N (%)	28 (23)	38 (30)
Previous Agricultural experience in months Mean (SD)	20 (18)	8 (8)
Domestic animals N (%)	27 (22)	34 (27)
Shared room with domestic animals	7 (6)	10 (8)
Pesticide use N (%)		
For household pests[a]	52 (43)	60 (50)
For mosquito control	23 (19)	28 (22)
Previous diseases N (%)		
Chest injury/operation	1 (0.8)	0
Bronchitis	9 (7.4)	12 (9.5)
Pneumonia	3 (2.5)	4 (3.2)
Pulmonary TB	1 (0.8)	2 (1.6)
Asthma	4 (3.3)	3 (2.4)
Smoking		
Current & Previous smokers	None	None

IGH: Inside Greenhouse; OGH: Outside Greenhouse; *Pearson chi-square test, P < 0.001; [a]Fleas, bed bugs, lice, mice.

Endotoxin exposure measurements

The personal endotoxin exposure ranged from < LOD to 180 EU/m^3 with a geometric mean of 22.8 EU/m^3 (Table 3). Only one of the samples exceeded the Dutch recommended health-based exposure limit value for endotoxins in inhalable dust of 90 EU/m^3 [26]. The endotoxin exposure inside the greenhouses was significantly higher than outside the greenhouses ($p < 0.05$) (Table 3). Workers in Farm I had significantly higher endotoxin exposure than workers in Farm II (GM = 29.2 Vs. 17.3 EU/m^3; $P < 0.01$). The greenhouse workers in Farm I were the subgroup with the highest endotoxin exposure (GM = 37.8 EU/m^3) (Table 3).

The day-to-day endotoxin exposure variability (within workers) was higher than the between worker variability (Table 4). In a mixed-effects model analysis, the fixed

Table 3 Personal endotoxin exposure among female flower farm workers according to farm (I or II) and workstation (inside vs. outside greenhouse)

Farm ID	Workstation	Nw	Ns	Ns <LOD	Endotoxin (EU/m3)		
					AM	Range[a]	GM (GSD)
Farm I	IGH	10	19	2	47.3	9.2 – 180	37.8 (2.0)*[b]
	OGH	15	20	8	28.2	10.0– 64.6	22.9 (2.0)
	Total	25	39	10	37.5	9.2 – 180	29.2 (2.1)**[c]
Farm II	IGH	12	19	8	24.9	8.7 – 60.9	18.9 (2.1)[ns,b]
	OGH	9	17	9	17.1	9.1 – 34.7	15.8 (1.5)
	Total	21	36	17	21.3	8.7 – 60.9	17.3 (1.9)
Total	IGH	22	38	10	36.1	8.7 – 180	26.7 (2.2)*[b]
	OGH	24	37	17	23.1	9.1 – 64.6	19.3 (1.8)
	Total	46	75	27	29.7	8.7 – 180	22.8 (2.1)

Independent sample t-tests were used to compare groups.
EU/m^3: Endotoxin Units per cubic meter; Nw: Number of workers; Ns: Number of sample; <LOD: Below Limit of Detection; AM: Arithmetic Mean; GM: Geometric Mean; GSD: Geometric Standard Deviation; IGH: Inside Greenhouse; OGH: Outside Greenhouse (packhouse); **P < 0.01, *P < 0.05, ns = not significant, [a]The lowest exposure in all subgroups are estimated values for results below LOD; [b]Comparing samples inside and outside greenhouses; [c]Comparing Farm I and Farm II.

factors workstation and farm, explained 17% of the total variance in endotoxin exposure (Table 4). The fixed factors explained parts of the between-worker variance only. Work in Farm I was associated with 1.7 times higher personal exposure to endotoxin compared to Farm II, while those working inside the greenhouse had 1.4 times higher exposure than those working outside.

Use of Personal Protective Devices (PPD)

None of the female workers in any of the four flower farms used any type of Respiratory Protective Devices (RPD). Almost all (99.6%) of the workers indicated the reason for not using RPD was because it is unavailable or not provided at the work place. Gloves at work were used by 64% of all female workers (78% and 50% among inside and outside greenhouse workers respectively) with significant differences between the farms (p < 0.01). The reported reason for not using gloves was mainly because gloves were not available or provided.

Prevalence of chronic respiratory symptoms

Among all invited workers in the four farms shortness of breath (53%), chest tightness (27%) and morning cough (25%) were the most frequently reported symptoms (Table 5). Morning cough, runny nose and blocked nose were significantly higher among greenhouse workers compared to those working outside (Table 5). When adjusting for education by logistic regression analyses, only the prevalence of blocked nose remained significantly higher among workers inside greenhouses. The prevalence of morning cough and day/night time cough with sputum were significantly different among the four flower farms (p = 0.009 & 0.028 respectively), while the other symptoms did not differ among these groups. Farm I had the highest prevalence for most of the symptoms (results not shown). When comparing results of Farm I & II, where we also have measurements of personal endotoxin exposure and Fractional exhaled Nitric Oxide (FeNO), Farm I has relatively higher prevalence for most of the symptoms. The prevalence inside the greenhouse was higher than outside for most of the symptoms. Due to small numbers, the groups inside and outside the greenhouse in these two farms were not statistically compared after stratification by farm.

Fractional exhaled Nitric Oxide (FeNO)

A total of 114 female flower workers from Farm I & II participated in measurements of Fractional exhaled Nitric Oxide (FeNO), and valid results were obtained from 108 of these.

Among all participants FeNO ranged from 5 to166 ppb with a GM of 14 ppb (Table 6). Only two workers (1.8%) had FeNO concentration greater than 50 ppb, a level often used to indicate the presence of asthma [27]. The mean FeNO of those working inside and outside the greenhouses did not differ significantly, either among workers in Farm I and Farm II together or within each

Table 4 Linear mixed-effects model for the $\log_e$-transformed personal endotoxin exposure levels of female workers

	Endotoxin (EU/m^3)		
	Random-effects Model β (SE)	Mixed-effects Model β (SE)	Effect (e^{β})
Intercept	3.14 (0.09)**	2.67 (0.15)**	
Workstation (OGH = 0 & IGH = 1)		0.35 (0.16)*	1.4
Farm ID (Farm II = 0 & Farm I = 1)		0.53 (0.16)**	1.7
WWδ (SE)	0.35 (0.09)	0.35 (0.09)	
BWδ (SE)	0.17 (0.09)	0.08 (0.08)	
% of explained variance		17%	

SE: Standard Error; β: Regression Coefficient; IGH: Inside Greenhouse; OGH: Outside Greenhouse; WWδ: Within Worker Variance; BWδ: Between Worker Variance; **P < 0.01, *P < 0.05.

Table 5 Prevalence of respiratory symptoms by workstation (inside vs. outside greenhouse)

	Workstation			Adjusted OR (95% CI)[a]
	Total	IGH	OGH	
	N = 248	N = 122	N = 126	
	n (%)	n (%)	n(%)	
Morning cough	63 (25)	38 (31)*	25 (20)	1.19 (0.63, 2.26)
Cough day/night time	41 (17)	23 (19)	18 (14)	1.08 (0.53, 2.21)
Cough 4–6 days a week	47 (19)	29 (24)	18 (14)	1.31 (0.66, 2.64)
Cough more days in 3 months	18 (7)	11 (9)	7 (6)	1.11 (0.39, 3.13)
Morning cough with sputum	39 (16)	22 (18)	17 (14)	1.03 (0.49, 2.14)
Cough day/night time with sputum	19 (8)	11 (9)	8 (6)	1.15 (0.43, 3.09)
Cough 4–6 days a week with sputum	25 (10)	15 (13)	10 (8)	0.99 (0.39, 2.45)
Cough more days in 3 months with sputum	11 (4)	7 (6)	4 (3)	1.01 (0.27, 3.79)
Shortness of breath walking on level ground/slight hill	131 (53)	60 (49)	71 (56)	0.65 (0.38, 1.09)
Shortness breath walking own pace	38 (15)	22 (18)	16 (13)	1.16 (0.56, 2.43)
Wheezing	40 (16)	20 (16)	20 (16)	0.69 (0.33, 1.46)
Chest tightness	66 (27)	34 (28)	32 (25)	0.89 (0.49, 1.62)
Sneezing	70 (29)	32 (26)	38 (30)	0.74 (0.42, 1.33)
Runny nose	48 (19)	30 (25)*	18 (14)	1.74 (0.89, 3.39)
Blocked nose	36 (15)	25 (21)**	11 (9)	2.36 (1.08, 5.17)

The groups were compared using chi-square tests and logistic regression, while adjusting for education.
N: Total number of samples; n: number of cases with the symptom; **P < 0.01 & *P < 0.05 (unadjusted chi-square tests); [a]95 percent confidence interval.

of the farms (Table 6). Workers in Farm I had significantly higher mean FeNO than in Farm II (GM = 15.8 ppb and 11.8 ppb; P = 0.009) respectively (Table 6). When excluding the two values above 50 ppb, the statistical differences between the groups did not change.

Discussion

Our study indicated that endotoxin exposure and FeNO levels were low while there were high prevalences of self-reported respiratory symptoms among the female workers in the flower farms. Greenhouse workers had significantly higher endotoxin exposure and reported more symptoms than workers outside greenhouses. However, after adjusting for education, only blocked nose remained significant. FeNO levels differed significantly between the farms but there was no difference comparing inside vs. outside greenhouse workers.

Table 6 Mean FeNO level according to workstation (inside vs. outside greenhouse) and farm among the female flower farm workers

Farm ID	Workstation	N	AM	Range	Ns > 50 ppb	GM	GSD
Farm I	IGH	26	16.5		0	15.3	1.47
	OGH	37	21.4		1	16.2	1.93
	Total[a]	63	19.4	5-166	1	15.8*	1.75
Farm II	IGH	23	17.2		1	12.8	1.95
	OGH	22	12.3		0	10.8	1.65
	Total[a]	45	14.8	5-107	1	11.8*	1.82
Total	IGH	49	16.8		1	14.1	1.72
	OGH	59	18.0		1	13.9	1.88
	Total	108	17.5	5-166	2	13.9	1.81

[a]Independent *t*-test; *P < 0.01 when comparing Farm I and II; Ns: Number of samples; IGH: Inside Greenhouse; OGH: Outside Greenhouse (packhouse).

All the endotoxin samples, except one, were below the Dutch recommended health-based exposure limit value (90 EU/m^3) [26]. Nevertheless, the mean endotoxin exposure was higher than reported for flower/ornamental growers inside European greenhouses (GM = 2.9; range 0.4-101.4 EU/m^3) [28]. Studies among Dutch and Danish flower growers in greenhouses reported similar or slightly higher endotoxin exposure (GM = 27 & 44 EU/m^3 respectively) [20,29]. In those studies they used inhalable dust samplers which have been reported to sample 1.5-4 times more dust by mass than the "total" dust samplers used in the present study [30]. Thus, it is difficult to directly compare the obtained results with other studies and with the Dutch limit value since the total dust samplers in our study presumably collected lower levels of endotoxins than were present in the inhalable dust fraction. A study among cucumber and tomato employees in greenhouses reported considerably higher endotoxin exposure (median = 320 EU/m^3) which might be partly due to the larger leaf areas of these plants [9]. Greenhouse workers in Farm I had the highest endotoxin exposure of all the groups in both farms.

Use of biological pest control method in Farm I might have contributed to the higher exposure, as this is the only apparent difference between the farms. One may speculate whether biological pest control combined with less use of pesticides could be related to this differences in exposure.

The day-to-day variance was higher than the between worker variance for the endotoxin exposure. One reason might be temporary relocation of workers to other greenhouses during spraying. However, we did not systematically register the relocation times. The fixed factors in the mixed-effects model only explains the between-worker variability in endotoxin exposure, which is logical since the individual worker did not change workstation (inside/outside greenhouse) or farm.

The greenhouse workers had higher prevalence for most symptoms than workers outside. However, when we adjust for education, only the prevalence of blocked nose, which is most likely a symptom of rhinitis, was significantly higher. This is similar to the findings in Croatia that female greenhouse workers had higher prevalence of respiratory symptoms than controls [2]. However, the prevalence of rhinitis in the Croatian study was higher (42%) than for blocked nose in the present study (21%). This difference may be explained by the use of different terms describing nose symptoms. The term rhinitis is broad, and more people may have reported this symptom than the more specific symptom blocked nose. Rhinitis is known to precede asthmatic conditions [31], which might mean that the workers inside greenhouses could be at risk of developing asthma. However, only surveys over a longer time can support this. The results in the present study are also partly consistent with our previous study [13], showing high prevalence of respiratory symptoms, including blocked nose. However, in that study a different control group was used. The low endotoxin exposure in the present study is not likely to explain the respiratory symptoms, and might rather be related to other components in the bioaerosol including fungi or pesticides [3,15]. Studies on greenhouse workers in Oman [32] and Turkey [33] reported prevalence of cough of 30% and 31%, respectively. The higher prevalence in these two studies than in the present study (19% of day/night time cough), might be explained by the higher age (78% over 30 years), cigarette smoking (19.8%) and longer work experience (73% over 7 years) of the workers in the Oman study. It might be possible that longer work experience with longer exposure time cause more respiratory health problems than we have been able to demonstrate.

This relatively high prevalence of shortness of breath, chest tightness and wheezing, even in the young worker population in our study, might be partly due to unknown factors such as reporting errors or living conditions. Over a quarter of the workers had domestic animals, which may also expose them to dust and allergens.

The mean FeNO in our study was GM = 13.9 ppb, which is considered to be low [34]. A study among endotoxin exposed female agricultural workers also found to be low FeNO (GM = 11.4 ppb) [35]. Previous studies of asthmatics have shown elevated FeNO levels [36,37]. Although we found low FeNO level in our study, it may not necessarily mean that these workers do not have any risk of asthma or other respiratory problems.

Strength and limitation

Strengths of the present study are that objective measurements were done both for endotoxin exposure and FeNO. Moreover, the subgroups (inside vs. outside greenhouses) were comparable for most variables except education, which we controlled for in the analysis.

However, it is a weakness that we only measured endotoxin exposure during one summer (rainy and wet). This may not represent the winter (sunny and dry) exposure. A high fraction of the endotoxin samples had values below the limit of quantification at the laboratory. The high fraction of these low levels has presumably influenced the estimates of mean exposures and the fixed factors in the mixed-effects model, but presumably they did not affect the main findings. Pesticides and fertilizers of different types were widely used in the flower farms [13], but we were unable to measure these exposures in this study. There might be a healthy worker effect as most workers had short work experience due to high turnover. In addition, the administration may have picked the healthiest workers for examination. However, the administrative personnel was not likely to know all the details of the workers' health.

Conclusion

Greenhouse workers in flower plants had higher prevalence of blocked nose than those outside greenhouses, which may indicate the presence of rhinitis. Endotoxin exposure was low, but the levels were highest inside the greenhouses. There were few workers with objective signs of airway inflammation, but most workers had only been working in the greenhouses for two years. Further studies should be performed in the rose farms to evaluate the effect of longer employment and exposure time as well as to investigate possible occupational exposure to pesticides and other components in the bioaerosol.

Abbreviations

FeNO: Fractional exhaled nitric oxide; GM: Geometric mean; BMRC: British medical research council; TB: Tuberculosis; PPB: Parts per billion; NO: Nitric oxide; LOQ: Limit of quantification; LOD: Level of detaction; EU/m^3: Endotoxin unit per cubic meter; RPD: Respiratory protective devices.

Competing interests
The authors declare that they have no competing interests.

Authors' contributions
AWN has contributed to the conception, planning and design of the study, data collection, analysis and interpretation, drafting and revising the manuscript. BEM contributed to the planning and design of the study, data collection, analysis and interpretation of the data and critical reviewing of the manuscript. MB contributed to the planning and design of the study, analysis and interpretation of the data and critical reviewing of the manuscript. WD contributed to the planning of the study, data collection and critical reviewing of the manuscript. All authors read and approved the final manuscript.

Authors' information
AWN: PhD Candidate, Occupational and Environmental Medicine Research Group, Bergen University, Norway. BEM: MD, PhD; Director of Center for International Health, Bergen University, Norway. MB: PhD, Occupational and Environmental Health Research Group, Bergen University, Norway. WD: PhD, Head of Public Health Faculty, Addis Ababa University, Ethiopia.

Acknowledgements
We are very grateful to the flower farm workers and the farm managements for their willingness to participate and cooperate in this study. We are grateful to Lennart Larsson and Christina Pehrson who analyzed the endotoxin samples for us. We also acknowledge the Norwegian Education Fund for the financial support to conduct the study.

Author details
[1]Department of Global Public Health and Primary Care, University of Bergen, Bergen, Norway. [2]School of Public Health, Addis Ababa University, Addis Ababa, Ethiopia.

References
1. Sutton JaNK: An Enterprise Map of Ethiopia. International Growth Centre 2010:205. http://personal.lse.ac.uk/sutton/Enterprise_Map_Ethiopia_Book.pdf
2. Zuskin E, Schachter EN, Mustajbegovic J. Respiratory function in greenhouse workers. Int Arch Occup Environ Health. 1993;64(7):521–6.
3. Hernandez AF, Casado I, Pena G, Gil F, Villanueva E, Pla A. Low level of exposure to pesticides leads to lung dysfunction in occupationally exposed subjects. Inhal Toxicol. 2008;20(9):839–49.
4. Adhikari A, Gupta J, Wilkins JR, Olds 3rd RL, Indugula R, Cho KJ, et al. Airborne microorganisms, endotoxin, and (1→3)-beta-D-glucan exposure in greenhouses and assessment of respiratory symptoms among workers. Ann Occup Hyg. 2011;55(3):272–85.
5. Sahle A, Potting J. Environmental life cycle assessment of Ethiopian rose cultivation. Sci Total Environ. 2013;443:163–72.
6. Lee SA, Adhikari A, Grinshpun SA, McKay R, Shukla R, Reponen T. Personal exposure to airborne dust and microorganisms in agricultural environments. J Occup Environ Hyg. 2006;3(3):118–30.
7. Mekonnen Y, Ejigu D. Plasma cholinesterase level of Ethiopian farm workers exposed to chemical pesticide. Occup Med. 2005;55(6):504–5.
8. Watterson A. Pesticide health and safety and the work and impact of international agencies: partial successes and major failures. Int J Occup Environ Health. 2001;7(4):339–47.
9. Madsen AM, Hansen VM, Nielsen SH, Olsen TT. Exposure to dust and endotoxin of employees in cucumber and tomato nurseries. Ann Occup Hyg. 2009;53(2):129–38.
10. Tual S, Clin B, Leveque-Morlais N, Raherison C, Baldi I, Lebailly P. Agricultural exposures and chronic bronchitis: findings from the AGRICAN (AGRIculture and CANcer) cohort. Ann Epidemiol. 2013;23(9):539–45.
11. Monso E. Occupational asthma in greenhouse workers. Curr Opin Pulm Med. 2004;10(2):147–50.
12. Mekonnen Y, Agonafir T. Effects of pesticide applications on respiratory health of Ethiopian farm workers. Int J Occup Environ Health. 2002;8(1):35–40.
13. Hanssen VM, Nigatu AW, Zeleke ZK, Moen BE, Bratveit M. High prevalence of respiratory and dermal symptoms among Ethiopian flower farm workers. Arch Environ Occup Health. 2014;15:15.
14. Madsen AM. Airborne endotoxin in different background environments and seasons. Ann Agric Environ Med. 2006;13(1):81–6.
15. Hansen VM, Winding A, Madsen AM. Exposure to bioaerosols during the growth season of tomatoes in an organic greenhouse using Supresivit (Trichoderma harzianum) and Mycostop (Streptomyces griseoviridis). Appl Environ Microbiol. 2010;76(17):5874–81.
16. Paba E, Tranfo G, Corsetti F, Marcelloni AM, Iavicoli S. Indoor exposure to airborne endotoxin: a review of the literature on sampling and analysis methods. Ind Health. 2013;51(3):237–55.
17. Dutkiewicz J, Cisak E, Sroka J, Wojcik-Fatla A, Zajac V. Biological agents as occupational hazards - selected issues. Ann Agric Environ Med. 2011;18(2):286–93.
18. Quirce S, Lemiere C, de Blay F, del Pozo V, Gerth Van Wijk R, Maestrelli P, et al. Noninvasive methods for assessment of airway inflammation in occupational settings. Allergy. 2010;65(4):445–58.
19. Khalili B, Boggs PB, Bahna SL. Reliability of a new hand-held device for the measurement of exhaled nitric oxide. Allergy. 2007;62(10):1171–4.
20. Spaan S, Wouters IM, Oosting I, Doekes G, Heederik D. Exposure to inhalable dust and endotoxins in agricultural industries. J Environ Monit. 2006;8(1):63–72.
21. Wasserfallen JB, Gold K, Schulman KA, Baraniuk JN. Development and validation of a rhinoconjunctivitis and asthma symptom score for use as an outcome measure in clinical trials. J Allergy Clin Immunol. 1997;100(1):16–22.
22. Alving K, Janson C, Nordvall L. Performance of a new hand-held device for exhaled nitric oxide measurement in adults and children. Respir Res. 2006;7:67.
23. ATS/ERS. Recommendations for standardized procedures for the online and offline measurement of exhaled lower respiratory nitric oxide and nasal nitric oxide, 2005. Am J Respir Crit Care Med. 2005;171(8):912–30.
24. Rappaport SM, Kupper LL. Interpreting Levels of Exposures to Chemical Agents. In: Patty's Industrial Hygiene. edn.: John Wiley & Sons, Inc.; 2001
25. Hornung RW, Reed LD. Estimation of Average Concentration in the Presence of Nondetectable Values. Appl Occup Environ Hyg. 1990;5(1):46–51.
26. Health Council of the Netherlands. Endotoxins. Health-Based Recommended Occupational Exposure Limit. The Hague: Health Council of the Netherlands; 2010.
27. Olin AC, Bake B, Toren K. Fraction of exhaled nitric oxide at 50 mL/s: reference values for adult lifelong never-smokers. Chest. 2007;131(6):1852–6.
28. Radon K, Danuser B, Iversen M, Monso E, Weber C, Hartung J, et al. Air contaminants in different European farming environments. Ann Agric Environ Med. 2002;9(1):41–8.
29. Thilsing T, Madsen AM, Basinas I, Schlunssen V, Tendal K, Baelum J. Dust, endotoxin, fungi, and bacteria exposure as determined by work task, season, and type of plant in a flower greenhouse. Ann Occup Hyg. 2014;59:142.
30. Martin JRJ, Martin DMD. Comparison of total dust/inhalable dust sampling methods for the evaluation of airborne wood dust. Appl Occup Environ Hyg. 1998;13(3):177–82.
31. Storaas T, Steinsvåg SK, Florvaag E, Irgens A, Aasen TB. Occupational rhinitis: diagnostic critera, relation to lower airway symptoms and IgE sensitization in bakery workers. Acta Otolaryngol. 2005;125(11):1211–7.
32. Esechie JO, Ibitayo OO. Pesticide use and related health problems among greenhouse workers in Batinah Coastal Region of Oman. J Forensic Leg Med. 2011;18(5):198–203.
33. Ergonen AT, Salacin S, Ozdemir MH. Pesticide use among greenhouse workers in Turkey. J Clin Forensic Med. 2005;12(4):205–8.
34. Dweik RA, Boggs PB, Erzurum SC, Irvin CG, Leigh MW, Lundberg JO, et al. An official ATS clinical practice guideline: interpretation of exhaled nitric oxide levels (FENO) for clinical applications. Am J Respir Crit Care Med. 2011;184(5):602–15.
35. Smit LA, Heederik D, Doekes G, Wouters IM. Exhaled nitric oxide in endotoxin-exposed adults: effect modification by smoking and atopy. Occup Environ Med. 2009;66(4):251–5.
36. Alving K, Weitzberg E, Lundberg JM. Increased amount of nitric oxide in exhaled air of asthmatics. Eur Respir J. 1993;6:1368–70.
37. Gratziou C, Lignos M, Dassiou M, Roussos C. Influence of atopy on exhaled nitric oxide in patients with stable asthma and rhinitis. Eur Respir J. 1999;14:897–901.

17

Prioritizing industries for occupational injury prevention and research in the Services Sector in Washington State, 2002–2010

Naomi J Anderson*, David K Bonauto and Darrin Adams

Abstract

Background: The Services Sector, as defined by the National Occupational Research Agenda (NORA), is comprised of a diverse industry mix and its workers face a variety of occupational exposures and hazards. The objective of this study was to identify high-risk industry groups within the Services Sector for prevention targeting.

Methods: Compensable Washington State workers' compensation claims from the Services Sector from 2002 through 2010 were analyzed. A "prevention index" (PI), the average of the rank orders of claim count and claim incidence rate, was used to rank 87 Services Sector industry groups by seven injury types: Work- Related Musculoskeletal Disorders (WMSDs), Fall to Lower Level, Fall on Same Level, Struck By/Against, Caught In/Under/Between, Motor Vehicle, and Overexertion. In the PI rankings, industry groups with high injury burdens appear higher ranked than industry groups with low counts or low rates of injury, indicating a need for prioritizing injury prevention efforts in these groups.

Results: In the Services Sector, these 7 injury types account for 84% of compensable claims in WA. The industry groups highest ranked by PI across the injury types included: Services to Buildings and Dwellings; Executive, Legislative, and Other General Government Support; and Waste Collection. WMSDs had the highest compensable claims rates.

Conclusions: Services is a large sector of the economy, and the substantial number, rate, and cost of occupational injuries within this sector should be addressed. Several Services Sector industry groups are at high risk for a variety of occupational injuries. Using a PI to rank industry groups based on their injury risk provides information with which to guide prevention efforts.

Keywords: Surveillance, NORA sector, Workers' compensation, Traumatic injury, Work related musculoskeletal disorder, Falls, Motor vehicle, Occupational health, Safety

Background

Occupational injuries and illnesses are common, costly, and a burden to workers and employers. Resources for prevention are limited, and there is a need for information to better focus research and prevention activities to maximize their impact. Other than the Bureau of Labor Statistics Survey of Occupational Injuries and Illnesses [1], there is relatively little published surveillance data comparing occupational injury and illness rates across industries [2-5]. In order to effectively prevent occupational injuries, employers, policymakers, healthcare providers, and researchers must know which injuries are occurring, where, and to what extent (magnitude, associated costs and time-loss). Analyzing injuries by industry can identify workers at high-risk for occupational injuries, and industry groups with the greatest need for prevention activities, safety and health programs, and further research.

The second-decade National Occupational Research Agenda (NORA) [6] is a partnership program between the National Institute for Occupational Safety and Health (NIOSH) [7] and businesses, universities, labor and other stakeholders, to promote and improve occupational health and safety research and workplace practices. The North American Industry Classification System (NAICS) classifies establishments into industries based on their business activities (and similarity in processes used to produce

* Correspondence: naomi.anderson@lni.wa.gov
Washington State Department of Labor & Industries, Safety & Health Assessment & Research for Prevention (SHARP) Program, PO Box 44330, Olympia, WA 98504-4330, USA

goods or services) [8]. NORA aggregates the 20 NAICS 2-digit Industry sectors into 10 Sector groups [9].

The Services Sector, as defined by NORA, includes diverse industries that face a range of exposures and hazards (e.g. offices, banks, educational establishments, auto repair shops, science and technical work, restaurants, fast food, hotels and motels, waste collection and the performing arts) and vary in establishment size and work organization. The Services Sector encompassed approximately 65 million workers in 2011, or more than 50% of the total U.S. workforce [10]. The scope and diversity of this Sector makes targeting occupational safety, prevention and research efforts difficult. Workers in the Services Sector may also face a higher burden of occupational injury and illness [5] and of occupational fatalities [11].

Previous efforts in Washington State (WA) used workers' compensation (WC) data to prioritize WA industries for injury prevention by 'prevention index' (PI) rankings for common costly occupational injury types and identified several NAICS industry groups that ranked highly on the prevention index [2,12]. The prevention index is calculated as the average of the industry's rank order of WC compensable claim count and compensable claims rate. In other words, the PI ranks industries by equally weighting how common injuries are and how high a worker's risk for injury is. Industry groups that are ranked higher by PI are those with a greater burden or risk of injuries. PI rankings indicate which industry groups should be prioritized in targeting research and prevention.

In one study, Anderson, Bonauto, and Adams [12] used PI methodology to rank all industry groups in WA (limited to State Fund claims) between 2002–2010. Of the 262 industry groups that met the inclusion criteria, 5 of the top 25 industry groups represented were from the Services Sector (Table 1). Two Services Sector industry groups, Services to Buildings and Dwellings (NAICS 5617) and Waste Collection (NAICS 5621) were in the top 5 by claim rate or count overall. These findings identified the Services Sector as a candidate for more in-depth characterization.

This study uses the established PI methodology to rank industry groups within the Services Sector by injury type for compensable WC claims between 2002 and 2010. The objective of this study was to identify and prioritize high-risk industry groups in the Services Sector by seven common, high-cost injury types for research and prevention efforts. Looking at PIs for each injury type allows for further tailoring of prevention efforts, as some industry groups may be at high-risk for specific injury types and not others. Industry groups that rank highly by PI across several injury types should be a top priority for those engaged in occupational health and safety.

Materials and methods

Washington's workers' compensation system

In Washington State, non-federal employers are required to obtain workers' compensation insurance through the Department of Labor and Industries' (L&I) industrial insurance system, unless they qualify to self-insure, or are covered by an alternative WC system (e.g. Longshore and Harbor Workers' Compensation Program). L&I administers the State Fund (SF), an industrial insurance program that provides coverage for approximately two-thirds of the 3.3 million workers in WA. The SF generally does not mandate WC insurance for self-employed workers, though elective coverage is available. Outside of the SF, there are approximately 450 self-insured (SI) entities (individual companies or groups of companies) that are not included in the State Fund insurance pool who employ nearly one-third of the workforce. Data from both SF and SI programs are collected and maintained in centralized databases at L&I.

Claim coding & data

In WA, a physician and worker initiate a WC claim by filing a Report of Industrial Injury or Occupational Disease (RIIOD) form, which includes the workers' demographic information, employment and wage information, and a brief description of the incident. The physician provides a medical diagnosis (with ICD-9) code, subjective and objective information regarding the diagnosis, and a diagnostic and treatment plan.

Workers' compensation administrative data include: codes characterizing the injury or illness; costs associated with disability payments, wage replacement, and pensions; billing information for health care providers, procedures, and treatment; and physician diagnosis codes. Information on SI claims is often incomplete; therefore cost data is only reported for SF claims in this analysis.

Claim costs for closed claims reflect actual paid costs. For claims that are not closed, costs reflect actual totals paid to date plus actuarial estimates for future costs associated with the claim. Indirect costs (to the employer and worker, e.g. lost or reduced productivity, employee turnover, and morale) and the administrative costs of managing claims are not included in the claim costs.

All WA WC SF claims are coded for nature, part of body affected, source and secondary source, and event or exposure leading to injury or illness according to the Occupational Injury and Illness Classification System (OIICS) [13] from the information on the RIIOD form. OIICS codes are only assigned at the beginning of a claim, and represent a description of the injury or illness at that point in time.

Each employer is assigned a NAICS 2002 code [14] identifying the firm's industry. NAICS groups 'economic activity' into 20 *sectors* (two digit code), 100 *subsectors*

Table 1 Top 25 NAICS industry groups by prevention index for WA State fund (all sectors, all injury types), 2002-2010

NORA sector	4-digit NAICS (Industry group)	NAICS industry group description	FTE	# Compensable claims (COUNT)	Compensable claim rate/10,000 FTE (RATE)	Median compensable cost	Median days TL	Severity TL (days/10,000 FTE)	Rate rank (All SF)	Count rank (All SF)	Overall SF PI rank
C	2381	Foundation, structure, and building exterior contractors	137,685	9,312	676.3	$13,196	68	161,159	2	3	1
C	2361	Residential building construction	186,292	9,792	525.6	$11,280	57	129,804	10	2	2
C	2383	Building finishing contractors	160,942	8,281	514.5	$13,697	71	136,950	11	4	3
U	4841	General freight trucking	89,627	4,985	556.2	$10,779	55	137,877	8	11	4
C	2382	Building equipment contractors	276,061	12,495	452.6	$17,782	77	105,487	18	1	4
H	6232	Residential mental retardation, mental health and substance abuse facilities	48,764	3,251	666.7	$6,354	33	115,168	3	19	6
A	1133	Logging	35,322	2,642	748.0	$14,347	66	204,306	1	26	7
C	2389	Other specialty trade contractors	123,197	5,456	442.9	$13,214	62	111,986	21	9	8
U	4842	Specialized freight trucking	46,765	2,685	574.2	$9,130	49	116,432	7	25	9
S	**5617**	**Services to buildings and dwellings**	**192,258**	**7,860**	**408.8**	**$7,489**	**43**	**82,849**	**30**	**5**	**10**
H	6231	Nursing care facilities	122,719	4,437	361.6	$6,649	33	63,675	41	12	11
S	**5621**	**Waste collection**	**21,310**	**1,316**	**617.6**	**$7,665**	**34**	**90,504**	**5**	**53**	**12**
M	3219	Other wood product manufacturing	48,441	2,032	419.5	$8,869	30	74,729	26	32	12
C	2373	Highway, street, and bridge construction	45,004	1,880	417.7	$30,101	108	109,069	27	35	14
H	6243	Vocational rehabilitation services	55,612	2,179	391.8	$5,206	28	60,168	35	30	15
C	2371	Utility system construction	57,242	2,147	375.1	$19,443	78	96,020	38	31	16
C	2362	Nonresidential building construction	108,886	3,580	328.8	$25,025	94	72,752	54	16	17
S	**9221**	**Justice, public order, and safety activities**	**137,032**	**4,149**	**302.8**	**$9,360**	**30**	**37,377**	**65**	**13**	**18**
M	3211	Sawmills and wood preservation	26,888	1,131	420.6	$9,902	34	83,822	24	58	19

Table 1 Top 25 NAICS industry groups by prevention index for WA State fund (all sectors, all injury types), 2002-2010 *(Continued)*

S	**8111**	**Automotive repair and maintenance**	**132,964**	**3,730**	**280.5**	**$10,053**	**45**	**65,058**	**73**	**15**	**20**
T	4244	Grocery and related product merchant wholesalers	194,917	5,187	266.1	$9,441	43	48,304	81	10	21
M	3323	Architectural and structural metals manufacturing	45,395	1,572	346.3	$10,914	41	57,173	49	44	22
H	6233	Community care facilities for the elderly	96,742	2,740	283.2	$7,686	39	56,851	71	24	23
U	2213	Water, sewage and other systems	109,958	3,060	278.3	$9,755	26	30,818	74	22	24
S	**5613**	**Employment services**	**245,383**	**6,118**	**249.3**	**$5,687**	**42**	**44,743**	**92**	**8**	**25**

NORA Sector key: *A* = Agriculture, Forestry & Fishing; *C* = Construction; *H* = Healthcare & Social Assistance; *M* = Manufacturing; *S* = Services; *U* = Transportation, Warehousing & Utilities; *T* = Wholesale & Retail Trade.
Services Sector industry groups (bold).
There were 262 NAICS Industry Groups ranked in the PI for All Injury Types (State Fund only).
FTE = (hours/2000); Severity TL = (TL days/10,000 FTE).

(three digit code) and 317 NAICS *industry groups* (four digit code) [14]. The Services Sector, as defined by NORA, is comprised of industries within 11 NAICS Sectors: Information (NAICS 51); Finance and Insurance (NAICS 52); Real Estate, Rental, Leasing (NAICS 53); Professional, Scientific, and Technical (NAICS 54); Management of Companies and Entities (NAICS 55); Administrative Support and Waste Management (NAICS 56); Education (NAICS 61); Arts, Entertainment and Recreations (NAICS 71); Accommodations and Food Services (NAICS 72); Other Services (NAICS 81); and Public Administration (NAICS 92).

In WA, the Services Sector accounted for 48.5% of the SF workforce between 2002 and 2010 [12]. The 2010 BLS Geographic Profile of Employment & Unemployment for Washington State provides percentages of employment by certain industry groups; an estimated 62.2% of the WA workforce in 2010 was employed in the Services Sector (based on aggregate estimates from the industry groups that comprise the Services Sector as defined by NORA) [15].

Data ascertainment

We identified all WC claims within the Services Sector with dates of injury or illness from January 1, 2002 through December 31, 2010. Claims were extracted on December 19, 2012. Data extracted for each claim included claim identification number, claim status (medical only; compensable), OIICS codes for nature, part of body, source, and event or exposure of injury or illness, costs associated with the claim and time loss information. In WA, WC premiums are based on hours of exposure. Employers report hours on a quarterly basis for premium payment. Hours by NAICS industry group were obtained by WC account aggregated over the nine year study period.

A claim is considered a 'compensable' claim if it is categorized by the WC system as a 'compensable', 'kept on salary', 'total permanent disability', 'fatal' or 'loss of earning power' claim. A claim qualifies as 'compensable' if it involves payment for time lost from work. Wage replacement payments for time loss commence on the first missed workday following a three day waiting period which does not include the day of injury.

Injury type

Using OIICS codes, injuries were described by event code (alone or in combination with OIICS nature or body part affected codes and/or ICD-9 codes) and grouped into seven aggregated injury types, which have been described previously [12]. When referring to these aggregated injury type groups in this report, the term "injury type" is used. Claims were analyzed by 7 common injury types that were previously identified as accounting for the majority of compensable claims across all sectors and having significant costs. The injury types were: 1) Work- Related Musculoskeletal Disorders (WMSDs), 2) Fall to Lower Level, 3) Fall on Same Level, 4) Struck By/Against, 5). Caught In/Under/Between, 6) Motor Vehicle, and 7) Overexertion.

Certain injury types were excluded because they each comprised less than 2% of compensable claims (Exposure to Loud Noises; Extreme Temperatures; Bodily Reaction; Abraded; Electrical; Explosion; and Violence). Claims assigned an injury type of 'Other' tend to be poorly defined as 'unclassified/insufficient data', or 'accident type not elsewhere classified', and were also excluded from analysis. SI claims were more frequently coded as 'Other'. The term "All Injury Types" refers to all injuries, outside of categorization by injury types.

Data analysis

Descriptive analyses were conducted on compensable claims. A full time equivalent employee (FTE) was defined as working 2,000 hours per year (40 hours per week for 50 weeks per year). Claim rates are expressed as cases per 10,000 FTE. In some instances, a rate of time loss days (TL) per 10,000 FTE was included as a severity measure.

We utilized a prevention index (PI) to rank industries within the Services Sector for prevention and intervention purposes, by 7 high-cost, common occupational injury types. The PI evaluates the frequency and prevalence of claims within an industry group: claim count - how common are the injuries, and claim incidence rate - how high is the worker risk within that industry. The PI is the average of the rank orders of the claim count and claim incidence rate:

$$PI = \frac{\text{Frequency Rank} + \text{Incidence Rank}}{2}$$

In case of tie, rate rank was used as the tiebreaker. Industry groups that have high counts and rates (higher injury burden) appear higher ranked in the resultant tables than industry groups with lower counts and rates (lower injury burden).

For determination of the PI for each injury type and to avoid unstable estimates, NAICS industry groups were limited to those who had reported hours in 6 or more years of the study period, with ≥45 compensable WC claims over the period of the study and ≥100 FTE per year during the study period, from 2002 to 2010. There were 87 NAICS Service Sector Industry Groups that met the criteria for inclusion for 'All Injury Types.' The top 25 industry groups are presented for 'All Injury Types', and the Top 15 are presented for the remaining injury types.

Results

Overall description (data not shown)

Between 2002–2010 there were 410,006 compensable claims in WA WC data. Of these 410,006 compensable claims, 267,581 were in the State Fund. Compensable claims in the WA SF between 2002–2010 amounted to $9,923,849,314 dollars in direct WC costs.

Seven common, high cost injury types were analyzed – WMSD, Fall to Lower Level, Fall on Same Level, Struck By/Against, Caught In/Under/Between, Motor Vehicle and Overexertion. These 7 injury types account for 86% of all (SF) compensable claims and 89% of all compensable claim costs (SF only). In the Services Sector, these 7 injury types account for 84% of (combined SF and SI) compensable claims in WA.

In the 87 industry groups that met the ranking criteria in the Services Sector, there were 132,673 compensable claims during the study period. There were 85,183 State Fund compensable claims accounting for 15,937,396 days of time loss (TL) with a median cost of $7,753 (mean cost $35,259). There were 47,490 self-insured compensable claims during the study period.

All injury types

Within the study period, there were 87 industry groups (4-digit NAICS) within the Services Sector that met the inclusion criteria for ranking for All Injury Types. The top 5 industry groups ranked for All Injury Types (Table 2) were Executive, Legislative, and Other General Government Support (NAICS 9211); Services to Buildings and Dwellings (NAICS 5617); Waste Collection (NAICS 5621); Justice, Public Order, and Safety Activities (NAICS 9221); and Employment Services (NAICS 5613). These were followed closely (tie for 5th rank) by Automotive Repair and Maintenance (NAICS 8111). These industry groups were consistently ranked in the top 12 by PI for all 7 injury types.

Waste Collection (NAICS 5621) had the highest compensable claim rate per 10,000 FTE for All Injury Types (580.9; Table 2) and the highest severity rate (TL days/10,000 FTE). For SF compensable claims, Remediation and Other Waste Management Services (NAICS 5629) had the highest median cost per compensable claim, $14,560 and highest median time loss (Table 2).

Work-Related Musculoskeletal Disorder (WMSD)

WMSDs (Table 3) account for approximately 41% of compensable claims in the Services Sector, and had the highest compensable claim rates. For WMSD compensable claims, there were 79 industry groups that met the inclusion criteria. Executive, Legislative, and Other General Government Support (NAICS 9211) was ranked the highest for WMSD compensable claims. Waste Collection (NAICS 5621) had the highest compensable claim rate per 10,000 FTE. In SF compensable claims, the highest median compensable claim cost, median days TL, and severity rate were all found in Remediation and Other Waste Management Services (NAICS 5629) (data not shown). Both Waste Collection and Remediation fall in the 3-digit NAICS subsector 562 - Waste Management and Remediation Services. Subsector 811 - Repair and Maintenance, also has several industry groups, including Automotive Repair and Maintenance, ranked in the Top 15 for WMSD.

Fall to lower level

For Fall to Lower Level compensable claims (Table 4), there were 39 industry groups that met the inclusion criteria. The median costs, median days TL, and severity rates were higher in Fall to Lower Level than in the other 6 injury types (data not shown), particularly in Personal and Household Goods Repair and Maintenance (NAICS 8114), which includes workers engaged in repair and maintenance of home and garden equipment, appliances, upholstery and furniture, and footwear and leather goods. Both NAICS 811 - Repair and Maintenance and NAICS 531 - Real Estate, which includes renting/leasing real estate and property management and appraisal services, had multiple industry groups represented in Fall to Lower Level.

Fall on Same Level

For Fall on Same Level (Table 5) compensable claims, there were 50 industry groups that met the inclusion criteria. Services to Buildings and Dwellings (NAICS 5617) was ranked highest overall by PI and for claim rate. NAICS Subsector 722 - Food Services and Drinking Places and NAICS 561 - Administrative and Support Services (which includes Employment Services and Investigative and Security Services) are the subsectors with the most representation in the Top 15 for Fall on Same Level.

Struck By/Against

For Struck By/Against (Table 6) compensable claims, there were 48 industry groups that met the inclusion criteria. Employment Services (NAICS 5613) was ranked the highest for Struck By/Against compensable claims, followed by Services to Buildings and Dwellings (NAICS 5617); these groups are both in the NAICS 561 - Administrative and Support Services subsector. NAICS Subsector 722 - Food Services and Drinking Places was also represented by 3 industry groups in the Top 15.

Fall on Same Level and Struck By/Against are widely distributed, and were the most common occupational injury types following WMSD, making up approximately 13% of compensable claims respectively. These injury

Table 2 Top 15 industry groups by prevention index for all injury types within the services sector in WA (SF + SI), 2002 - 2010

4-digit NAICS (industry group) & industry group description		State fund only			All (State fund + Self insured)					
		Median comp claim cost (SF Only)	Median days TL (SF only)	Severity TL (days/10,000 FTE)	FTE (SF + SI)	# Compensable claims (COUNT) (SF + SI)	Compensable claim rate/10,000 FTE (RATE) (SF + SI)	Count rank (SF + SI)	Rate rank (SF + SI)	PI rank
9211	Executive, legislative, and other general government support	$9,049.00	36	28533.8	655654	24136	368.1	1	4	1
5617	Services to buildings and dwellings	$6,760.00	43	84570	215906	8696	402.8	3	3	2
5621	Waste collection	$6,576.00	34	92058.3	38768	2252	580.9	10	1	3
9221	Justice, public order, and safety activities	$8,618.00	29	38268	137032	4155	303.2	7	8	4
5613	Employment services	$5,031.00	42	45339.6	289788	7315	252.4	6	11	5
8111	Automotive Repair and maintenance	$9,095.00	45	66582.6	132964	3732	280.7	8	9	5
5311	Lessors of real estate	$8,764.00	46	50760.4	78429	1888	240.7	12	12	7
6111	Elementary and secondary schools	$9,596.00	37	20605.4	875087	16169	184.8	2	22	7
7211	Traveler accommodation	$5,792.00	38	43325.8	162269	3497	215.5	9	17	9
7221	Full-Service restaurants	$4,371.00	24	24673	499789	7879	157.6	4	32	10
5629	Remediation and other waste management services	$14,560.00	72	89842.2	95755	1764	184.2	13	23	10
7139	Other amusement and recreation industries	$6,329.00	33	26585.7	120372	2068	171.8	11	26	12
8113	Commercial and industrial machinery and equipment (except automotive and electronic) repair and maintenance	$8,447.00	43	74734.6	27780	876	315.3	31	7	13
7223	Special food services	$6,427.00	37	47563.6	56334	1223	217.1	24	16	14
7112	Spectator sports	$8,258.00	63	77654.1	13226	649	490.7	41	2	15
5622	**Waste treatment and disposal**	**$6,804.00**	**31**	**65461.2**	**13378**	**484**	**361.8**	**45**	**5**	**18**
7222	**Limited-Service eating places**	**$4,578.00**	**27**	**15293.1**	**722327**	**7681**	**106.3**	**5**	**49**	**20**

There were 87 NAICS Industry Groups ranked in the PI for All Injury Types.
FTE = (hours/2000); Severity TL = (TL days/10,000 FTE).
Included are industry groups in the Top 5 by Count or Rate Rank (bold) but not in the Top 15 by Prevention Index.

Table 3 Top 15 industry groups by prevention index for Work-Related Musculoskeletal Disorders (WMSD) within the services sector in WA (SF + SI), 2002 - 2010

4-digit NAICS (industry group) & industry group description		FTE	# Compensable claims (COUNT)	Compensable claim rate/10,000 FTE (RATE)	Count rank	Rate rank	PI rank
9211	Executive, legislative, and other general government support	655,654	10,247	156.3	1	4	1
5617	Services to buildings and dwellings	215,906	3,393	157.2	3	3	2
5621	Waste collection	38,768	1,031	265.9	10	1	3
9221	Justice, public order, and safety activities	137,032	1,735	126.6	7	8	4
5613	Employment services	289,788	3,003	103.6	4	13	5
8111	Automotive repair and maintenance	132,964	1,566	117.8	9	10	6
5311	Lessors of real estate	78,429	846	107.9	11	12	7
7211	Traveler accommodation	162,269	1,574	97.0	8	15	7
6111	Elementary and secondary schools	875,087	6,345	72.5	2	26	9
5629	Remediation and other waste management services	95,755	845	88.2	12	18	10
8121	Personal care services	76,800	690	89.8	16	17	11
7223	Special food services	56,334	522	92.7	23	16	12
8123	Drycleaning and laundry services	32,347	364	112.5	31	11	13
8113	Commercial and industrial machinery and equipment (except automotive and electronic) repair and maintenance	27,780	345	124.2	33	9	13
8114	Personal and household goods repair and maintenance	20,813	301	144.6	38	5	15
7112	**Spectator sports**	**13,226**	**215**	**162.6**	**44**	**2**	**17**
7222	**Limited-service eating places**	**722,327**	**2,897**	**40.1**	**5**	**52**	**23**

There were 79 NAICS Industry Groups ranked in the PI for Work-Related Musculoskeletal Disorders.
FTE = (hours/2000).
Included are industry groups in the Top 5 by Count or Rate Rank (bold) but not in the Top 15 by Prevention Index.

types (Tables 5 and 6) also had the 2nd and 3rd highest numbers of industry groups that met the inclusion criteria (groups that report these injury types regularly).

Caught in/under/between

For Caught In/Under/Between (Table 7) compensable claims, there were 13 industry groups that met the inclusion criteria. Rates and counts for these claims were the lowest among the 7 identified injury types. Employment Services (NAICS 5613) was ranked the highest for Caught/In/Under Between compensable claims overall and by count. Waste Collection (NAICS 5621) ranked the highest by compensable claim rate.

Motor vehicle

For Motor Vehicle (Table 8) compensable claims, there were 20 industry groups that met the inclusion criteria. Executive, Legislative, and Other General Government Support (NAICS 9211) was ranked the highest for Motor Vehicle compensable claims. Automotive Equipment Rental and Leasing (NAICS 5321) had the highest compensable claim rate.

Overexertion

For Overexertion (Table 9) compensable claims, there were 24 industry groups that met the inclusion criteria. Services to Buildings and Dwellings (NAICS 5617) ranked the highest overall. Waste Collection (NAICS 5621) had the highest compensable claim rate. The NAICS 811 subsector - Repair and Maintenance - was highly represented in the Top 15 for Overexertion.

Complete tables of industry group rankings for All Injury Types and each injury type, as well as expanded tables with compensable claim costs, time loss, and severity rates (SF compensable claims data only) are available upon request.

Discussion

Using the PI to rank industry groups within the Services Sector in WA identified industry groups that may most benefit from research and prevention activities. These injury types account for the majority of compensable claims, claims costs, and time loss. Industry groups or subsectors that appear highly ranked by PI across injury types have a higher burden of occupational injury. These

Table 4 Top 15 industry groups by prevention index for fall to lower level within the services sector in WA (SF + SI), 2002 - 2010

4-digit NAICS (industry group) & industry group description		FTE	# Compensable claims (COUNT)	Compensable claim Rate/10,000 FTE (RATE)	Count rank	Rate rank	PI rank
5617	Services to buildings and dwellings	215,906	918	42.5	2	2	1
9211	Executive, legislative, and other general government support	655,654	1,169	17.8	1	10	2
8111	Automotive repair and maintenance	132,964	256	19.3	7	8	3
5311	Lessors of real estate	78,429	186	23.7	11	5	4
5613	Employment services	289,788	464	16.0	4	14	5
5313	Activities related to real estate	110,988	200	18.0	10	9	6
9221	Justice, public order, and safety activities	137,032	236	17.2	8	12	7
5621	Waste collection	38,768	126	32.5	18	4	8
6111	Elementary and secondary schools	875,087	877	10.0	3	20	9
7211	Traveler accommodation	162,269	227	14.0	9	16	10
7139	Other amusement and recreation industries	120,372	171	14.2	12	15	11
8114	Personal and household goods repair and maintenance	20,813	75	36.0	25	3	12
7112	Spectator sports	13,226	69	52.2	28	1	13
5616	Investigation and security services	83,931	135	16.1	16	13	13
5324	Commercial and industrial machinery and equipment rental and leasing	36,810	79	21.5	24	7	15
7222	**Limited-service eating places**	**722,327**	**355**	**4.9**	**5**	**37**	**19**

There were 39 NAICS Industry Groups ranked in the PI for Fall to Lower Level.
FTE = (hours/2000).
Included are industry groups in the Top 5 by Count or Rate Rank (bold) but not in the Top 15 by Prevention Index.

Table 5 Top 15 industry groups by prevention index for fall on same level within the services sector in WA, 2002 - 2010

4-digit NAICS (industry group) & industry group description		FTE	# Compensable claims (COUNT)	Compensable claim rate/10,000 FTE (RATE)	Count rank	Rate rank	PI rank
5617	Services to buildings and dwellings	215,906	1,006	46.6	5	1	1
7211	Traveler accommodation	162,269	617	38.0	6	4	2
9211	Executive, legislative, and other general government support	655,654	2,180	33.2	2	8	2
6111	Elementary and secondary schools	875,087	2,629	30.0	1	10	4
9221	Justice, public order, and safety activities	137,032	536	39.1	8	3	4
7221	Full-service restaurants	499,789	1,526	30.5	3	9	6
7139	Other amusement and recreation industries	120,372	361	30.0	9	11	7
7223	Special food services	56,334	193	34.3	18	6	8
5621	Waste collection	38,768	160	41.3	23	2	9
8111	Automotive repair and maintenance	132,964	324	24.4	10	16	10
5613	Employment services	289,788	597	20.6	7	20	11
5616	Investigation and security services	83,931	206	24.5	15	15	12
5313	Activities related to real estate	110,988	235	21.2	12	18	12
5311	Lessors of real estate	78,429	204	26.0	16	14	12
7222	Limited-service eating places	722,327	1,329	18.4	4	26	12
5321	**Automotive equipment rental and leasing**	**25,744**	**93**	**36.1**	**34**	**5**	**17**

There were 50 NAICS Industry Groups ranked in the PI for Fall on Same Level. SF Data not shown for SF industry groups that do not meet the inclusion criteria alone (without the addition of SI data).
FTE = (hours/2000).
Included are industry groups in the Top 5 by Count or Rate Rank (bold) but not in the Top 15 by Prevention Index.

Table 6 Top 15 industry groups by prevention index for struck by/against within the services sector in WA, 2002 - 2010

4-digit NAICS (industry group) & industry group description		FTE	# Compensable claims (COUNT)	Compensable claim rate/10,000 FTE (RATE)	Count rank	Rate rank	PI rank
5613	Employment services	289,788	1,515	52.3	4	5	1
5617	Services to buildings and dwellings	215,906	1,363	63.1	5	4	1
9211	Executive, legislative, and other general government support	655,654	2,222	33.9	1	12	3
5621	Waste collection	38,768	274	70.7	11	2	3
8111	Automotive repair and maintenance	132,964	651	49.0	7	8	5
7221	Full-service restaurants	499,789	1,537	30.8	3	14	6
8113	Commercial and industrial machinery and equipment (except automotive and electronic) repair and maintenance	27,780	185	66.6	16	3	7
5311	Lessors of real estate	78,429	269	34.3	13	10	8
9221	Justice, public order, and safety activities	137,032	382	27.9	9	16	9
7211	Traveler accommodation	162,269	430	26.5	8	17	9
7112	Spectator sports	13,226	134	101.3	26	1	11
6111	Elementary and secondary schools	875,087	1,681	19.2	2	25	11
7139	Other amusement and recreation industries	120,372	305	25.3	10	19	13
7223	Special food services	56,334	184	32.7	17	13	14
7224	Drinking places (alcoholic beverages)	67,862	199	29.3	15	15	14

There were 48 NAICS Industry Groups ranked in the PI for Struck By/Against.
FTE = (hours/2000).

injuries can be personally devastating and are associated with high costs, both in direct workers' compensation claim costs and time loss wage replacement, and in costs to the worker, employer, health-care systems, and society. Several industry groups were consistently ranked highly (Table 10) across injury types, indicating that they warrant priority focus in overall injury prevention, including: Services to Buildings and Dwellings (NAICS 5617), Executive, Legislative, and Other General Government Support (NAICS 9211), Waste Collection (NAICS 5621), Employment Services (NAICS 5613) and Automotive Repair and Maintenance (NAICS 8111).

Table 7 Industry groups by prevention index for caught in/under/between within the services sector in WA, 2002 - 2010

4-digit NAICS (industry group) & industry group description		FTE	# Compensable claims (COUNT)	Compensable claim rate/10,000 FTE (RATE)	Count rank	Rate rank	PI rank
5613	Employment services	289,788	422	14.6	1	2	1
5617	Services to buildings and dwellings	215,906	243	11.3	3	3	2
9211	Executive, legislative, and other general government support	655,654	347	5.3	2	6	3
5621	Waste collection	38,768	71	18.3	8	1	4
8111	Automotive repair and maintenance	132,964	135	10.2	5	4	4
6111	Elementary and secondary schools	875,087	226	2.6	4	10	6
5111	Newspaper, periodical, book, and directory publishers	82,937	64	7.7	10	5	7
9221	Justice, public order, and safety activities	137,032	68	5.0	9	7	8
7222	Limited-service eating places	722,327	134	1.9	6	12	9
7221	Full-service restaurants	499,789	115	2.3	7	11	9
7139	Other amusement and recreation industries	120,372	55	4.6	11	8	11
7211	Traveler accommodation	162,269	52	3.2	12	9	12
5413	Architectural, engineering, and related services	262,812	46	1.8	13	13	13

There were 13 NAICS Industry Groups ranked in the PI for Caught In/Under/Between. SF Data not shown for SF industry groups that do not meet the inclusion criteria alone (without the addition of SI data).
FTE = (hours/2000).

Table 8 Top 15 industry groups by prevention index for motor vehicles within the services sector in WA SF, 2002 - 2010

4-digit NAICS (industry group) & industry group description		FTE	# Compensable claims (COUNT)	Compensable claim rate/10,000 FTE (RATE)	Count rank	Rate rank	PI rank
9211	Executive, legislative, and other general government support	655,654	1,367	20.8	1	3	1
5617	Services to buildings and dwellings	215,906	417	19.3	3	4	2
5621	Waste collection	38,768	96	24.8	8	2	3
9221	Justice, public order, and safety activities	137,032	172	12.6	4	6	3
5321	Automotive equipment rental and leasing	25,744	75	29.1	11	1	5
5616	Investigation and security services	83,931	98	11.7	6	7	6
6111	Elementary and secondary schools	875,087	436	5.0	2	12	7
8111	Automotive repair and maintenance	132,964	93	7.0	9	9	8
9261	Administration of economic program	50,494	67	13.3	13	5	8
5614	Business support services	168,586	78	4.6	10	13	10
7222	Limited-service eating places	722,327	166	2.3	5	18	10
5613	Employment services	289,788	97	3.3	7	16	10
9241	Administration of environmental quality programs	50,862	48	9.4	17	8	13
8129	Other personal services	90,669	51	5.6	16	10	14
5111	Newspaper, periodical, book, and directory publishers	82,937	46	5.5	18	11	15

There were 20 NAICS Industry Groups ranked in the PI for Motor Vehicle. SF Data not shown for SF industry groups that do not meet the inclusion criteria alone (without the addition of SI data).
FTE = (hours/2000).

Table 9 Top 15 industry groups by prevention index for overexertion within the services sector in WA, 2002 - 2010

4-digit NAICS (industry group) & industry group description		FTE	# Compensable claims (COUNT)	Compensable claim rate/10,000 FTE (RATE)	Count rank	Rate rank	PI rank
5617	Services to buildings and dwellings	215,906	357	16.5	3	4	1
9211	Executive, legislative, and other general government support	655,654	807	12.3	1	7	2
5621	Waste collection	38,768	111	28.6	9	1	3
5613	Employment services	289,788	353	12.2	4	8	4
8111	Automotive repair and maintenance	132,964	213	16.0	7	5	4
6111	Elementary and secondary schools	875,087	574	6.6	2	13	6
5311	Lessors of real estate	78,429	106	13.5	11	6	7
7211	Traveler accommodation	162,269	126	7.8	8	11	8
9221	Justice, public order, and safety activities	137,032	108	7.9	10	10	9
7221	Full-service restaurants	499,789	273	5.5	5	17	10
5313	Activities related to real estate	110,988	82	7.4	12	12	11
8113	Commercial and industrial machinery and equipment (except automotive and electronic) repair and maintenance	27,780	48	17.3	22	3	12
8114	Personal and household goods repair and maintenance	20,813	45	21.6	24	2	13
7223	Special food services	56,334	57	10.1	17	9	13
7222	Limited-service eating places	722,327	221	3.1	6	21	15

There were 24 NAICS Industry Groups ranked in the PI for Overexertion. SF Data not shown for SF industry groups that do not meet the inclusion criteria alone (without the addition of SI data).
FTE = (hours/2000).

Table 10 Top 15 services sector industry groups that were highest ranked by prevention index for 7 common injury types, WA, 2002 - 2010

4-digit NAICS (industry group) & industry group description		Average of PI ranks
5617	Services to buildings and dwellings*	1.6
9211	Executive, legislative, and other general government support*	2.1
5621	Waste collection*	4.9
5613	Employment services*	5.6
8111	Automotive repair and maintenance*	6.0
9221	Justice, public order, and safety activities*	6.6
6111	Elementary and secondary schools*	7.6
7211	Traveler accommodation	7.7
5311	Lessors of real estate	8.0
9261	Administration of economic program	9.0
5616	Investigation and security services	10.7
7223	Special food services	12.0
7221	Full service restaurants*	12.3
8113	Commercial and industrial machinery and equipment (except automotive and electronic) repair and maintenance	12.3
5313	Activities related to real estate	13.2
7139	**Other amusement and recreation industries***	**14.3**
7222	**Limited service eating places***	**15.9**

*Indicates that industry group was ranked in the Top 25 overall and for all seven injury types.
Included are industry groups (bold) not in the Top 15, but ranked in the Top 25 overall and for all seven injury types.

Services to Buildings and Dwellings (NAICS 5617) was ranked in the top 2 in all 7 injury types (Tables 3, 4, 5, 6, 7, 8 and 9) and ranked highest by average of PI ranks (Table 10). Workers in this industry group are at high risk for occupational injury across the board and would benefit substantially from injury prevention and safety improvements. The Services to Buildings and Dwellings industry group includes: Exterminating and Pest Control Services, Janitorial Services, Landscaping Services, Carpet and Upholstery Cleaning Services, and Other Services to Buildings and Dwellings (e.g. chimney cleaning, drain cleaning). These workers may encounter multiple hazards, work alone, or work with hazardous tools or chemicals. They may also face low wages, and other job stresses in addition to risks for a variety of occupational injuries and illnesses [16]. Workers in Services to Buildings and Dwellings also reported the greatest number of occupational traumatic injury fatalities of industry groups within the NORA Services Sector during 2003–2007 [5]. Services to Buildings and Dwellings has been previously identified in WA [2,12] as a high-risk industry group, and continued high rankings across injury types establish it as a group in need of prevention and intervention efforts.

Employment Services (NAICS 5613) includes establishments that provide staff or refer and/or place applicants, where work activities and control over workplace hazards is generally the responsibility of the hiring employer, but the workers compensation liability rests with the temporary agency. Temporary Help workers have been previously identified by WA as a group in need of research and prevention efforts, due to increased injury rates [17-19]. In the same NAICS Subsector (561), Investigative and Security Services (NAICS 5616), was also highly ranked by average of PI scores across injury types (Table 10) and was at high risk for Fall injuries and for Motor Vehicle incidents.

Two industry groups from NAICS 562 - Waste Management and Remediation Services, a subsector engaged in local hauling of waste materials, operating materials recovery facilities (including sorting), and providing remediation (cleaning contaminated buildings, mines, soil, water) and septic services, were identified as being especially high-risk for common and costly injuries. Waste Collection (NAICS 5621) had the highest rate and severity rate for All Injury Types and was consistently ranked highly (Table 10), especially by rate, for prevention efforts in each of the identified injury types. Waste Collection has been identified previously and is already targeted for research and prevention efforts in WA [12,20], which identified WMSDs as a primary injury type for the waste management industry and 'Containers' as the most common source of injury [20]. Both Waste Collection and Remediation and Other Waste Management Services, along with another in this subsector, Waste Treatment and Disposal (NAICS 5622), have also been identified in the top 5 Services Sector Industry Groups by average annual DAFW rates [5].

Automotive Repair and Maintenance (NAICS 8111), which includes body shops and collision repair work, was ranked highly across all 7 injury types and was ranked 5th overall by average PI rank (Table 10). Collision repair shops, in addition to ranking highly for these seven occupational injury types, have been previously identified in WA for occupational respiratory illness (isocyanates asthma) prevention activities [21].

Additional industry groups may be targeted by specific injury type(s), such as Fall to Lower Level, which remains a leading cause of injury. A study of occupational ladder fall injuries (using the Bureau of Labor Statistics Survey of Occupational Injuries and Illnesses (SOII) data) reported that 29% of workers with occupational ladder fall injuries were in a Services industry [22]. Fall on Same Level injuries are also widespread in the Services sector. Accommodation and Food Services workers (NAICS 72, included in the NORA Services Sector) experienced the highest number of falls over a five-year period and had higher Fall on Same Level rates than the construction industry based on United States Bureau of Labor Statistics data [23]. Fall to Lower Level and Fall on Same Level together accounted for approximately 20% of compensable claims in the WA Services Sector between 2002–2010.

Subsectors NAICS 562 - Waste Management and Remediation and NAICS 811 - Repair and Maintenance, have several industry groups in the Top 15 for WMSDs (Table 3), and Repair and Maintenance is also highly represented in the Top 15 for Overexertion (Table 9). WMSDs and Overexertion can be caused or aggravated by work exposures and activities such as material handling, awkward postures, and repetitive or forceful exertions; prevention efforts in industry groups in these subsectors should be directed towards reducing such exposures.

Another factor in the health of Services Sector workers is that many of these jobs are low or minimum wage work. Data from the Bureau of Labor Statistics (BLS) in 2012 show that the industry with the highest proportion of hourly paid workers at or below the federal minimum wage was "Leisure and Hospitality" [24] which would include workers in NAICS 72 - Accommodation and Food Services and 71 - Arts, Entertainment, and Recreation. Five industry groups that are high-ranking across injury types by average PI (Table 10) are found in NAICS 71–72. A study of low socio-economic status (SES) workers found that they reported more chronic diseases, increased risk behaviors, and worse health; were disproportionately younger, single, non-white and Spanish speaking; and clustered in low-wage industries, two of which are Services Sector industries - Accommodation and Food Services and Administrative and Waste Services [25]. In the same study, half of Services Sector industries had median annual wages below $35,000 in 2008; including: Accommodation and Food Services; Arts, Entertainment, and Recreation; Administrative and Waste Services; Other Services; and Real Estate and Rental and Leasing [25]. Using BLS Occupational Employment Wage Estimates from May 2010, for median hourly wage and mean annual wage for the U.S. (national, all occupations) [26] compared with those industries in the Service Sector [27], this pattern remained. Industry groups from these sectors - Accommodation and Food Services, Arts, Entertainment, and Recreation, Administrative and Waste Services, Other Services, and Real Estate and Rental and Leasing - made up the majority of industry groups that were highly ranked for prevention across injury types (Table 10); only 4 industry groups (3 from NAICS 92 - Public Administration, and one from NAICS 61 - Educational Services) were from industry sectors with higher median hourly/mean annual wages. Accommodation and Food Services includes workers in Traveler Accommodation (NAICS 7221) which was also ranked highly by PI across several injury types (Table 10). Traveler Accommodation includes Hotels and Motels, Casino Hotels, and Other Traveler Accommodations (bed and breakfast inns, guest houses, cabins and cottages, tourist homes, hostels). Hotel workers in particular, have been identified as having higher injury rates, especially for females, housekeepers, and those of Hispanic ethnicity [28]. These jobs have also been found to be associated with cleaning tasks and high physical effort (strain, muscle load, postures, repetitive movement), low wages and low job control, among other risks [28]. Workers in Services to Buildings and Dwellings who may face similar risks include Janitors and Cleaners and Landscaping workers.

While many industries in the Services Sector have much higher median hourly and mean annual wages, these industries are not as strongly represented in the PI rankings for work-related injuries in WA. Low socioeconomic status is also associated with job insecurity and work organization hazards [29]. In contrast, those ranked lowest by PI (data not shown) for All Injury Types were clustered in the Finance and Insurance, Information, and Professional, Scientific, and Technical Services industries, which were among the industries with the highest reported wages in the Services Sector, according to the 2010 BLS data [27].

There are relatively few studies in the literature that rank industries by some measure of risk, count or cost of occupational injury and illness. A previous study [3] ranking industries (using Standard Industrial Classification System (SIC) codes [30]) for estimated high-cost fatal and non-fatal injuries and illnesses in the United States identified many industries similar to the findings in the WA Services Sector: including Services to Buildings, Personnel Supply Services, and Automotive Repair Shops. Okun et al. [4] used a 'risk index score' and also identified (by SIC code) landscape and horticultural services (SIC 078), which may be comparable to some workers in NAICS 5617 Services to Buildings and Dwellings (e.g. NAICS 561730 Landscaping Services). However, the study's difference in classification system and the restriction to 'small-business' makes comparison difficult.

A recent study characterizing occupational injuries, illnesses and fatalities in Services Sector workers [5] using BLS data had results that were similar to the WA data. Industry groups were ranked by average annual rank of Days-Away-From-Work (DAFW) Injury Rates (for several years), and identified similar industry groups. The five highest ranked industry groups by DAFW were NAICS 5621 Waste Collection, 5622 Waste Treatment and Disposal, 5323 General Rental Centers, 5617 Services to Buildings and Dwellings, and 5629 Remediation and Other Waste Management [5]. The same study [5] also used a PI to rank Services Sector industry groups combining DAFW Injury and Illness Counts and Rates, and identified 5617 Services to Buildings and Dwellings and 5621 Waste Collection, ranked 1st and 3rd, respectively.

The PI results represent a portion of the data, and the difference between individual ranks does not reflect the magnitude of the actual difference in count or rate between industry groups. The difference between individual ranks is of less importance than which industry groups are consistently ranked highly (demonstrating higher burden of injury).

The particular combination of compensable claim rate and rank may suggest different prevention activities for the industry or industries at risk and facilitate decision making as to the approach for allocation of prevention resources. For example, in the WMSD PI (Table 3), Services to Buildings and Dwellings (NAICS 5617) has a high rate rank and high count rank, which indicates that it is a large, hazardous industry group that could benefit from an intensive multi-faceted approach using every available resource (consultation, enforcement, and education). In the same table (Table 3), Elementary and Secondary Schools (NAICS 6111) has the largest number of FTEs and is ranked 2nd for compensable claims but has one of the lower compensable claims rates of all the industry groups that met the inclusion criteria for this injury type. High count rank but low rate rank may indicate a large, but less hazardous, industry, with claims scattered across a large number of workplaces and it is unlikely that any single workplace has high risk; therefore, the industry group may be more suited to an education campaign in order to reach the large number of workplaces and employees. Conversely, smaller industry groups with low count but high rate, such as Waste Treatment and Disposal (NAICS 5622, Table 3) may be hazardous industries with concentrated risk; a focused inspection/consultation may be an effective approach. Industry groups with low claim count and low claim rate likely need minimal prevention resources or efforts, with injury and illness surveillance for any emerging hazards. Business size may also influence strategies for prevention, as employer size varies considerably in the Services Sector. Large organizations may have more resources to devote to occupational injury prevention, while small businesses may benefit from collaboration with intermediary organizations to help develop and spread health and safety interventions [31].

Several of the limitations associated with this PI methodology and the use of WC data have been previously discussed [2]. Generalizability of results is limited by the varying statutes of workers' compensation in the United States, as well as by variations in industry distribution. Another limitation to this report is that the injury and illness rates reported in this study are dependent on the completeness of reporting of cases and employee work hours to the WC system. These may be incomplete for a variety of reasons (e.g. employer reporting practices, fear of retribution, administrative barriers, or the use of alternative medical insurance providers). The extent of underreporting to the WA WC system is unknown. Additionally, data coding in large administrative databases such as the WA WC system is not always complete or accurate and there is a chance for miscoding (for example, OIICS coding takes place at the initial assessment of the claim, and the injury or illness may be poorly defined on the initial claim form, and thus the coding may not reflect the true nature of the injury or illness associated with the claim). Future efforts to rank industry groups for prevention and intervention activities may include other elements (an expanded PI approach) such as severity measures based on TL and cost data, to better capture the magnitude of the burden of injury.

PI rankings provide evidence as to where research and prevention efforts can be most effectively targeted for maximum benefit in reducing common and costly injuries. Ranking industries by PI overall and by specific injury types provides data to prioritize industry groups, guide prevention efforts, and inform the setting of policy and research agendas that reflect the particular needs of workers in industry groups within the Services Sector.

Competing interests

The authors declare that they have no competing interests.

Authors' contributions

All authors conceived of the study and participated in its design and coordination, and helped to draft the manuscript. DA and NA participated in data acquisition, management, and analysis. NA and DB participated in the interpretation and presentation of results and discussion. All authors read and approved the final manuscript.

Acknowledgements

This research was supported in part by Grant Number 5U60OH008487 from CDC – NIOSH. Its contents are solely the responsibility of the authors and do not necessarily represent the official views of NIOSH or the Centers for Disease Control and Prevention. The authors wish to thank Christina Rappin and Caroline Smith, MPH for their assistance in reviewing the manuscript.

References

1. U.S. Department of Labor, Bureau of Labor Statistics (BLS): **Survey of Occupational Injury and Illness (SOII).** [http://www.bls.gov/iif/]. Last accessed: August 1, 2014.
2. Bonauto D, Silverstein B, Adams D, Foley M: **Prioritizing industries for occupational injury and illness prevention and research, Washington State Workers' Compensation Claims, 1999–2003.** *J Occup Environ Med* 2006, **48**(8):840–851.
3. Leigh JP, Waehrer G, Miller TR, Keenan C: **Costs of occupational injury and illness across industries.** *Scand J Work Environ Health* 2004, **30**(3):199–205.
4. Okun A, Lentz TJ, Schulte P, Stayner L: **Identifying high-risk small business industries for occupational safety and health interventions.** *Am J Ind Med* 2001, **39**(3):301–311.
5. Utterback D, Charles L, Schnorr T, Tiesman H, Storey E, Vossenas P: **Occupational injuries, illnesses, and fatalities among workers in the services sector industries: 2003 to 2007.** *J Occup Environ Med* 2012, **54**(1):31–41.

6. **National Occupational Research Agenda (NORA).** [http://www.cdc.gov/niosh/nora/default.html]. Last accessed: August 1, 2014
7. **National Institute for Occupational Safety and Health (NIOSH).** [http://www.cdc.gov/niosh/]. Last accessed: August 1, 2014
8. United States Census Bureau: **North American Industrial Classification System (NAICS), FAQs.** [http://www.census.gov/eos/www/naics/faqs/faqs.html#q1]. Last accessed: August 1, 2014
9. National Occupational Research Agenda (NORA): **NORA Sector Programs.** [http://www.cdc.gov/niosh/nora/sectorprograms.html]. Last accessed: August 1, 2014
10. National Institute for Occupational Safety and Health (NIOSH): **Program Portfolio: Services: Sector Description.** [http://www.cdc.gov/niosh/programs/pps/]. Last accessed: August 1, 2014
11. Biddle EA: **Is the societal burden of fatal occupational injury different among NORA industry sectors?** *J Safety Res* 2013, **44**:7–16.
12. Anderson N, Bonauto D, Adams D: **Prioritizing Industries for Occupational Injury and Illness Prevention and Research, Washington State Workers' Compensation Claims Data, 2002–2010.** Washington State Department of Labor & Industries. Technical Report #64-1-2013. [http://www.lni.wa.gov/Safety/Research/Files/bd_3F.pdf]. Last accessed: August 1, 2014
13. U.S. Department of Labor, Bureau of Labor Statistics (BLS): *Occupational Injury and Illness Classification (OIICS) Manual.* 2007.
14. Executive Office of the President, Office of Management and Budget (OMB): **North American Industrial Classification System (NAICS), 2002 NAICS Sector Structure.** [http://www.census.gov/cgi-bin/sssd/naics/naicsrch?chart=2002.] Last accessed: August 1, 2014
15. U.S. Department of Labor, Bureau of Labor Statistics (BLS): **Geographic Profile of Employment and Unemployment, 2010. Table 20. States: percent distribution of employed persons by industry, sex, race, and Hispanic or Latino ethnicity, 2010 annual averages.** [http://www.bls.gov/opub/gp/laugp.htm]. Last accessed: August 1, 2014
16. Charles L, Loomis D, Demissie Z: **Occupational hazards experienced by cleaning workers and janitors: a review of the epidemiologic literature.** *Work* 2009, **34**:105–116.
17. Smith C, Silverstein B, Bonauto D, Adams D, Fan Z: **Temporary workers in Washington State.** *Am J Ind Med* 2010, **53**(2):135–145.
18. Foley M: **Flexible work, hazardous work: the impact of temporary work arrangements on occupational safety and health in Washington State, 1991–1999.** *Res Hum Cap Dev* 1998, **12**:123–147.
19. Foley M, Ruser J, Shor G, Shuford H, Sygnatur E: **Contingent workers: workers' compensation data analysis strategies and limitations.** *Am J Ind Med* 2014, **57**:764–775.
20. Rauser E, Foley M, Bonauto DK, Edwards SK, Spielholz P, Silverstein B: **Preventing Injuries in the Trucking Industry: Focus Report 199–2005.** Washington State Department of Labor & Industries. Technical Report #90-17-2008. [http://www.lni.wa.gov/Safety/Research/Files/Trucking/PreventingTruckingInjuries.pdf]. Last accessed: August 1, 2014
21. Whittaker SG, Reeb-Whitaker C: **Characterizing the health and safety needs of the collision repair industry.** *J Occup Environ Hyg* 2009, **6**(5):273–282.
22. Socias CM, Chaumont Menéndez CK, Collins JW, Simeonov P: **Occupational ladder fall injuries - United States, 2011.** *MMWR* 2014, **63**(16):341–346.
23. Yeoh HT, Lockhart TE, Wu X: **Non-fatal occupational falls on the same level.** *Ergonomics* 2013, **56**(2):153–165.
24. U.S. Department of Labor, Bureau of Labor Statistics (BLS). 2013. **Labor Force Statistics from the Current Population Survey - Characteristics of Minimum Wage Workers: 2012.** [http://www.bls.gov/cps/minwage2012.htm]. Last accessed: August 6, 2014
25. Harris JR, Huang Y, Hannon PA, Williams B: **Low-socioeconomic status workers: their health risks and how to reach them.** *J Occup Environ Med* 2011, **53**(2):132–138.
26. U.S. Department of Labor, Bureau of Labor Statistics (BLS). **Occupational Employment Statistics - May 2010 National Occupational Employment and Wage Estimates - United States.** [http://www.bls.gov/oes/2010/may/oes_nat.htm]. Last accessed: August 6, 2014
27. U.S. Department of Labor, Bureau of Labor Statistics (BLS). **Occupational Employment Statistics - May 2010 National Industry-Specific Occupational Employment and Wage Estimates.** [http://www.bls.gov/oes/2010/may/oessrci.htm#00]. Last accessed: August 6, 2014
28. Buchanan S, Vossenas P, Krause N, Moriarty J, Frumin E, Shimek JM, Mirer F, Orris P, Punnett L: **Occupational injury disparities in the US hotel industry.** *Am J Ind Med* 2010, **53**:116–125.
29. Landsbergis PA, Grzywacz JG, LaMontagne AD: **Work organization, job insecurity, and occupational health disparities.** *Am J Ind Med* 2014, **57**:495–515.
30. Occupational Safety and Health Administration (OSHA): **Standard Industrial Classification System (SIC) Manual.** [https://www.osha.gov/pls/imis/sic_manual.html]. Last accessed: August 1, 2014
31. Sinclair RC, Cunningham TR, Schulte PA: **A model for occupational safety and health intervention diffusion to small businesses.** *Am J Ind Med* 2013, **56**:1442–1451.

18

Job-related stress and work ability of dispatchers in a metropolitan fire department

Marcus Oldenburg[1*†], Dennis Wilken[2†], Ralf Wegner[1], Bernd Poschadel[1] and Xaver Baur[3]

Abstract

Background: Our aim was to assess psychomental stress and strain among dispatchers in fire departments, particularly during emergency instructions by phone and to evaluate their work ability.

Methods: 27 dispatchers and 20 controls were examined. In a protocol, participants recorded 1. phone instructions causing mental stress (event) 2. working time without phone instructions (non-event) 3. breaks. Continuous heart rate (variability), urine catecholamine, salivary cortisol and lymphocytes were measured. To assess the job-related burden, the Work Ability Index (WAI) was applied.

Results: Dispatchers demonstrated significantly higher heart rates and reduced standard deviation of all NN (heartbeat-to-heartbeat) intervals (SDNN) than the controls in all phases. WAI of dispatchers was significantly lower than that of the controls. Within the dispatchers, there was a significantly higher rate of inability to work during the past year.

Conclusions: The increased heart rate and reduced SDNN of examined dispatchers indicate chronic stress effects as a possible preliminary stage of a health disorder. In respect of the reduced work ability among dispatchers preventive measures are required to reduce the stress situation during their job-performance.

Keywords: Dispatchers, Emergency call, Stress and strain at the workplace, Work ability

Background

It has repeatedly been shown that emergency service personnel (such as fire fighters, policemen and dispatchers) experience more job-related stress than non-emergency workers [1,2]. Thus, it is assumed that this kind of stress can affect their social, psychological and emotional life [3].

The studies on fire fighters' workload mainly investigated the physical strain arising from the exposure to various noxious substances during different services with a focus on respiratory diseases [4,5]. But the psychological strain experienced by fire fighters also progressively moved into the focus of medical interest. Many studies deal with post-traumatic stress disorders as a result of fire-brigade operations and with the opportunities for prevention. In 1993, Boxer and Wild (1993) reported that between 33% and 51% of examined fire fighters were experiencing significant psychological distress [6].

Dispatchers in mixed emergency and fire systems of fire departments are involved at the beginning of the rescue chain. They play a key role in allocating the right resource to patients in emergencies and they must communicate vital information during critical phases of operations. Errors in communications, for example, a wrong treatment priority, will compromise safe and effective patient care. Dispatchers' failures may lead to a delay in care and may contribute to the patient's death [7]. Therefore, although the dispatchers are not at the forefront of the "hands on" rescue, they bear high work-related responsibility.

Dispatchers often use specific instruction protocols or computerized call-taking systems which can increase the sensitivity for detecting cardiac arrest, as an example, to 77% and the specificity to 99% [8]. In dispatcher-directed cardiopulmonary resuscitation (CPR), the same dispatcher who receives the emergency call not only co-ordinates the dispatch of professional rescuers (e.g. fire and/or police and emergency medical services), but is

* Correspondence: marcus.oldenburg@bgv.hamburg.de
†Equal contributors
[1]Institute for Occupational and Maritime Medicine, Hamburg State Department for Health and Consumer Protection, ZfAM, University Medical Center Hamburg-Eppendorf, Seewartenstrasse10, D-20459 Hamburg, Germany
Full list of author information is available at the end of the article

also trained to remain on the telephone and verbally assist bystanders with the initiation of early CPR. The dispatcher-assisted telephone CPR instructions are proven to increase survival rates as the chances of survival from cardiac arrest depend on early diagnosis and prompt initiation of CPR including defibrillation. A recent study revealed a three-month survival rate of 5% when a cardiac arrest was not recognized by the dispatchers as compared to 14% when it was recognized (p = 0.04) [9]. Dispatchers' failure to identify a cardiac arrest was largely caused by deviation from their instruction protocol [10].

The high proportion of technical components and the need for rapid information processing are special work demands placed on dispatchers in fire departments. In total, the mental stress and strain experienced by dispatchers in emergency centres and its impact on their personal health have not been investigated so far.

The aim of this study was to assess the psychomental stress and strain among dispatchers in fire departments, particularly during emergency instructions by phone, and to evaluate their work ability.

Based on the literature, it is assumed that dispatchers experience a higher stress level (compared to the reference group) - especially due to their emergency instructions by phone call. As described in several studies, a relevant high stress level can lead to an elevation in biometric stress parameters (such as heart rate or clinical laboratory indices) and may increase the risk for work disability [11-13]. According to a review on work-related stressors and strain, it was concluded that both subjective aspects and objective indices (from physical examinations) are required to assess the level of strain and to promote mental health [14].

Methods

Participants

In the present cross-sectional study, the employees from a control centre of a metropolitan fire department were examined in the time period from October 2009 to April 2010. They were responsible for 1.8 million inhabitants.

The study cohort comprised all dispatchers from this fire department who worked full time in rotating shifts. They were former fire fighters who performed an additional training to coordinate and provide appropriate phone instructions for first aid. The dispatchers worked in a mixed emergency and fire system; that means, after dialing 112, the Europe-wide emergency phone number, the public can reach the different emergency services (ambulances, fire and rescue service and the police). In 2002, on average 540 deployments per day were recorded in this fire department and increased to more than 700 per day six years later.

A total of 27 male dispatchers were included in the study and represented 100% of all available dispatchers in this control centre. 20 of 22 available persons (91%) who work at the same fire department agreed to serve as an internal control group. These fire fighters are performing administrative and coordinating tasks e.g. planning fire protection concepts for public buildings or rescue scenarios for major events. Others are responsible for the controlling of human and financial resources. As these controls just like dispatchers mainly perform tasks as office workers by using a computer and a telephone and doing this also without high physical activity (mainly in a sitting position), they appear as a suitable reference group.

All study participants were informed about the content and procedure of the study, the pseudonymized data analysis and the possibility of withdrawing from the study at any time. Prior to the examination all employees gave their written informed consent for participation in this voluntary study. None of the office participants withdrew their participation during the study period. The ethical review board of the Institute for Occupational and Maritime Medicine approved this study.

General questionnaire

Medical history

A detailed general and workplace-specific medical history was taken and one clinically experienced physician examined thoroughly each employee to rule out that diseases could affect the results.

Phase protocol

In several studies, the most demanding fire fighting and rescue tasks of emergency workers in fire departments were explored by means of questionnaires [15]. According to these studies, experiences such as hearing that children are in burning buildings, carrying out victims, fire suppression, resuscitation, catastrophic injury to self or co-workers were classified as heavy psycho-mental load [6,16].

All participants kept a log of events, non-events and breaks in phase protocols during each shift. Among dispatchers, an event was defined as an incoming emergency call characterized by

- Tasks that were objectively or subjectively perceived as psychologically stressful (in line with the above mentioned statements about most demanding rescue tasks), and/or
- Callers who were more difficult (because of language problems, aggression or hysteria).

In administrative workers, events were all situations that they perceived as stressful (e.g. conflicts with colleagues, problems with customers).

Instruments

The instruments we used to evaluate the theoretical construct of the study are listed in Table 1.

Mental/ physical strain

Physical strain

The participants' heart rate was continuously monitored and recorded by the portable telemetric beat-to-beat recorder Polar RS 800 with 1000 Hz sampling rate (Polar Electro, Oy-Kempele, Finland). This device was validated for the accurate measurement of NN intervals and for the purpose of the analysis of HRV [17]. As parameters of physical strain, the heart rate variability (HRV), the standard deviation of all NN intervals (SDNN) and the ratio of low- to high frequency power (LF/HF) were calculated. The NN intervals were visually inspected for artefacts. Occasional ectopic beats were identified and replaced with interpolated NN interval values (less than 1% of the data). HRV analyses were performed with Kubios HRV Version 2.

To assess the participants' energy expenditure, the SenseWear™ Armband (SWA) (BodyMedia, Inc. Pittsburgh, Pennsylvania) was used [18,19]. This is a physical activity and lifestyle monitor that objectively measures free-living energy balance [20,21]. The armband worn on the right upper arm utilized a 2-axis accelerometer, heat flux sensor, galvanic skin response sensor, skin temperature sensor and a near-body ambient temperature sensor to gather data about the activity and energy expenditure.

This device calculates energy expenditure, expressed as the metabolic equivalent of task (MET). This parameter reflects the energy cost of physical activities and is defined as the ratio of metabolic rate during a specific physical activity to a reference metabolic rate. 1 MET is considered as the resting metabolic rate obtained during quiet sitting. MET values of activities range from 0.9 (sleeping) to 18 (marathons).

Both the heart rate monitor and armband were attached to the participants and were worn during the entire examined work shift. The devices are comfortable to wear. The continuously measured physical parameters were analyzed separately for the different phases during the examined shift.

Table 1 Instruments used to evaluate the theoretical construct of the study

Construct	Instruments
Mental/physical strain	Heart rate, SDNN, LF/HF ratio
	Energy expenditure
	Clinical laboratory parameters
Work ability	WAI

Clinical laboratory parameters

For cortisol analysis all participants gave 5 salivary samples during the shift (due to the different shift lengths the sampling times were different -for the dispatchers 06:30, 09:15, 12:00, 14:45 and 17:30 and for the control group 08:00, 10:00, 12:00, 14:00 and 16:00). The samples were frozen after the end of each shift and stored at −20°C. The analysis was performed in a commercial laboratory using competitive enzyme immunoassay (ELISA).

Furthermore, urine samples were collected to determine adrenaline and noradrenaline levels, separately for the first and second part of the examined shift (dispatchers: from 06:30 to 11:59 and from 12:00 to 17:30; control group: from 07:30 to 11:59 and from 12:00 to 16:30).

After the shift, a blood sample was taken from all 27 dispatchers and from all 20 control subjects for the measurement of lymphocytes. The analysis was performed by flow cytometer (Becton Dickinson FACScalibur) in a commercial laboratory.

Work ability

Work ability index (WAI)

This standardized questionnaire reflects the ability to work based on the workers' self-perception. The WAI has also been validated in large international studies. It has a Cronbach's alpha between 0.72 and 0.80 [22]. The work ability index has strong predictive power with regard to the future course of work ability [23]. The higher the WAI scale (from 7 to 49), the better is the respondent's work ability; a good ability is assumed at a scale-score above 37. The WAI was repeatedly applied in research projects dealing with workplace health promotion in occupational health care.

Statistical analysis

Data was analyzed using SPSS for Windows (version 20.0 SPSS GmbH Software, Munich, Germany). Continuous variables were expressed as median (from min to max). The Mann Whitney test was performed for the comparison of unpaired groups. After adjustment for age and working hours per week, the linear regression analysis was applied for the metric values. All indicated p-values were two-sided, and an α-value of < 0.05 was regarded as statistically significant.

Results

General questionnaire

On average, the control group was slightly older than the dispatchers. There were no significant differences in all examined demographic data between the study groups. In addition, measurements of BMI and blood pressure revealed similar averages. The demographic, biometric and occupational data of both groups are listed in Table 2.

Based on the physical findings or underlying diseases no participant was excluded from the study. Cardiovascular diseases were present in 4 (14.8%) of the dispatchers and in 7 (35.0%) subjects from the control group. During the physical examination a hypertensive blood pressure was found in 1 (3.7%) dispatcher and in 2 (10.0%) control subjects. 12 (44.4%) dispatchers and 8 (40.0%) controls were suffering from diseases of the muscular-skeletal system. 5 dispatchers (2 controls) stated that they had diseases of the airways.

According to the general questionnaire, employment in the fire department was longer among control subjects than among dispatchers. However, on average, the dispatchers worked longer in their current position than the subjects from the control group (Table 2).

The occurrence of work disability within the last 12 months before the investigation was significantly ($p = 0.004$) higher among dispatchers. No difference was found in the number of disability days (Table 2). Considering the last quarter, 58% of dispatchers and 42% of control subjects reported a work disability in the past 3 months before the study.

Heart rate measurement

The stated medicines taken by the participants did not affect the measured physiological parameters. The real-time heart rate was measured during the complete investigated shift and separately analysed for the three phases "event", "non-event" and "breaks". The average heart rate and heart rate variability of the dispatchers and the control group in the different phases and the duration of the phases in the examined shift are shown in Table 3.

According to the phase protocol, the dispatchers had longer working days and longer breaks than the control group. The duration of stressful events due to phone calls in dispatchers or due to demanding situations in the control group was similar in spite of a significantly higher number of events in dispatchers (Table 3).

Although dispatchers showed no significant differences in heart rate between the different phases, in comparison to the control group they had significantly higher heart rates in all phases and a tendency of decreased heart rate variability in event and non-event phases. In addition, the LF/HF ratio reflecting the global sympatho-vagal balance was high, especially in dispatchers, but also in the control group, indicating a pronounced sympathetic response.

Energy expenditure

Energy costs of the dispatchers were assessed by means of the SenseWear armband. The mean metabolic equivalent of task (MET) of all participants during the shift was 1.39 (SD 0.43) without noticeable differences between dispatchers and control group.

Determination of salivary cortisol

On average, the course of the measured values corresponds to the expected circadian rhythm of cortisol with a peak value at 6:00 to 7:00. The values of the control group matched those of the dispatchers in the corresponding measurement period, with a slightly lower value at 14:00 (Figure 1). The mean values showed no significant differences between the study groups. Looking at the individual measurements, outliers from the normal course could be seen. In 50% of the cases, these

Table 2 Demographic, biometric and occupational data of the control group and the dispatchers

	Control group (n = 20)	Dispatchers (n = 27)
Demographic and biometric data		
Age, years (median (min.-max.))	46 (31–57)	39 (34–51)
Living in partnership, %	72.2%	84.0%
Presence of children, %	68.4%	84.0%
Current smoker, %	21.1%	12.0%
Body mass index (median (min.-max.))	27.7 (22.1-37.0)	27.5 (22.7-40.1)
Blood pressure, mmHg (median (min.-max.))	130 (110–170)/80 (70–90)	130 (100–160)/80 (60–110)
Occupational data (median (min.-max.))		
Employment at the fire department, years	23.0 (2.5-32)	16.5 (9–30)
Employment in the current position, years	1.0 (0.5-5.0)	2.5 (0.5-17)
Average working hours per week, hours	447,5 (20–61)	46 (34–79)
Work disability[a], yes/no (% yes)	42.1%	84.0%
Work disability[a], number of days (median (min.-max.))	14 (0–90)	14 (0–85)

[a]During the past year.

Table 3 Average heart rate (variability) and duration of the phases during the examined shift of the control group and the dispatchers

	Control group (n = 20)	Dispatchers(n = 27)	p[a] Control group vs. dispatchers
Event phases[b], (median (min.-max.))			
Cumulative duration, min	0 (0–60)	4.0 (0–47)	0.901
Number of events	0 (0–3)	0 (0–5)	**0.006**
beats/min	64.1 (57.5-69.8)	76.6 (72.2-87.4)	**0.001**
SDNN, ms	105.1 (58.8-159.7)	70.4 (40.4-152.9)	0.052
LF/HF	4.5 (1.3-14.9)	5.5 (0.4-30.1)	0.281
Non-event phases[c], (median (min.-max.))			
Cumulative duration, hours	6.7 (5.8-8.2)	9.1 (7.8-9.6)	**0.001**
beats/min	69.2 (59.9-79.3)	74.6 (56.4-89.8)	**0.034**
SDNN, ms	128.3 (59.2-357.6)	83.6 (65.1-158.6)	**0.034**
LF/HF	5.1 (2.6-14.2)	6.5 (1.2-11-0)	0.629
Breaks[d], (median (min.-max.))			
Cumulative duration, hours	0.5 (0–0.7)	1.5 (0.5-1.8)	**0.001**
beats/min	69.3 (64.0-82.3)	77.3 (60.3-89.3)	**0.036**
SDNN, ms	112.8 (56.1-155.9)	91.6 (53.8-267.0)	0.527
LF/HF	4.7 (1.8-9.8)	6.7 (1.7-30.1)	0.239

SDNN = standard deviation of all NN intervals.
LF/HF = ratio of low-high frequency power.
[a]Mann Whitney test.
[b]Time periods during which the dispatchers had marked a stressful call/ a difficult caller or the internal control group had marked a subjectively stressful situation on the phase protocol.
[c]Working hours without stressful events.
[d]Time outside working hours.
Significant findings are bold.

peaks correlated with phone calls marked as psychologically stressful in the phase protocol.

Determination of catecholamine in 24-hour urine

The adrenaline levels of the dispatchers (Table 4) were slightly lower than those of the control group (n.s.). Noradrenaline levels showed smaller differences between the groups.

Lymphocytes

There was no significant difference between dispatchers and the control group regarding the different subtypes

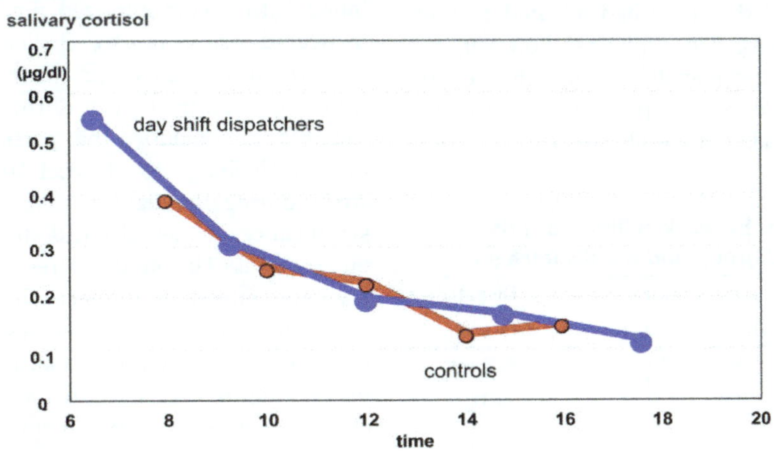

Figure 1 Salivary cortisol of dispatchers and controls.

Table 4 Laboratory parameters of the control group and the dispatchers

	Control group (n = 20)	*Dispatchers (n = 27)*	*Reference values*	*p*[a] Control group vs. dispatchers
Urine catecholamines separated for first and second half of the shift [μg/g creatinine] (median (min.-max.))				
Noradrenaline 1st half	27.8 (9.6-53.9)	30.5 (22.2-51.1)	n.a.	0.313
Noradrenaline 2nd half	32 (8.7-58.5)	23.3 (15.9-42)	n.a.	0.098
Adrenaline 1st half	7.4 (2.8-29.3)	6.45 (2.8-27.1)	n.a.	0.145
Adrenaline 2nd half	7.8 (3.2-16.9)	5.3 (2.1-17.5)	n.a.	0.144
Serum lymphocytes at the end of the shift (median (min.-max.))				
Lymphocytes (% of Leucocytes)	31.1 (15.8-46.9)	29.2 (19.3-55.9)	25-45	0.568
% T-Helper Lymphocytes (CD4+)	46.5 (24–58)	44 (31–70)	30-62	0.404
% NK-Cells (CD3-, CD16/56+)	16 (7–22)	13 (8–25)	5-29	0.237
% B-Lymphocytes (CD19+)	11.5 (6–22)	14 (5–20)	7-23	0.226

[a]Mann Whitney test.

of lymphocytes in blood samples. The same applies to the percentage of natural killer cells between the groups (Table 4).

Work ability index (WAI)

After adjustment for age and working hours per week, the dispatchers had a significantly lower work ability index than the control group (36.2 ± 6.4 and 40.1 ± 5.3 respectively; p = 0.009). More than 84% of the control group and only 45% of the dispatchers were classified as good or excellent according to the WAI work ability groups. Table 5 demonstrates the distribution of the WAI within the group of dispatchers and the control group.

Discussion

In this study, the average heart rate, its variability and laboratory parameters were measured as strain responses to job challenges. The fact that in all examined phases the average heart rate of the dispatchers was in the normal range may indicate that they had adapted to their job-related stress. During event phases, however, the average heart rates of the dispatchers and the control group were 78 and 65 beats/min (p = 0.001). As the dispatchers were not noticeably physically stressed (according to the armband monitor their MET was 1.41 on average), the significant differences in heart rate are assumed to be caused mainly by their chronic job-related mental stress. The increased heart rate among dispatchers compared to controls - although being in normal ranges - can indicate a preliminary stage of a health disorder and probably a higher risk for work disability [13].

Correspondingly, the heart rate variability was reduced particularly during the event phases, which also suggests chronic stress effects. In contrast, between the different phases no significant differences of heart rate, heart rate variability and laboratory findings (salivary cortisol, catecholamines in urine or lymphocytes in serum) were observed. Thus, during the examined shift only chronic stress effects (e.g. elevated heart rate at the beginning and during the shift) could be measured, but no acute responses.

In a recent study, fire fighters were examined, first under a single condition during exercise on a cycle ergometer and second during the same exercise combined with a computerized fire fighting strategical and tactical decision-making challenge [24]. Since the fire fighters' heart rates and their serum catecholamines were significantly higher during the second condition, the authors concluded that particularly the addition of a mental challenge to physical stress alters responses to stress during fire fighting. These findings highlight the significance of mental stress due to decision-making in emergencies. This kind of stress (coordination of imaginary emergency tasks) reflects the typical job-demands of dispatchers to a high degree, also in contrast to the job demands of the examined control group working in the office. Among call centre workers as office workers who also don't experience this mental stress due to decision-making (similar to the present control group) a higher work-related stress was described as a risk factor for

Table 5 Distribution into the work ability index (WAI) categories of the control group and the dispatchers

WAI scale for work ability	Control group (n = 20)	Dispatchers (n = 27)
Poor (7–27)	5.3%	8.3%
Moderate (28–36)	10.5%	45.8%
Good (37–43)	52.6%	33.3%
Excellent (44–49)	31.6%	12.5%

psychological health, and especially for a lower self-assessed work ability (WAI) [25].

Although they are not subjected to high physical exertion - as shown in the present study - the mental stress caused by the coordination of rescue tasks during emergency calls under these specific conditions is obviously very high for dispatchers. In addition, after emergencies, fire fighters have the opportunity to exchange their emotions regarding the mutually experienced rescue actions as a team process when they return to their fire department. Dispatchers, however, often have to manage different emergencies in quick succession without having an opportunity to cope with their emotions and speak with others about their feelings. Compared to the internal controls, a higher frequency of short-term events was confirmed in this study.

Furthermore, this study revealed significantly lower WAI among dispatchers than in the examined control group. In line with this self-assessment, a significantly higher frequency of disabilities had occurred objectively in dispatchers during the past year. In both study groups we found an equal number of disability days (on average 22 days per year) in the past year, but the dispatchers reported more acute, short-term disabilities (as a possible early sign of burnout) and less often chronic diseases (correspondingly, the control group distinctly more often stated cardiovascular diseases). The level of disability is extraordinarily high compared to the German general working population (12.8 disability days per year) [26].

It is plausible that the observed impaired work ability of dispatchers in comparison to the control group might be due to their high mental stress at the worksite [27]. This kind of stress can lead to a decreased well-being and consequently to a higher number of disability days [11] - also without a corresponding elevation of objective stress parameters (such as heart frequency) [12,28]. Most of available studies on work ability using the WAI haven't included biometric measurements [13]. Sometimes contradicting findings were described concerning work ability and objective variables [28,29]. In line with the present results, some studies revealed that disabled employees didn't demonstrate increased biometric stress parameters [11]. Parkka et al. [11] found only modest, but significant correlations between self-assessed stress level and physiological variables (such as heart rate or activity) among people participating in a work ability rehabilitation program. Furthermore, the authors described conflicting correlations at individual level. Therefore, psychological instruments, such as WAI, appear to be more sensitive to determine work ability than biometric parameters [12].

As a limitation of this study, the number of examined participants was low so that some possible relations between job-related stressors and outcome variables may not be clearly shown. However, in spite of the small number, some significant differences became evident, e.g. the strong relationship between the investigated occupational group and self-assessed work ability. A further limitation of this study is a selection bias which could have influenced the study results: it can't be excluded that some individuals with working ability restrictions were employed in the rescue coordination centre due to transfers from other fire fighting services. It is also possible that voluntarily recruited dispatchers had already accumulated work-related health complaints and had a higher tendency towards health problems. Moreover, as all study participants were only examined once, it is unclear to what degree the stress load varies from day to day. To reduce this shortcoming the participants were examined randomly on different weekdays in a 7-month time period.

We recommend the development or establishment of more precise dispatch protocols and specified training programs for dispatchers in the communities to improve their performance. The implementation of such standardized protocols for the assessment of the patient's health status is reported to increase the detection of health impairments by emergency medical dispatchers and thus to improve the treatment [30-32]. Furthermore, the dispatchers should have suitable opportunities for coping with their emotions and exchanging their feelings and impressions at regular intervals to reduce their observed chronic stress level.

Dispatchers' competence in CPR via phone is described as being dependent on re-training and a feedback on patient outcome [33]. Avoiding vague language, giving specific instructions for checking a patient, and finally reminding the caller to perform the explained procedures led to a high rate of successful communications. In addition, Dowdall-Thomae et al. (2009) presented a Peer Support Action Plan for several different intervention techniques as a coaching and support strategy in order to correct behaviours and keep the rescue workers at their optimum level of functioning and performance (problem-focused and seeking social support) [34]. Other authors also confirmed that (emotional) social support is a crucial measure to cope with job-related stress in emergency personnel [35-37].

Furthermore, video communication through mobile phones nowadays principally available in many situations can improve communication and avoid misunderstanding. This may provide a new basis for dispatcher assistance and can contribute to improved rescuer compliance [38].

Conclusions

The dispatchers' participating in this study had an elevated heart rate and reduced heart rate variability at the beginning and during the examined shift compared to the control group, probably indicating a higher level of chronic work-related stress. Additionally, they showed a significantly increased risk of work disability compared to the control group. Further studies are required to explore dispatchers' stress load and to draw conclusions concerning the effectiveness of appropriate intervention measures.

Abbreviations

CPR: Cardiopulmonary resuscitation; HRV: Heart rate and its variability; LF/HF: Ratio of low-high frequency power; MET: Metabolic equivalent of task; NN interval: Heartbeat-to-heartbeat interval; SD: Standard deviation; SDNN: Standard deviation of all NN intervals; SWA: SenseWear™ Armband; WAI: Work ability index.

Competing interests

Our work has been funded by a grant of the Hamburg fire department. The grant has been given to the Institute for Occupational and Maritime Medicine, ZfAM, University Medical Centre Hamburg-Eppendorf. No author has personally received any funding. Representatives of the fire department or any other external institution have neither influenced the measurements, the data collection and analysis nor the preparation of the manuscript. The authors declare that they have no conflict of interest.

Authors' contributions

All authors had full access to all data. XB and RW had the original idea for the paper and vouch for the integrity of the analysis. MO and DW performed medical examinations and took samples for laboratory analysis at the worksite. MO, BP, RW and DW analysed the data. MO and DW wrote and edited the manuscript. All authors collaborated in interpreting the data and have read and approved the final manuscript.

Acknowledgements

The authors thank all participants of the Hamburg fire department for participation in this study. Furthermore, we express our gratitude to Robina Mick and Hanna Graef for their support on the spot. We also thank Dr. Alexander Jaroslaw Galach for his technical support.

Author details

[1]Institute for Occupational and Maritime Medicine, Hamburg State Department for Health and Consumer Protection, ZfAM, University Medical Center Hamburg-Eppendorf, Seewartenstrasse10, D-20459 Hamburg, Germany. [2]Department of Pulmonary Medicine, Asklepios Hospital Harburg, Hamburg, Germany. [3]Institute for Occupational Medicine, Charité University Medicine Berlin and EOM Society, Berlin, Germany.

References

1. al Naser F, Everly GS Jr, Ibrahim, al Khulaifi MI: **Overcoming the effects of disasters: a rationale for the Kuwaiti CISM Program.** *Int J EmergMent Health* 2001, **3**:11–13.
2. Berger W, Coutinho ES, Figueira I, Marques-Portella C, Luz MP, Neylan TC, Marmar CR, Mendlowicz MV: **Rescuers at risk: a systematic review and meta-regression analysis of the worldwide current prevalence and correlates of PTSD in rescue workers.** *Soc Psychiatry PsychiatrEpidemiol* 2012, **47**:1001–1011.
3. al-Naser F, Everly GS Jr: **Prevalence of posttraumatic stress disorder among Kuwaiti firefighters.** *Int J EmergMent Health* 1999, **1**:99–101.
4. Fent KW, Evans DE: **Assessing the risk to firefighters from chemical vapors and gases during vehicle fire suppression.** *J Environ Monit* 2011, **13**:536–543.
5. De Vos AJ, Cook A, Devine B, Thompson PJ, Weinstein P: **Effect of protective filters on fire fighter respiratory health during simulated bushfire smoke exposure.** *Am J Ind Med* 2006, **49**:740–750.
6. Boxer PA, Wild D: **Psychological distress and alcohol use among fire fighters.** *Scand J Work Environ Health* 1993, **19**:121–125.
7. Greenwood MJ, Heninger JR: **Structured communication for patient safety in emergency medical services: a legal case report.** *PrehospEmerg Care* 2010, **14**:345–348.
8. Flynn J, Archer F, Morgans A: **Sensitivity and specificity of the medical priority dispatch system in detecting cardiac arrest emergency calls in Melbourne.** *Prehosp Disaster Med* 2006, **21**:72–76.
9. Berdowski J, Beekhuis F, Zwinderman AH, Tijssen JG, Koster RW: **Importance of the first link: description and recognition of an out-of-hospital cardiac arrest in an emergency call.** *Circulation* 2009, **119**:2096–2102.
10. Hallstrom AP, Cobb LA, Johnson E, Copass MK: **Dispatcher assisted CPR: implementation and potential benefit. A 12-year study.** *Resuscitation* 2003, **57**:123–129.
11. Parkka J, Merilahti J, Mattila EM, Malm E, Antila K, Tuomisto MT, Saarinen AV, van Gils M, Korhonen I: **Relationship of psychological and physiological variables in long-term self-monitored data during work ability rehabilitation program.** *IEEE Trans InfTechnol Biomed* 2009, **13**:141–151.
12. Gupta N, Jensen BS, Sogaard K, Carneiro IG, Christiansen CS, Hanisch C, Holtermann A: **Face validity of the single work ability item: comparison with objectively measured heart rate reserve over several days.** *Int J Environ Res Public Health* 2014, **11**:5333–5348.
13. Lindholm H, Sinisalo J, Ahlberg J, Hirvonen A, Hublin C, Partinen M, Savolainen A: **Attenuation of vagal recovery during sleep and reduction of cortisol/melatonin ratio in late afternoon associate with prolonged daytime sleepiness among media workers with irregular shift work.** *Am J Ind Med* 2012, **55**:643–649.
14. Ezoe S, Morimoto K: **Quantitative assessment of stressors and stress reaction: a review.** *Sangyo Igaku* 1994, **36**:397–405.
15. Bugajska J, Zuzewicz K, Szmauz-Dybko M, Konarska M: **Cardiovascular stress, energy expenditure and subjective perceived ratings of fire fighters during typical fire suppression and rescue tasks.** *Int J OccupSaf Ergon* 2007, **13**:323–331.
16. Beaton R, Murphy S, Johnson C, Pike K, Corneil W: **Exposure to duty-related incident stressors in urban firefighters and paramedics.** *J Trauma Stress* 1998, **11**:821–828.
17. Cassirame J, Tordi N, Mourot L, Rakobowchuk M, Regnard J: **Using of new beat to beat recorder system for traditional analysis of heart rate variability.** *Sci Sport* 2007, **22**:238–242.
18. Miwa H, Sasahara S, Matsui T: **Roll-over detection and sleep quality measurement using a wearable sensor.** *Conf Proc IEEE Eng Med BiolSoc* 2007, **2007**:1507–1510.
19. Al Otair H, Al-Shamiri M, Bahobail M, Sharif MM, BaHammam AS: **Assessment of sleep patterns, energy expenditure and circadian rhythms of skin temperature in patients with acute coronary syndrome.** *Med SciMonit* 2011, **17**:CR397–CR403.
20. Shuger SL, Barry VW, Sui X, McClain A, Hand GA, Wilcox S, Meriwether RA, Hardin JW, Blair SN: **Electronic feedback in a diet- and physical activity-based lifestyle intervention for weight loss: a randomized controlled trial.** *Int J BehavNutr Phys Act* 2011, **8**:41.
21. Sunseri M, Liden CB, Farringdon J, Pelletier R, Safier S, Stivoric J, Teller A, Vishnubhatla S: *The SenseWear armband as a Sleep Detection Device.* 2012. http://sensewearbodymediacom/SenseWear-Studies/SW-Whitepapers/The-SenseWear-armband-as-a-Sleep-Detection-Device Accessed at May 2012.
22. Tuomi K, Huuhtanen P, Nykyri E, Ilmarinen J: **Promotion of work ability, the quality of work and retirement.** *Occup Med (Lond)* 2001, **51**:318–324.
23. Hasselhorn H, Freude G: *Der Work Ability Index-ein Leitfaden.* Dortmund, Berlin, Dresden: Schriftenreihe der Bundesanstalt für Arbeitsschutz und Arbeitsmedizin: Sonderschrift; 2007:87.
24. Huang CJ, Webb HE, Garten RS, Kamimori GH, Evans RK, Acevedo EO: **Stress hormones and immunological responses to a dual challenge in professional firefighters.** *Int J Psychophysiol* 2010, **75**:312–318.
25. Conway PM, Campanini P, Punzi S, Fichera GP, Camerino D, Francioli L, Neri L, Costa G: **Work stress, common mental disorders and work ability index among call center workers of an Italian company.** *EpidemiolPrev* 2013, **37**:17–28.
26. Bundesanstalt für Arbeitsschutz und Arbeitsmedizin: **Volkswirtschaftliche Kosten durch Arbeitsunfähigkeit 2010.** In *Book Volkswirtschaftliche Kosten durch Arbeitsunfähigkeit 2010.* Berlin: BAuA; 2012.
27. Hagglund KM, Helsing C, Sandmark H: **Assistant nurses working in care of older people: associations with sustainable work ability.** *Scand J Caring Sci* 2011, **25**:325–332.
28. Nygard CH, Eskelinen L, Suvanto S, Tuomi K, Ilmarinen J: **Associations between functional capacity and work ability among elderly municipal employees.** *Scand J Work Environ Health* 1991, **17**(1):122–127.

29. Kaewboonchoo O, Saleekul S, Usathaporn S: **Factors related to work ability among Thai workers.** *Southeast Asian J Trop Med Public Health* 2011, **42**:225–230.
30. Roppolo LP, Westfall A, Pepe PE, Nobel LL, Cowan J, Kay JJ, Idris AH: **Dispatcher assessments for agonal breathing improve detection of cardiac arrest.** *Resuscitation* 2009, **80**:769–772.
31. Buck BH, Starkman S, Eckstein M, Kidwell CS, Haines J, Huang R, Colby D, Saver JL: **Dispatcher recognition of stroke using the national academy medical priority dispatch system.** *Stroke* 2009, **40**:2027–2030.
32. Tonje L, Elisabeth S, Lars W: **Handling of drug-related emergencies: an evaluation of emergency medical dispatch.** *Eur J Emerg Med* 2009, **16**:37–42.
33. Bang A, Ortgren PO, Herlitz J, Wahrborg P: **Dispatcher-assisted telephone CPR: a qualitative study exploring how dispatchers perceive their experiences.** *Resuscitation* 2002, **53**:135–151.
34. Dowdall-Thomae C, Culliney S, Piechura J: **Peer support action plan: northwest fire and rescue.** *Int J EmergMent, Health* 2009, **11**:177–183.
35. Dudek B, Koniarek J: **Social support as a modifier of response to stress: theoretical aspects and measurement.** *Med Pr* 2003, **54**:427–435.
36. Farnsworth JK, Sewell KW: **Fear of emotion as a moderator between PTSD and firefighter social interactions.** *J Trauma Stress* 2011, **24**:444–450.
37. Fullerton CS, McCarroll JE, Ursano RJ, Wright KM: **Psychological responses of rescue workers: fire fighters and trauma.** *Am J Orthopsychiatry* 1992, **62**:371–378.
38. Johnsen E, Bolle SR: **To see or not to see-better dispatcher-assisted CPR with video-calls? a qualitative study based on simulated trials.** *Resuscitation* 2008, **78**:320–326.

Tuberculosis in healthcare workers – a narrative review from a German perspective

Albert Nienhaus[1,2*], Anja Schablon[1], Alexandra M Preisser[3], Felix C Ringshausen[4] and Roland Diel[5,6]

Abstract

Introduction: Despite the decline of tuberculosis in the population at large, healthcare workers (HCW) are still at risk of infection.

Methods: In a narrative review the TB risk in HCW and preventive measures are described, with the focus on epidemiology and Occupational Safety and Health (OSH) regulations in Germany.

Results: There is an increased risk of infection not only in pneumology and laboratories with regular contact with tuberculosis patients or infectious materials. Epidemiological studies have also verified an increased risk of infection from activities that involve close contact with patients' breath (e.g. bronchoscopy, intubation) or close contact with patients in need of care in geriatric medicine or geriatric nursing. In occupational disease claim proceedings on account of tuberculosis, the burden of proof can be eased for insured persons who work in these or other comparable fields. Forgoing evidence of an index person as a source of infection has led to a doubling of the rate of cases of tuberculosis recognised as an occupational disease and has halved the duration of occupational disease claim proceedings in Germany. For several years now, it has been possible to use the new interferon-y release assays (IGRAs) to diagnose a latent tuberculosis infection (LTBI) with significantly greater validity than with the traditional tuberculin skin test (TST). However, variability of the IGRAs around the cut-off poses problems especially in serial testing of HCWs. At around 10%, LTBI prevalence in German healthcare workers is lower than had been assumed. It can make sense to treat a recent LTBI in a young healthcare worker so as to prevent progression into active tuberculosis. If the LTBI is occupational in origin, the provider of statutory accident insurance can cover the costs of preventive treatment. However, little is known about disease progression in HCWs with positive IGRA sofar.

Conclusion: TB screening in HCWs will remain an important issue in the near future even in low incidence, high income countries, as active TB in HCWs is often due to workplace exposure. The IGRAs facilitate these screenings. However, variability of IGRA results in serial testing of HCWs need further investigations.

Keywords: Tuberculosis, Provision, Occupational disease, Assessment, Healthcare, Prevention

Introduction

Tuberculosis (TB) is the second most frequent work-related infectious disease among German healthcare workers (HCW) [1]. Understanding the dynamics of infection risks for HCWs and developing an adequate Occupational Safety and Health (OSH) system is crucial to protect HCW from TB and to limit the spread of infections from HCWs to patients. In this narrative review we describe the German perspective and experience with TB in HCWs. As Germany has an elaborate system for occupational disease prevention and rehabilitation, telling the story from a German perspective might encourage other countries with less developed OSH systems [2] to improve infection control in HCWs.

* Correspondence: a.nienhaus@uke.de
[1]Institute for Health Service Research in Dermatology and Nursing (IVDP), Center of Excellence for Epidemiology and Health Service Research for Healthcare Professionals (CVcare), University Medical Center Hamburg-Eppendorf, Martinistraße 52, Hamburg 20246, Germany
[2]Principles of Prevention and Rehabilitation Department (GPR), Institute for Statutory Accident Insurance and Prevention in the Health and Welfare Services (BGW), Hamburg, Germany
Full list of author information is available at the end of the article

Epidemiology of tuberculosis in Germany

According to information provided by the Robert Koch Institute (RKI), in 2011 a total of 4,317 cases of tuberculosis were registered in Germany (previous year: 4,388), equivalent to an incidence of 5.3 (previous year: 5.3) new cases per 100,000 inhabitants [3]. The clear downward trend observed in Germany in recent years thus almost ground to a halt (Figure 1). The lung was the organ most frequently affected by TB, accounting 79.6% (3,346) of cases. Around one third (33.9%) of lung tuberculosis were of the infectious, microscopically positive type. The success of treatment in higher age groups declined continuously to just 63.3% in patients aged 70 and over. The incidence of TB among citizens with a migration background is approximately four times higher than among German nationals (5.3 versus 21.5/100,000).

Transmission paths and clinical picture of TB

Bacteria of the *Mycobacterium tuberculosis* (MTB) complex are transmitted from person to person by droplet infection and rarely via smear infections on skin and mucous membranes, via contaminated dust particles or cuts and stab wounds involving contaminated cannulae or scalpels [4]. Environmental factors, hygiene conditions, the amount of germs discharged and the virulence of the pathogens determine the degree of infection risk. Personal factors such as nutritional condition, age, immune status and comorbidity determine susceptibility of infection and the progression of the disease.

Primary tuberculosis or latent TB infection (LTBI)

The risk of infection increases with the duration and closeness of contact with the source of infection. However, brief occasional contacts – even a single conversational contact – can also lead to infection [5]. After an incubation period of five to six weeks on average (maximum 8 weeks), an inflammatory reaction occurs in the lung (primary focus) and possibly in the regional lymph nodes (primary complex). In most cases, this process heals without significant clinical symptoms. Sometimes calcification takes place, so that the primary focus and possibly also the associated lymph nodes remain radiologically identifiable at a later date (Ghon foci). However, it is also possible that active tuberculosis will develop immediately, with a progressive, infiltrative and cavitating process and/or with bronchogenic, haematogenous or lymphogenous spread, leading to further organ manifestations.

In the primary complex, which often cannot be rendered visible, viable mycobacteria capable of replication and proliferation may remain for years or decades. This leads to sensitisation of monocytes circulating in the peripheral blood. The presence of these sensitised monocytes can be measured by means of a tuberculin skin test (TST) or with the interferon-γ release assays (IGRAs) that have recently become available. Both tests are based on the cell-mediated immune response to *M. tuberculosis* antigens. However, the IGRA is considerably more specific than the TST, since it works with only two or three *M. tuberculosis* antigens instead of approximately 200 antigens as in the tuberculin for the TST [6,7]. Therefore, a positive TST should be validated by an IGRA so as to rule out non-specific reactions, e.g. to a Bacillus Calmette-Guerin (BCG) vaccination or to environmental non-tuberculous mycobacteria (NTM). Two different IGRAs are commercially available, the ELISA-based QuantiFERON-TB Gold In-Tube® and the ELISPOT-based T-SPOT.TB®.

Since IGRAs are *in vitro* tests, the problem of boosting that occurs in serial testing with TST is avoided. The IGRA correlates better than the TST with exposure to infectious patients and shows higher sensitivity to active TB than the TST [6-9]. Moreover, IGRAs have a higher

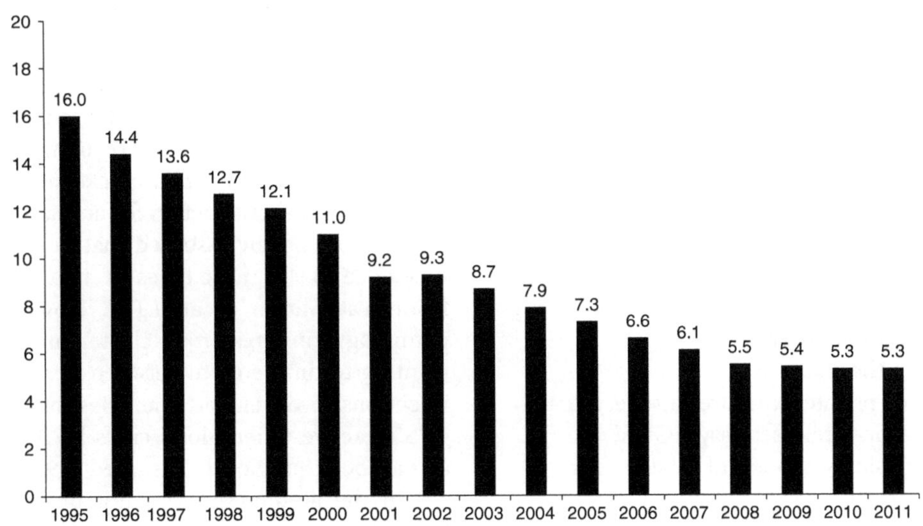

Figure 1 Incidence of TB in Germany in the years 2000 to 2011 [3].

predictive value in contact tracings of persons with close contact to infectious patients in low-incidence countries as regards the progression of the disease [10,11]. Even though only one study reported progression risk in HCWs based on four cases [11], IGRAs are likely to improve both the effectiveness and the efficiency of TB screening in HCWs [12]. However, as yet no consensus exists on the interpretation of IGRA results in serial testing [6,7,13]. In serial testing especially, it is important to state IGRA results not only qualitatively but also quantitatively.

Some more water needs to be purred into the wine. As IGRA are not able to distinguish LTBI from active TB, IGRA are no reliable test for the diagnosis of active TB [14].

A conversion – when a previously negative test result becomes positive when measured again – indicates a fresh infection with *M. tuberculosis.* Reversion of immunological tests from positive to negative is possible if MTB is successfully eliminated (transient infection) or if there is so little MTB activity in the primary complex that T-cells are no longer sensitised [15].

Post-primary tuberculosis

In the generalisation phase, the mycobacteria spread through the blood or lymph, developing a focus in the lung or other organs. Initially, this is usually silent. If such foci are reactivated – in the lungs, usually in the apex area – active tuberculosis of the lung, or for example of the kidney, genitals or bone, may develop months or even decades later, requiring treatment. As mentioned above, around one-third of new cases are extra-pulmonary [3]. These forms of tuberculosis result from the reactivation of primary tuberculosis, or may be caused by re-infection.

Diagnosis

Diagnosing TB is sometimes difficult due to the diverse forms of manifestation. In addition, diagnosis is often belated because there are no specific symptoms and the possibility of TB is too rarely considered in differential diagnosis.

Symptoms or circumstances that indicate the presence of TB are:

- Clinical symptoms such as coughs, phlegm, weight loss, tiredness, nocturnal sweating, fever, breathing-dependent pain in the thorax
- Tuberculosis in the anamnesis
- Occupational or private exposure to tuberculosis
- Positive interferon-γ release assay (IGRA)
- X-ray results raising suspicion of tuberculosis

The diagnosis is confirmed by evidence of tuberculosis pathogens in test materials such as sputum, bronchial secretions, gastric juice, urine or pus from an abscess. The quickest method is microscopic examination. However, this is crude and only shows positive results at approx. 10^4–10^5 bacteria/ml of material. Since only acid-fast bacilli (AFB) can be verified under the microscope, the diagnosis of TB is not confirmed. Only a positive culture confirms TB. Cultural verification is possible with only around 50–100 bacteria/ml in the test material. Alternatively, TB can be confirmed by molecular biology methods (e.g. polymerase chain reaction, PCR) to verify TB-specific DNA or RNA.

Welcome progress has been made in developing these methods further in recent years. In an attempt to create an easy-to-use, low-cost test, the Xpert MTB/RIF system has become prevalent. The WHO has been recommending the use of the test since 2010 for initial diagnosis where tuberculosis is suspected, primarily in high-prevalence countries with a high proportion of HIV patients and where multi-drug-resistant (MDR) tuberculosis is suspected. The Xpert MTB/RIF offers a fully automatic real-time PCR for *M. tuberculosis* complex-specific DNA and a sub-unit of bacterial RNA polymerase beta (rpoB), which is observed in 95% of resistance to Rifampicin. It is easy to handle and takes about 20 minutes of active work, with a result available in two hours. Admittedly, the Xpert MTB/RIF is not sensitive enough to be the sole method used in developed countries. The role of Xpert MTB/RIF in the diagnosis of TB in high income, low TB incidence countries is currently under study [16].

Risk factors for tuberculosis

The WHO assumes that 30% of the world's population is infected with *M. tuberculosis.* These latent TB infections (LTBIs) lead to active TB in 10% of those affected during the course of their lives. In around half, active TB develops within the first two years after infection. Children are more likely than adults to develop active TB after infection (around 30%) [10]. Malnutrition, homelessness and alcoholism, along with HIV infection and other diseases that weaken the immune system, or immunosuppressive therapies (in which TNF-alpha blockers are especially significant) are typical risk factors for activation of LTBI.

It was previously assumed that in countries with a low incidence of TB most cases of active tuberculosis result from reactivation of an LTBI. However, infection epidemiology findings from cluster analyses using fingerprinting to differentiate between strains suggest that new infections in developed countries may account for up to 40% of active tuberculosis cases [17,18], rather than 10% as had been previously assumed [19]. An LTBI or active TB in the anamnesis does not protect against reinfection. Depending on the country and study, reinfections are responsible for 10% to 75% of all second episodes of tuberculosis [20]. However, it can also be shown that targeted prevention measures can significantly reduce transmissions of *M. tuberculosis* [21,22].

Tuberculosis risks in healthcare

Healthcare workers are at increased risk of LTBI and active tuberculosis [22-25]. However, in countries with a low incidence of TB, it can be difficult to verify this increased risk of infection since the customary risk factors for both infection and for active TB are less prevalent than among the general population, and not all healthcare workers have contact with TB patients. Moreover, appropriate preventive action (see below) can be taken to minimise the risk of infection when caring for patients known to be suffering from tuberculosis [24].

Fingerprinting and the supplementary molecular biology methods for differentiating between strains of *M. tuberculosis* improve the possibility of discovering infection pathways. Individuals with different strains of TB cannot have infected each other. Individuals with the same strain of TB may be part of a common infection pathway. In molecular epidemiology, patients with the same strain of TB are known as clusters (Figure 2). However, belonging to a cluster cannot be equated with confirmed transmission of TB. Rather, an appropriate infectious contact needs to be ascertained as probable by interviewing the members of the cluster. Three molecular epidemiology studies on the occupational risk of infection have been published so far [4,26,27].

In the Hamburg fingerprint study [4], mycobacteria cultures have been used continuously since 1997 to generate fingerprints of all individuals with notifiable TB. The study covers 848 cases where IS6110 fingerprinting was carried out. Ten study participants with TB were healthcare workers. Through fingerprinting and a subsequent survey, it was possible to prove occupation-related transmission in eight of those individuals. Thus the proportion of occupation-related tuberculosis in healthcare workers was 80% (95%CI 44%–97%). Of eight occupation-related transmissions, six were unknown prior to fingerprinting.

A fingerprint study on the infection risk among healthcare workers in the Netherlands found that in 28 out of 67 (43%) persons with active TB, transmission from patient to staff was proved [26]. The main reason for transmission was belated diagnosis of index cases, especially among older patients. Ten (out of 28) index cases were older people with comorbidity whose tuberculosis had not been diagnosed promptly, as a result of which no appropriate preventive measures had been taken.

The most up-to-date molecular epidemiology study on the occupational infection risk included all TB cases reported in San Francisco from 1993 to 2003 [27]. In all, there were 2,510 TB cases. Fingerprinting was then performed for 1,852 patients. Thirty-one patients (1.2% of the total) were healthcare workers. Occupationally related TB was confirmed in ten (32%) of the 31 healthcare workers.

LTBI prevalence in healthcare workers

LTBI is assumed when the IGRA is positive and active TB is excluded by X-ray. In German HCWs LTBI prevalence depends on the age of employees. It increases from 2.6% among the under-25 s to 22.2% among the over-55 s (Table 1) [28-31]. The prevalence of LTBI is the same for men and women. The reason for investigation pursuant to the German regulation on occupational healthcare provisions (ArbMedVV) (see below) also has no influence on the prevalence of LTBI. Likewise, there are no differences between doctors and nurses. LTBI prevalence is higher among geriatric care nurses, otherwise no differences were described between the different occupational groups and activities in Germany [29-31]. About 15% of German HCWs are foreign born and their prevalence of LTBI is more than two times higher than in German born HCWs [30].

LTBI prevalence among healthcare workers in Germany is considerably lower than had been assumed on the basis of studies based on TST [29]. Moreover, the prevalence of LTBI in Germany is significantly lower than in France or Portugal (10%, 19%, 33%) [32,33]. As yet, no comparative data on the prevalence of LTBI in the unaffected population is available for Germany.

Prevention of tuberculosis

The most effective measures for preventing TB infection are early identification of cases and isolation. It is therefore important for hospitals to consider the possibility of TB when corresponding symptoms arise. The risk of

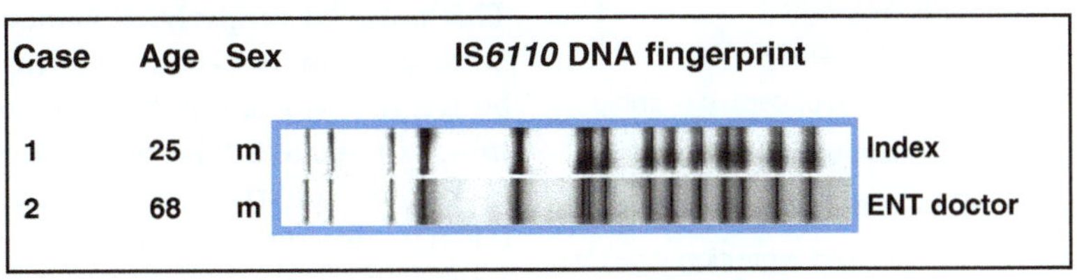

Figure 2 Example of two identical fingerprints from the Hamburg fingerprint study [4].

Table 1 Latent TB infections (positive IGRA) among healthcare workers according to the German TB network of occupational health physicians, following [28-31]

Variable	N = 3,823 n (%)	IGRA	
Age		Negative n (%)	Positive n (%)
< 25 years	494 (12.9)	481 (97.4)	13 (2.6)
25-35 years	926 (24.2)	878 (94.8)	48 (5.2)
35-45 years	1,057 (27.6)	982 (92.9)	75 (7.1)
45-55 years	974 (25.5)	867 (89.0)	107 (11.0)
>55 years	372 (9.7)	297(79.8)	75 (20.2)
Gender			
Female	2,959 (77.4)	2,716 (91.8)	243 (8.2)
Male	864 (22.6)	789 (91.3)	75 (8.7)
Reason for screening			
Regular contact with TB patients or infectious material (obligatory)	2,533 (66.3)	2,310 (91.2)	223 (8.8)
Contact tracing (optional)	1,290 (33.7)	1,195 (92.6)	95 (7.4)
Profession			
Physician	583 (15.2)	538 (92.3)	45 (7.7)
Nurse	1,962 (51.3)	1,804 (91.9)	158 (8.1)

progression from LTBI to active TB can be reduced by preventive chemotherapy [34].

Table 2 summarises the main protective measures for effective control of tuberculosis in the clinical field. Various studies proved that implementing these measures to prevent infection contributes substantially toward reducing the risk for healthcare workers [34-36]. However, it is not possible to make any specific deductions as to the significance of individual sub-aspects. Clearly, organisational and administrative measures are very important, followed by technical and individual preventive measures. Ultimately, only the interaction of various preventive measures can reduce the risk of infection to a minimum.

Table 2 Tuberculosis prevention measures in the inpatient sector, following [35]

Organisational/administrative measures	- Early establishment of a diagnosis
	- Isolation
	- Early initiation of appropriate therapy
Patient	- Information and clarification
	- Cough hygiene
	- Mouth and nose protection
Employee	- General hygiene
	- Respiratory protection
	- If necessary, protective clothing
	- Education and training
	- Operational monitoring
Workplace	- Correct room ventilation
	- Suitable disinfection

Isolation

The decision whether to isolate must be made on a case-by-case basis. Isolation is indicated as a matter of principle when open, and therefore infectious, tuberculosis of the respiratory tract is suspected or confirmed. The decision whether to isolate patients with negative sputum microscopy must be made individually. Isolation in special tuberculosis wards is not necessary, but the patient should be in a single room. Cohort isolation should only be effected when direct infection chains are assumed (e.g. mother–child). Tests and transfers to other departments for diagnostic or therapeutic purposes that can be postponed should be deferred if possible until the patient can be assumed to be no longer infectious.

As a rule, isolation measures are not necessary in cases of extrapulmonary tuberculosis, though infectious material must be treated with appropriate caution [37].

The decision whether to discontinue isolation depends primarily on the microscopically verifiable decrease in the secretion of pathogens in sputum and on the clinical and radiological response to therapy. Three microscopically negative sputum results are necessary. In most cases, sputum conversion takes place three weeks after the start of an effective therapy. In individual cases (cavernous processes, absence of bacteriological and/or clinical evidence that therapy has been successful, drug resistance, immunosuppression, lack of compliance), however, a longer period of isolation may be necessary. In such cases, the date for ceasing isolation must be determined individually. Decisions on the need for treatment as an inpatient must be taken individually, taking into account factors such as the severity of the tuberculosis, underlying diseases or comorbidity, problems with therapy and patient cooperation. If the appropriate framework conditions are in place (medical care, patient reliability, home circumstances), clinically stable tuberculosis patients can be treated as outpatients [37].

Therapy adherence

The most important prerequisite for treatment to succeed is reliable, regular intake of anti-tuberculosis drugs. This must be properly explained to patients. They must be told in understandable terms why tuberculosis must be treated with a combination of drugs for such a long time. If reliable intake of medication is not assured or is in doubt, the treatment must be supervised directly (DOT = directly observed treatment). As a matter of principle, medicines must be taken under supervision during a stay in hospital.

The obligation under the German Prevention and Control of Infectious Diseases Act (Infektionsschutzgesetz, IfSG) to notify refusal or premature withdrawal from treatment is intended to facilitate the identification of patients in need of active support and possibly also close supervision during their treatment.

General hygiene

Patients must be encouraged to adopt hygienic behaviour (coughing into a paper handkerchief, turning away from other people) and to wear a mask over mouth and nose. In a recent study, it was shown for the first time that the MTB concentration in the air of the patient's room is lower if the patient wears a mask [38]. When contamination of the hands with pathogen-containing material is to be feared (e.g. during oral hygiene, aspiration, catheter maintenance and urine disposal in tuberculosis of the urinary tract, and bandage changing or wound dressing when skin secretions contain pathogens), personnel must wear protective gloves and, in the event of aerosol-generating procedures, a respirator mask (see below). Personnel at risk, fellow patients and other contact persons must be given detailed, understandable instructions about possible paths of infection and the necessary protective measures.

Ventilation

Adequate ventilation of rooms where infectious tuberculosis patients are accommodated is of crucial importance, as it helps to dilute or eliminate infectious aerosols and minimise the further spread of germs into the environment (no recirculation of air containing bacteria, air flow towards the patient's room and from there to outside) [34,36,39]. If a ventilating and air-conditioning system (with negative air pressure in the isolation room and positive air pressure in the anteroom) is used, there should be a change of air at least four to six times per hour. Some authors call for a frequency of nine to twelve times an hour. No scientific arguments could be found for a precise minimum frequency of air change [35].

Respiratory protection

There is no evidence-based proof of the effectiveness of respiratory masks in preventing *M. tuberculosis* infection. Given that diagnosis, therapy, and the control and infection prevention measures outlined above already significantly reduce the risk of transmission via known or suspected tuberculosis cases, respiratory masks make a limited contribution toward risk reduction. However, where there is exposure to higher concentrations of aerosols, it makes sense to wear one.

Like the masks worn in industry, better fitting, particle-filtering half masks with improved filtration are available for medical needs (filtering face piece = FFP). The FFPs currently available are classified according to European standards (EN 149). The total leakage from a mask is made up of leakages around the face, leakage around the exhalation valve (if there is one) and leakage from the actual filter penetration. The average total leakage for Class 1 respiratory masks must not exceed 22% under test conditions. That of Class 2 masks must not exceed 8% and Class 3 must not exceed 2% (with an average particle diameter of 0.6 µm). FFP2 masks (or equivalent) are recommended as a personal protective measure for preventing infection in case of tuberculosis. The wearer must be instructed and the fit must be checked, as the protective effect of the respirator can only be reliable if it fits properly and is used correctly [40].

In the presence of other persons, patients should wear at least conventional mouth and nose covering masks inside and always outside the isolation room so as to reduce the spread of aerosol (see above).

In order to ascertain the need for personnel to use respiratory masks, a risk analysis should be undertaken for the relevant institution or relevant department and the specific patient. FFP2 masks are used either where exposure to the coughing of patients suffering from suspected or confirmed open tuberculosis is unavoidable, or where a high concentration of aerosol must be assumed. In special situations, a specific risk assessment must be carried out to identify suitable respiratory protection.

Disinfection and sterilisation

Thermal disinfection is always preferable to chemical disinfection, as it is safer, more reliable (inter alia because of the possibility of automation) and less harmful (allergies resulting from chemical disinfectants, environmental pollution). Industry has developed devices for different fields of medicine that enable thermal disinfection of a variety of instruments, respiratory accessories, etc. [37].

Surfaces should be disinfected by standard hygienic methods. Spray disinfection is not sufficiently effective. Although microorganisms, and thus also tuberculosis bacteria, can be detected on surfaces such as walls, floors and furniture, they are very rarely a real infection risk for humans because no aerosols are formed.

Special disinfection of urine or stool is not necessary. If pathogen-containing excretions are collected, they can be disposed of by thermal disinfection (with customary cleaning and disinfection equipment).

Disinfectant cleaning of surfaces that may be contaminated with pathogen-containing particles should also be carried out in the home. Clothing should be washed at a minimum of 60°C with customary laundry detergents and carpets should be cleaned to remove dust particles as far as possible, if need be by spray extraction. The spraying of formaldehyde is no longer permitted.

Precautions against tuberculosis

Contact tracings by health authorities pursuant to IfSG serve to identify at an early stage cases of TB and individuals who can benefit from preventive chemotherapy. TB screening by occupational health physicians serves the same purpose.

As the TB incidence in Germany decreased over recent decades (Figure 1), in order to avoid unnecessary X-ray examinations due to a false positive TB test there was a paradigm shift to optional checks as warranted by accidental occupational exposure to *M. tuberculosis*. According to the German regulation on occupational healthcare provisions (ArbMedVV), employees must be offered tests 'if as a result of exposure to biological agents a serious infection or disease can be expected and post-exposure prophylactic (prevention) measures are possible'. This applies to TB.

In contrast, obligatory checks pursuant to the ArbMedVV are only provided for in the case of employees in tuberculosis departments and other pneumological facilities or research institutes and laboratories who have regular contact with infectious patients or materials. If regular obligatory checks are performed, there is no need for an additional test after unprotected contact with an infectious patient or infectious materials.

Participation in an optional check or obligatory occupational health check in accordance with ArbMedVV replaces contact investigations pursuant to IfSG. In order to avoid duplicate tests, it makes sense for occupational health physicians to conduct their tests in consultation with public health authorities and to use the appropriate formula for checks as per the German Central Committee to Combat Tuberculosis (Deutsches Zentralkomitee zur Bekämpfung der Tuberkulose, DZK) recommendation for contact investigations [5]. If an employee fails take up the option of a test, the local public health authority is responsible for performing the contact investigation in accordance with IfSG.

The aim of TB screenings is to identify employees with a recent LTBI, as they will benefit most from preventive chemotherapy. It is therefore not expedient to examine all possible contact persons. Instead, only 'close contact persons' should be tested, as the proportion of recent infections among them will be higher in close contacts.

The probability of transmission depends on the patient's infectiousness (microscopically positive or negative), proximity to the infectious source, and the duration of contact. This suggests the following criteria for selecting contact persons [5]:

A) brief but intensive contact with a coughing, sputum-positive patient without protection,
B) cumulative contact duration of at least eight hours with a patient with microscopic evidence of AFB in a direct specimen of sputum,
C) cumulative contact duration of at least 40 hours with a patient with only culturally or molecular biologically confirmed evidence of tuberculosis.

In practice, this rule is often difficult to apply because the contact duration cannot be reliably estimated or because uncertainty among employees may lead them to want a check-up. Hence the above-mentioned criteria should be seen only as guides to the selection of contact persons.

In the case of optional checks, an IGRA should be carried out only eight weeks after the last contact with the index patient or the infectious materials, so as to leave sufficient time for the immunological reaction to develop. A chest X-ray after a positive IGRA should be done only three months after the last contact with the possible source of infection, since development of active TB is unlikely before then. The flow chart below is based on the recommendations for contact investigations [5].

Preventive check-ups in accordance with ArbMedVV are repeated regularly (obligatory test) or as warranted after unprotected contact. This raises the question how different IGRA results in serial tests are to be interpreted. The variability of IGRA in serial tests is not yet sufficiently understood [6,13,41]. Reversion of positive IGRA results into negative results is more frequent than conversion of negative IGRA results into positive ones. More significant is the fact that the probability of conversion or reversion depends on the quantitative test results of the first IGRA. Thus a grey area could be helpful in separating genuine conversions and reversions and chance deviations. The Center for Disease Control and Prevention (CDC) and the European Centre for Disease Prevention and Control have proposed a grey area in the range 5–7 spot forming cells (SFC) for T-SPOT.TB [42]. As yet, however, no consensus has been reached on a grey area for QuantiFERON-TB Gold In-Tube (QFT). A grey area of 0.2 and 0.7 IU/mL and defining conversion and reversion as overstepping this grey area minimise the rate of conversion and reversion and keep the proportion of employees whose QFT values are within this grey area relatively low [43-45].

Since the reversion rate with IGRA is higher than expected [6,13], 'once positive, always positive', the statement that used to apply to TST, is obsolete. All healthcare workers should be re-tested with the IGRA in a planned routine screening. This reduces the number of chest X-rays needed, since no further medical check is necessary if the IGRA reverts to negative and there are no recognisable clinical signs of active TB. Chemoprevention (see below) in employees with fluctuating test results requires further discussion. Assuming that recent exposure to *M. tuberculosis* is probable, the simplest approach would be to rule out lung tuberculosis if the IGRA result is positive and not to carry out any further medical examination if the test result is negative and there are no recognisable clinical symptoms of tuberculosis. The same applies to employees with results in the grey area. If they have no clinical symptoms, no further medical examination is necessary. However, more data on progression to the disease is needed in order to deduce evidence-based recommendations for chemotherapy treatment for employees with an IGRA conversion or reversion, and for employees with IGRA results in the grey area.

Employees whose anamnesis includes chemotherapy for LTBI or those with repeat positive IGRA results should not be re-tested in subsequent preventive checks since the IGRA results would not be revealing. If one of these employees is part of a cohort with a low risk of progression (e.g. no active tuberculosis among hospital personnel in recent years), a chest X-ray should only be taken if there are suspicious clinical symptoms. Figure 3 shows a decision tree for repeat preventive checks for healthcare workers in accordance with ArbMedVV. However, it should be noted that further research is needed to prove the usefulness of this approach in countries with low TB incidence and high hygiene standards [46]. Furthermore it needs to be pointed out that this recommendation seems helpful for countries like Germany with currently low TB incidence but history of high TB incidence and high prevalence of BCG vaccination in HCWs. In countries with a long history of low TB incidence and no BCG vaccination policy and therefore low rates of positive TST results in HCWs other conclusions might be drawn as is shown in the Canadian recommendations. In Canada for serial testing of HCWs the TST is recommended because compared to TST unexplained variability of the IGRA seems to be higher [47,48].

Chemoprevention

The probability of developing active TB during the first two years following a positive IGRA is significantly lower for healthcare workers than for close contacts in the general population [10,11]. This can probably be explained by the fact that healthcare workers do not have the typical risk factors for developing active TB (alcoholism, homelessness, etc.) and that a positive IGRA in healthcare workers is often caused by an remote LTBI with a low risk of progression. This should be taken into account when selecting individuals to be treated with preventive chemotherapy. Chemoprevention should only be considered if the employee is under 50 and the IGRA is positive after recent exposure to *M. tuberculosis* [5].

Before initiating chemoprevention, a chest X-ray must be taken to rule out active TB and a further check must be carried out after completing chemoprevention so as not to overlook a disease that may be developing despite chemoprevention.

Chemoprevention involves taking Isoniazid (INH) 300 mg daily for six or preferably nine months. This therapy for the treatment of LTBI can achieve 90% protection [49]. In practice, however, effectiveness is significantly lower, mainly because of insufficiently regular intake of the medication for this long period.

If the MTB of the index case is resistant to INH, or the contact (i.e. the HCW) is unable to tolerate INH, as

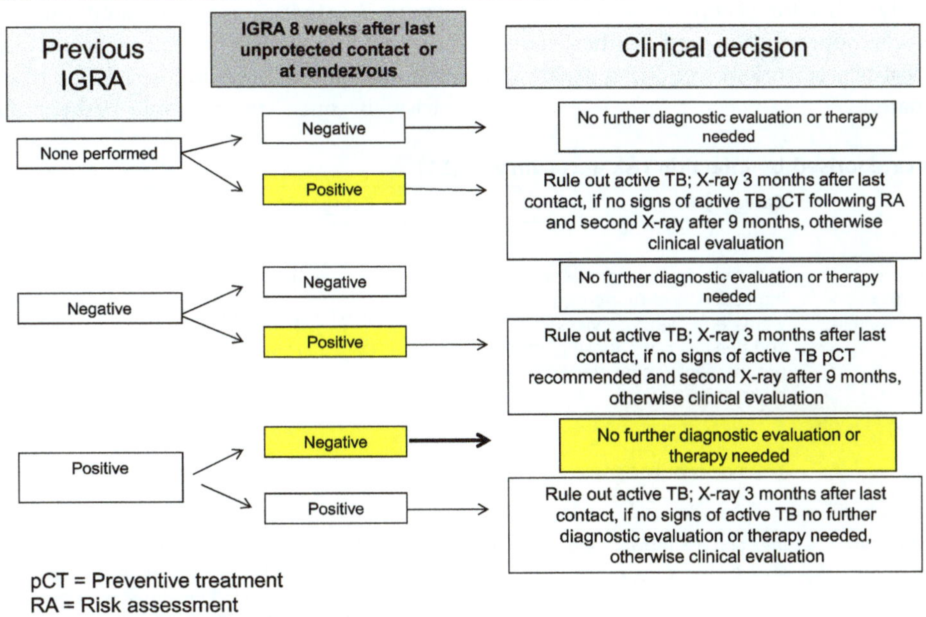

Figure 3 Decision tree for repeated IGRA according to [46].

an alternative 600 mg Rifampicin (RMP) can be taken for four months, or a combination of INH and RMP for three to four months for chemoprevention [50]. However, the effectiveness of these two alternatives has been less well researched.

Hepatotoxicity of chemoprevention with INH

Acceptance of chemoprevention is reduced by the fear of possible liver damage. Until now, only two meta-analyses have dealt with the number of INH-induced hepatitis in adults. According to these analyses, the probability of INH-associated hepatitis is 0.6%. Occasionally, however, significantly higher rates of up to 5% were described [49,51]. Because of the hepatotoxic side effect of INH, regular laboratory controls (after two and four weeks, then monthly) are necessary. If there is a significantly raised level of liver enzymes, chemoprevention should be discontinued.

New treatment regime in chemotherapy

Significantly shorter treatment periods and considerably fewer tablets than with previous offers are the key elements for improving the results of preventive treatment in persons with freshly diagnosed LTBI. Two recently published, extensive and randomly controlled studies provide evidence that the combined therapy of INH and Rifapentin (RPT) administered once a week for twelve weeks is less toxic than classic INH therapy and equally effective [52,53]. In the United States, therefore, the CDC recommends this combination therapy [54].

Should the new regime become established, this will make it considerably easier for occupational health physicians to advise chemoprevention and further reduce the number of healthcare workers requiring treatment for TB at a later date.

Tuberculosis as an occupational disease in Germany

Unlike in other European countries such as France [55], it is not generally assumed in Germany that healthcare workers with patient contact run a greater risk of TB infection, and therefore of contracting the disease. Therefore, according to number 3101 of the German Ordinance on Occupational Diseases (Berufskrankheitenverordnung, BKV), tuberculosis in a healthcare worker can only be recognised as an occupational disease if an increased occupational risk of infection can be proven and if there is no (competing) risk of infection outside work [56]. According to BKV, both tuberculosis in HCWs and silico-tuberculosis in workers exposed to silica dust can be recognised as occupational diseases. Furthermore, active TB as the result of an accident can be compensated by statutory accident insurance schemes. In addition to work postings to countries with a high incidence of TB, this is also relevant in the case of occupational exposure to *M. tuberculosis*, i.e. contact to a college with active TB outside the healthcare sector. Transmission of M. tuberculosis can be considered an accident as it takes place within 24 hours, the juridical definition for the relationship of cause and effect in the realm of the social accident insurance legislation in Germany.

As shown in Table 3, in addition to close contact with a known index person (infectious patient), healthcare workers run an increased risk of infection from work in specialist lung clinics and laboratories (Category A) if they regularly come into contact with tuberculosis patients or sputum samples. However, a raised risk of infection can also be explained epidemiologically (Category B) [25,31].

There is a special risk from unknown, or belatedly recognised, tuberculosis. Often, but not necessarily, Category B activities are associated with close contact with the air the patient exhales (bronchoscopy, intubation, extubation, etc.). An increased risk of infection may also arise if once in a while tuberculosis patients are

Table 3 Activities categorised by infection risk according to [51]

Category A	Category B	Category C	Category D
Activity, Area			
TB ward, specialist lung clinic, specialist lung doctors, microbiology laboratories that examine sputum	Bronchoscopies, laryngoscopy, emergency intubation, post mortems, work in infection wards, emergency services, A & E, geriatrics and geriatric care*, looking after at-risk groups, deployment abroad in areas with a high incidence	General hospitals General practitioners Dental practices	All other health service and welfare work
Easing of burden of proof			
Yes, index not necessary	Yes, index not necessary	No, index necessary, exceptions are possible	Index necessary
Reasons			
Infection risk due to particular patients or materials	Infection risk proven by epidemiological studies	Infection risk insufficiently proven by epidemiological studies. Index may be dispensed with if there are several patients with open TB in the work area.	Infection risk not proven by epidemiological studies

*If there is close contact with patients in need of care.

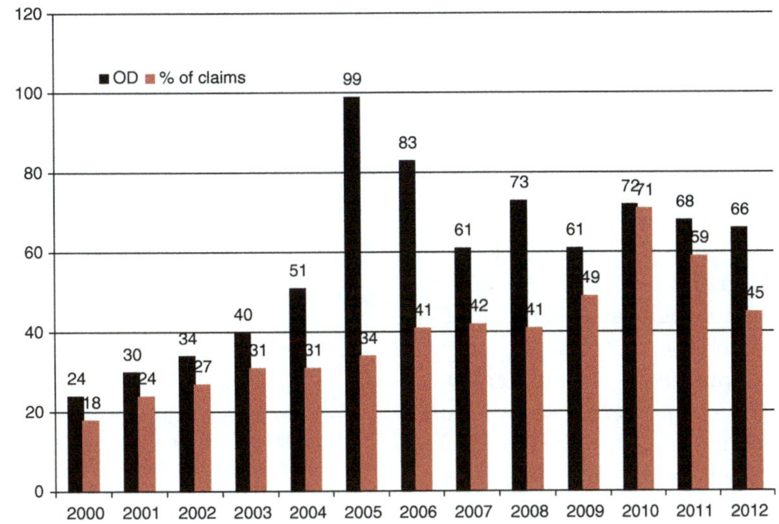

Figure 4 Number of active TB cases compensated as occupational disease (OD) and percentage of recognized claims in the years 2000 to 2012 according to [1].

diagnosed and treated in a particular area (Category C). Even if it is out of the question that the known patient is the index person, e.g. because there was no personal contact with the particular patient, in such institutions one can expect the rate of unrecognised TB cases in this group of patients to be higher than in the population at large. Typical institutions are e.g. general practices and general hospitals without infection wards.

Category D includes institutions where there is no indication of an increased rate of tuberculosis among patients. This category includes all institutions that do not fall under Category A to C, such as dermatologists, surgeons (except chest surgeons), rehab clinics, psychotherapy practices and physiotherapists (as long as they do not carry out respiration therapy).

In assessing the circumstances in occupational disease claim proceedings there is no need to look for an index person in Categories A and B. Instead, the typical clientele of patients (Category A) or epidemiological data (Category B) make it easier to find proof. In Category C it is possible to recognise the causal links even if no index person could be found. However, judgement must be passed on a case-by-case basis. No general statement can be made as to the number of TB cases per year from which there is an increased risk of infection. In Category D, recognition as an occupational disease is only possible if a plausible index person can be identified.

Since the publication of the new recognition criteria for the first time in 2003 [56], there has been a rise both in the number of tuberculosis cases reported and in the number recognised as occupational diseases at the Institute for Statutory Accident Insurance and Prevention in the Health and Welfare Services (Berufsgenossenschaft für Gesundheitsdienst und Wohlfahrtspflege, BGW) (Figure 4). In 2000, 24 HCWs with tuberculosis were recognised as having an occupational disease. In 2012, the number was 66. The rate of recognition among the decided claims rose from 18% in 2000 to 45% in 2012.

Since the risk of infection in the healthcare sector has not risen in recent years, one can assume that the increase in tuberculosis as an occupational disease is attributable to the extension of criteria that ease the burden of proof. An analysis of 150 expert opinions in claim proceedings cases found that it had been recommended that the burden of proof be eased in every second case (52%). Easing the burden of proof has halved

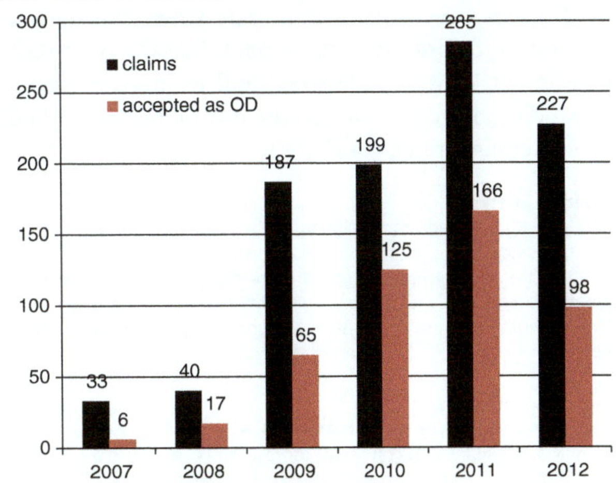

Figure 5 Number of latent tuberculosis infections (LTBIs) reported and recognised as occupational diseases in the years 2007 to 2012 at BGW according to [1].

the average time taken by occupational disease proceedings in Germany [56].

In addition to active tuberculosis, an LTBI can be reported as an occupational disease. The number of LTBIs reported as occupational diseases has risen significantly in the last few years (Figure 5). This increase, too, cannot be explained by an increase in the risk of infection in recent years. Rather, the increased reporting is based on the fact that for some years the above-mentioned IGRA has rendered the diagnosis of LTBI more valid in a population of HCWs with a high prevalence of BCG vaccination. It makes sense to report LTBI as an occupational disease especially if preventive chemotherapy is being considered. Preventive chemotherapy makes sense if a young healthcare worker (e.g. below the age of 35) has a positive IGRA eight weeks after close contact with a microscopically positive patient (see above). In this case, it is probable that the cause of the LTBI was occupational. There is no need for laborious investigations in occupational disease claim proceedings and the costs of consultation with and treatment by a pneumologist can be paid by the statutory accident insurance scheme under Paragraph 3 (Prevention) of the Ordinance on Occupational Diseases (BKV).

Conclusion

TB in HCW and nosocomial transmission of TB will remain a challenge for OSH experts as the downward trend in TB incidence in the general population has seemingly come to a halt and the TB incidence in migrants is still high in Germany. Furthermore, the pool of LTBI in HCW is large, especially in those who started work during the decades when TB incidence in Germany was higher. IGRAs allow for a better assessment of the infection risk than TSTs. However, they do not permit a distinction between remote and recent infection. Therefore evaluation of recent exposure remains important when choosing the target group for preventive treatment. Variability of IGRA results is not jet well understood and we need epidemiologic studies in order to decide the most effective and efficient screening strategy in HCWs.

Competing interest

RD received a travel grant from Qaigen/Cellestis and Oxford Immunotech and an unrestricted research fund from Qaigen/Cellestis. All other authors declare that they do not have any direct or indirect personal relationship, affiliation or association with any party with whom they deal in their day-to-day work that would give rise to any actual or perceived competing interest.

Authors' contributions

AN drafted the first version of the manuscript. AS, AMP, FCR and RD made substantial suggestions and comments for revision of the first draft. All authors read and approved the final version of the manuscript.

Author details

[1]Institute for Health Service Research in Dermatology and Nursing (IVDP), Center of Excellence for Epidemiology and Health Service Research for Healthcare Professionals (CVcare), University Medical Center Hamburg-Eppendorf, Martinistraße 52, Hamburg 20246, Germany. [2]Principles of Prevention and Rehabilitation Department (GPR), Institute for Statutory Accident Insurance and Prevention in the Health and Welfare Services (BGW), Hamburg, Germany. [3]Institute for Occupational and Maritime Medicine, University Medical Center Hamburg-Eppendorf (UKE), Hamburg, Germany. [4]Department of Respiratory Medicine, Hanover Medical School, Hanover, Germany. [5]Institute of Epidemiology, University Medical Center Schleswig-Holstein (UKSH), Kiel Campus, Kiel, Germany. [6]Lung Clinic Grosshansdorf, Member of the German Center for Lung Research (DZL), Grosshansdorf, Germany.

References

1. Nienhaus A, Kesavachandran C, Wendeler D, Haamann F, Dulon M: **Infectious diseases in healthcare workers - an analysis of the standardised data set of a German compensation board.** *J Occup Med Toxicol* 2012, **7**:8.
2. Von Hirschberg KR, Kähler B, Nienhaus A: **Social care and changes in occupational accidents and diseases – The situation in Eastern Europe in general and for skin diseases in particular.** *J Occup Med Toxicol* 2009, **4**:28.
3. RKI (Robert Koch Institut): *Report on the epidemiology of tuberculosis in Germany for the year 2011 [Bericht zur Epidemiologie der Tuberkulose in Deutschland für 2011, report in German].* Berlin: Robert Koch Institut; 2013.
4. Diel R, Seidler A, Nienhaus A, Rusch-Gerdes S, Niemann S: **Occupational risk of tuberculosis transmission in a low incidence area.** *Respir Res* 2005, **6**(1):35–45.
5. Diel R, Loytved G, Nienhaus A, Castell S, Detjen A, Geerdes-Fenge H, Haas W, Hauer B, Konigstein B, Maffei D, Magdorf K, Priwitzer M, Zellweger JP, Loddenkemper R: **New recommendations for contact tracing in tuberculosis [Neue Empfehlungen für die Umgebungsuntersuchungen bei Tuberkulose, article in German].** *Pneumologie* 2011, **65**:359–378.
6. Zwerling A, van den Hof S, Scholten J, Cobelens F, Menzies D, Pai M: **Interferon-gamma release assays for tuberculosis screening of healthcare workers: a systematic review.** *Thorax* 2012, **67**(1):62–70.
7. Nienhaus A, Ringshausen FC, Torres Costa J, Schablon A, Tripodi D: **Interferon-Y release assay vs. Tuberculin skin test for monitoring TB infection in healthcare workers.** *Expert Rev of Anti Infect Ther* 2013, **11**(1):37–43.
8. Diel R, Goletti D, Ferrara G, Bothamley G, Cirillo D, Kampmann B, Lange C, Losi M, Markova R, Migliori GB, Nienhaus A, Ruhwald M, Wagner D, Zellweger JP, Huitric E, Sandgren A, Manissero D: **Interferon-γ release assays for the diagnosis of latent M. tuberculosis infection: A systematic review and meta-analysis.** *Eur Respir J* 2011, **37**:88–99.
9. Diel R, Loddenkemper R, Nienhaus A: **Evidence-based comparison of commercial interferon-gamma release assays for detecting active TB: a meta-analysis.** *Chest* 2010, **137**(4):952–968.
10. Diel R, Loddenkemper R, Niemann S, Meywald-Walter K, Nienhaus A: **Negative and positive predictive value of a whole-blood IGRA for developing active TB - an update.** *AmJ Respir Crit Care Med* 2011, **183**:88–95.
11. Torres Costa J, Silva R, Ringshausen F, Nienhaus A: **Screening for tuberculosis and prediction of disease in Portuguese healthcare workers.** *J Occup Med Toxicol* 2011, **6**:19.
12. Nienhaus A, Schablon A, Costa JT, Diel R: **Systematic review of cost and cost-effectiveness of different TB-screening strategies.** *BMC Health Serv Res* 2011, **11**:247.
13. Ringshausen FC, Schablon A, Nienhaus A: **Interferon-gamma release assays for the tuberculosis serial testing of health care workers: a systematic review.** *J Occup Med Toxico* 2012, **7**(1):6.
14. Metcalfe JZ, Cattamanchi A, McCulloch CE, Lew JD, Ha NP, Graviss EA: **Test variability of the QuantiFERON-TB gold in-tube assay in clinical practice.** *Am J Respir Crit Care Med* 2013, **187**(2):206–211.
15. Andersen P, Doherty TM, Pai M, Weldingh K: **The prognosis of latent tuberculosis: can disease be predicted?** *Trends Mol Med* 2007, **13**(5):175–182.
16. Steingart KR, Flores LL, Dendukuri N, Schiller I, Laal S, Ramsay A, Hopewell PC, Pai M: **Commercial serological tests for the diagnosis of active pulmonary and extrapulmonary tuberculosis: An updated systematic review and meta-analysis.** *PLoS Med* 2011, **8**(8):e1001062.
17. Borgdorff MW, Nagelkerke NJ, de Haas PE, van Soolingen D: **Transmission of Mycobacterium tuberculosis depending on the age and sex of source cases.** *Am J Epidemiol* 2001, **154**(10):934–43.

18. Diel R, Schneider S, Meywald-Walter K, Ruf CM, Rüsch-Gerdes S, Niemann S: **Epidemiology of tuberculosis in Hamburg, Germany: long-term population-based analysis applying classical and molecular epidemiological techniques.** *J Clin Microbiol* 2002, **40**:532–539.
19. CDC - Centers for Disease Control: **The use of preventive therapy for tuberculosis infection in the United States – Recommendations of the Advisory Committee for Elimination of Tuberculosis.** *MMWR* 1990, **39**(RR-8):9–12.
20. Seidler A, Nienhaus A, Diel R: **The transmission of tuberculosis in the light of new molecular biological approaches.** *Occup Environ Med* 2004, **61**:96–102.
21. Cattamanchi A, Hopewell PC, Gonzalez LC, Osmond DH, Kawamura LM, Daley CL: **A 13-year molecular epidemiological analysis of tuberculosis in San Francisco.** *Int J Tuberc Lung Dis* 2006, **10**(3):297–304.
22. Baussano I, Bugiani M, Carosso A, Mariano D, Pia Barocelli A, Tagna M, Cascio V, Piccioni P, Arossa W: **Risk of tuberculin conversation among healthcare workers and the adoption of preventive measures.** *Occup Environ Med* 2007, **64**:61–66.
23. Baussano I, Nunn P, Williams B, Pivetta E, Bugiani M, Scano F: **Tuberculosis among health care workers.** *Emerg Infect Dis* 2011, **17**(3):488–494.
24. Menzies D, Joshi R, Pai M: **Risk of tuberculosis infection and disease associated with work in health care settings.** *Int J Tuberc Lung Dis* 2007, **11**(6):593–605.
25. Seidler A, Nienhaus A, Diel R: **Review of epidemiological studies on the occupational risk of tuberculosis in low-incidence areas.** *Respiration* 2005, **72**(4):431–446.
26. De Vries G, Sebek MMGG, Lambregts-van W: **Healthcare workers with tuberculosis infected during work.** *Eur Respir J* 2006, **28**:1216–1221.
27. Ong A, Rudoy I, Gonzalez LC, Creasman J, Kawamura LM, Daley C: **Tuberculosis in healthcare workers: a molecular epidemiologic study in San Francisco.** *Infect Control Hosp Epidemiol* 2007, **27**:453–458.
28. Schablon A, Peters C, Diel R, Diner G, Anskr U, Pankow W, Ringshausen FC, Nienhaus A: **Serial IGRA testing of trainees in the healthcare sector in a country with low incidence for tuberculosis - a prospective cohort study.** *GMS Hygiene and Infection Control* 2013, **8**(2):1–5.
29. Nienhaus A, Schablon A, Siano B, le Bacle C, Diel R: **Evaluation of the interferon-gamma release assay in healthcare workers.** *Int Arch Occup Environ Health* 2008, **81**:295–300.
30. Schablon A, Harling M, Diel R, Nienhaus A: **Risk of latent TB infection in individuals employed in the healthcare sector in Germany: a multicentre prevalence study.** *BMC Infect Dis* 2010, **10**:107.
31. Nienhaus A, Schablon A, Loddenkemper R, Hauer B, Wolf N, Diel R: **Prevalence of latent tuberculosis infection in healthcare workers in geriatric care [Erhöhte Prävalenz der latenten Tuberkulose-Infektion bei Beschäftigten in der Geriatrie].** *Pneumologie* 2007, **61**(9):613–616.
32. Torres Costa J, Sá R, Cardoso MJ, Silva R, Ferreira J, Ribeiro C, Miranda M, Plácido JL, Nienhaus A: **Tuberculosis screening in Portuguese healthcare workers using the tuberculin skin test and the interferon-gamma release assay.** *Eur Respir J* 2009, **34**:1423–8.
33. Tripodi D, Brunet-Courtois B, Nael V, Audrain M, Chailleux E, Germaud P, Naudin F, Muller JY, Bourrut-Lacouture M, Durand-Perdriel MH, Gordeeff C, Guillaumin G, Houdebine M, Raffi F, Boutoille D, Biron C, Potel G, Roedlich C, Geraut C, Schablon A, Nienhaus A: **Evaluation of the tuberculin skin test and the interferon-gamma release assay for TB screening in French healthcare workers.** *J Occup Med Toxicol* 2009, **4**:30.
34. Jensen PA, Lambert LA, Iademarco MF, Ridzon R: **Guidelines for preventing the transmission of Mycobacterium tuberculosis in Healthcare Settings.** *MMWR* 2005, **54**(RR-17):1–141.
35. WHO: **WHO policy on TB infection control in health-care facilities, congregate settings and household.** *WHO/HTM/TB* 2009, 419.
36. IUATLD - International Union against Tuberculosis and Lung Disease and the Tuberculosis Programme of the World Health Organization (WHO): **Control of tuberculosis in health care settings.** *Tuberc Lung Dis* 1994, **75**:94–95.
37. Ziegler R, Just HM, Castell S, Diel R, Gastmeier P, Haas W, Hauer B, Loytved G, Mielke M, Moser I, Nienhaus A, Richter E, Ruden H, Rusch-Gerdes S, Schaberg T, Wischnewski N, Loddenkemper R: **Tuberculosis Infection Control - Recommendations of the DZK [Infektionsprävention bei Tuberkulose - Empfehlungen des DZK. Article in German].** *Pneumologie* 2012, **6**:269–282.
38. Dharmadhikari AS, Mphahlele M, Stoltz A, Venter K, Mathebula R, Masotla T, Lubbe W, Pagano M, First M, Jensen PA, van der Walt M, Nardell EA: **Surgical face masks worn by patients with multidrug-resistant tuberculosis impact on infectivity of air on a hospital ward.** *Am J Respir Crit Care Med* 2012, **185**:1104–1109.
39. Menzies D, Fanning A, Yuan L, FitzGerald JM: **Canadian Collaborative Group in Nosocomial Transmission of Tuberculosis (2000). Hospital ventilation and risk of tuberculous infection in Canadian health care workers.** *Ann Intern Med* 2000, **133**:779–789.
40. Coffey CC, Lawrence RB, Zhuang Z: **Comparison of five methods for fit-testing N95 filtering-facepice respirators.** *Appl Occup Environ Hyg* 2002, **17**:723–730.
41. Zwerling A, Benedetti A, Cojocariu M, McIntosh F, Pietrangelo F, Behr MA, Schwartzmann K, Menzies D, Pai m: **Repeat IGRA testing in Canadian health workers: conversions or unexplained variability?** *PLoS One* 2013, **8**(1):e54748.
42. European Centre for Disease Prevention and Control: *Use of Interferon-Gamma Release Assays in Support of TB Diagnosis.* Stockholm: ECDC; 2011.
43. Schablon A, Harling M, Diel R, Ringshausen FC, Torres CJ, Nienhaus A: **Serial testing with an interferon-gamma release assay in German healthcare workers.** *GMS Hyg Infect Control* 2010, **5**(2).
44. Torres Costa J, Silva R, Sa R, Cardoso MJ, Nienhaus A: **Serial testing with the interferon-gamma release assay in Portuguese healthcare workers.** *Int Arch Occup Environ Health* 2011, **84**(4):461–469.
45. Moucaut A, Nienhaus A, Courtois B, Nael V, Longuenesse C, Ripault B, Rucay P, Moisan S, Roquelaure Y, Tripodi D: **The effect of introducing IGRA to screen French healthcare workers for tuberculosis and potential conclusions for the work organisation.** *J Occup Med Toxicol* 2013, **8**:12.
46. Nienhaus A, Schablon A, Ringshausen FC, Torres Costa J, Tripodi D, Diel R: **TB as an occupational disease. In Lange C, Migliori GB (Eds.), *Tuberculosis* (pp. 72–83).** *Eur Respir Soc* 2012, **58**:219–229.
47. Slater ML, Welland G, Pai M, Parsonnet J, Banaei N: **Challenges with QuantiFERON-TB Gold assay for large-scale, routine screening of U.S. healthcare workers.** *Am J Respir Crit Care Med* 2013, **188**(8):1005–10.
48. Ogunremi T, Menzies D, Embil J: **Canadian Tuberculosis Standards, Chapter 15 Prevention and control of tuberculosis transmission in healthcare and other settings – 7th edition.** *Can Thorac Soc* 2013. www.respiratoryguidelines.ca.
49. Smieja MJ, Marchetti CA, Cook DJ, Smaill FM: **Isoniazid for preventing tuberculosis in non-HIV infected persons.** *Cochrane Database Syst* 1999, **1**, CD0011363.
50. Schaberg T, Bauer T, Castell S, Dalhoff K, Detjen A, Diel R, Greinert U, Hauer B, Lange C, Magdorf K, Loddenkemper R: **Recommendations for Therapy, Chemoprevention and Chemoprophylaxis of Tuberculosis in Adults and Children, German Central Committee against Tuberculosis (DZK), German Respiratory Society (DGP) [Empfehlungen zur Therapie, Chemoprävention und Chemoprophylaxe der Tuberkulose bei Erwachsenen und Kindern. Deutsches Zentralinstitut zur Bekämpfung der Tuberkulose (DZK), Deutsche Gesellschaft für Pneumologie (DGP) Article in German].** *Pneumologie* 2012, **66**:133–171.
51. Steele MA, Burk RF, DesPrez RM: **Toxic hepatitis with isoniazid and rifampin- a meta-analysis.** *Chest* 1991, **99**:465–471.
52. Masandjwa R, Hausler H, Ram M, McIntrye JA, Gray GE, Chaisson RE: **New regimens to prevent tuberculosis in adults with HIV infection.** *N Engl J Med* 2011, **365**:11–20.
53. Shang N, Gordin F, Bliven-Sizemore E, Hackman J, Hamilton CD, Menzies D, Kerrigan A, Weis SE, Weiner M, Wing D, Conde MB, Bozeman L, Horsburgh CR Jr, Chaisson RE, TB Trials Consortium PREVENT TB Study Team: **Three months of once-weekly rifapentine and isoniazid for M tuberculosis infection.** *N Engl J Med* 2011, **2011**(365):2155–2166.
54. CDC - Centers for Disease Control and Prevention: **Recommendations for use of an isoniazid-rifapentine regimen with direct observation to treat latent Mycobacterium tuberculosis infection.** *MMWR* 2011, **60**:1650–1653.
55. INRS – Institut National de Recherche et Sécurité: *Les maladies professionelle.* Paris: INRS; 2012.
56. Nienhaus A: **Tuberculosis as occupational disease in healthcare workers [Tuberkulose als Berufskrankheit bei Beschäftigten im Gesundheitswesen, article in German].** *Med Sach* 2012, **108**(6):236–241.

Psychological stress and strain on employees in dialysis facilities: a cross-sectional study with the Copenhagen Psychosocial Questionnaire

Maren Kersten[1*], Agnessa Kozak[2], Dana Wendeler[1], Lara Paderow[3], Matthias Nübling[4] and Albert Nienhaus[1,2]

Abstract

Background: Work in dialysis facilities involves long term contact with chronically ill patients. International comparisons make it clear that dialysis work is being concentrated, staff is being reduced and more patients are being treated. It is more than 20 years since the last German publication on job strains and job satisfaction experienced by dialysis staff was published. The present study examines the stress and strain currently experienced by the staff of German dialysis facilities.

Methods: The staff of 20 dialysis facilities were surveyed with the Copenhagen Psychosocial Questionnaire (COPSOQ). The questionnaire was extended by adding dialysis-specific questions. The data from the dialysis facilities were assessed by comparison with other professions in medical care - nurses and geriatric nurses - using data recorded in the German COPSOQ database.

Results: A total of 367 employees took part in the study, corresponding to a response rate of 55%. For almost all psychosocial aspects, the dialysis staff regarded the stress and strain as being more critical than did the geriatric nurses. There were some positive differences in comparison to hospital nursing, including less conflict between work and private life. However, there were also negative differences, such as fewer possibilities of influencing the work.

Conclusions: The results of the study show that dialysis work exhibits both positive and negative aspects in comparison with other healthcare professions. The results in the different facilities were highly variable, indicating that the deficits found in the individual scales are not inevitable consequences of working in dialysis in general, but are influenced and might be favourably altered by the individual facilities.

Keywords: Stress, Strain, Dialysis staff, Health occupations, Psychosocial factors, COPSOQ

Zusammenfassung

Hintergrund: Die Arbeit in Dialyse-Einrichtungen ist geprägt durch langfristige Kontakte zu chronisch kranken Patienten. Die Verdichtung der Arbeit in der Dialysetätigkeit, Personalkürzungen sowie die steigende Zahl der Patienten zeigen sich in internationalen Vergleichen. Die letzte deutsche Veröffentlichung zum Thema Arbeitsbeanspruchungen und Arbeitszufriedenheit bei Dialysebeschäftigten ist vor mehr als 20 Jahren publiziert worden. Die vorliegende Studie untersucht die derzeitige Belastungs- und Beanspruchungssituation der Beschäftigten in Dialyse-Einrichtungen in Deutschland.

(Continued on next page)

* Correspondence: maren.kersten@bgw-online.de
[1]Institution for Statutory Accident Insurance and Prevention in the Healthcare and Welfare Services, Pappelallee 33-37, 22089 Hamburg, Germany
Full list of author information is available at the end of the article

(Continued from previous page)

Methoden: Eine Befragung von 20 Dialyse-Einrichtungen mit dem Copenhagen Psychosocial Questionnaire (COPSOQ) wurde durchgeführt. Der Fragebogen wurde um sieben dialysespezifische Fragen erweitert. Die gewonnenen Daten aus den Dialyse-Einrichtungen wurden zur besseren Einordnung mit denen anderer Pflegeberufen (Krankenpflege und Altenpflege) verglichen, welche in der COPSOQ-Datenbank erfasst sind.

Ergebnisse: Insgesamt nahmen 367 Beschäftigten an der Studie teil (Responserate 55%). Die Dialysebeschäftigten schätzten in fast allen psychosozialen Aspekten die Belastungs- und Beanspruchungssituation kritischer ein als diejenigen in der Altenpflege. Im Vergleich zu der stationären Krankenpflege gibt es zum Teil positive Unterschiede, z.B. geringere Konflikte zwischen Arbeit und Privatleben als auch kritischere Bewertungen, wie z.B. geringere Einflussmöglichkeiten bei der Arbeit.

Schlussfolgerungen: Die Ergebnisse der Studie weisen sowohl positive als auch negative Arbeitsaspekte der Dialysetätigkeit gegenüber den anderen Pflegeberufen auf. Die hohe Variabilität der Ergebnisse beim Vergleich zwischen den Einrichtungen deutet darauf hin, dass die beobachteten Defizite in einzelnen Skalen nicht zwingend dialysespezifisch sind, sondern von den konkreten Arbeitsbedingungen in den einzelnen Einrichtungen abhängen und von diesen beeinflusst werden können.

Schlüsselwörter: Belastung, Beanspruchung, Dialyse-Beschäftigte, Gesundheitsberufe, psychosoziale Arbeitsbedingungen, COPSOQ

Background

Work in dialysis facilities is marked by intensive and long-term contact with chronically ill patients [1,2], who are frequently frustrated or depressive [3]. This confrontation with suffering and death is very demanding for the medical care personnel in dialysis facilities [2,4-6]. There are also problems with staff reductions [7,8] and in mastering new modern technology [5,9,10].

In recent years, there have been numerous studies on the psychological stress and strain to which nurses and geriatric nurses are exposed [11-14], but little work has been done on the staff in dialysis facilities [15].

In work science and also in norms for measuring psychological stress, for instance ISO 10075 - one distinguishes between work load and stress (entirety of measurable external influence e.g. social working environment) and strain (effects of the stress on employee depending on his/her individual conditions e.g. emotional exhaustion) as well as the consequences of strain (e.g. disease).

A systematic review on stress and strain in employees in dialysis facilities [16] reported heterogeneous study results on stress, working conditions, strain and burnout. Current scientific knowledge indicates that there are positive aspects of this work, including high job satisfaction [1,7]. Moreover, nurses in dialysis facilities perceived their work as worthwhile and were very interested in professional details [17]. They enjoyed the high responsibility [1], as well as the chance to do things for people, the freedom to use their own judgement and the job security [15]. The negative aspects of dialysis work, as described in the literature, include low involvement in decision making [1,17], pressure at work, lack of time for individual patients, monotonous work and fear of blood-borne diseases [17]. Other negative aspects were the low salary and the general working conditions [15]. "Contact with other staff members could be a stressor as well as a resource for the nurses" [18]. Taken together, the data in the review indicate that the level of burnout is moderate for dialysis employees compared with different groups. In the systematic review seven studies were identified that used the same measurement (Maslach's Burnout Inventory). Three of these are comparable, because they used the same number of response scales and items. In the study by Klersy et al., burnout is moderate for dialysis employees (nurses and physicians) compared to healthcare workers and the general population in Italy [19]. In a further study, Arikan et al. found moderate burnout levels in comparison with intensive care units and ward nurses [20]. The study of Lewis et al. [5] used the medical workers (nurses and physicians) as reference group. In this study, the burnout level was slightly higher for the dialysis staff than in the reference groups.

The number of patients with chronic renal failure will rise in future, one reason being the increasing number of patients with diabetes. In 2012, about 90,000 persons required dialysis in Germany [21]. It can be expected that dialysis staff will be exposed to increasing stress, as staff numbers are being reduced and the number of patients is increasing, partially due to increased life expectancy [1,8]. It is therefore of the greatest importance that staff in dialysis facilities should be motivated and healthy and stay in their profession for as long as possible.

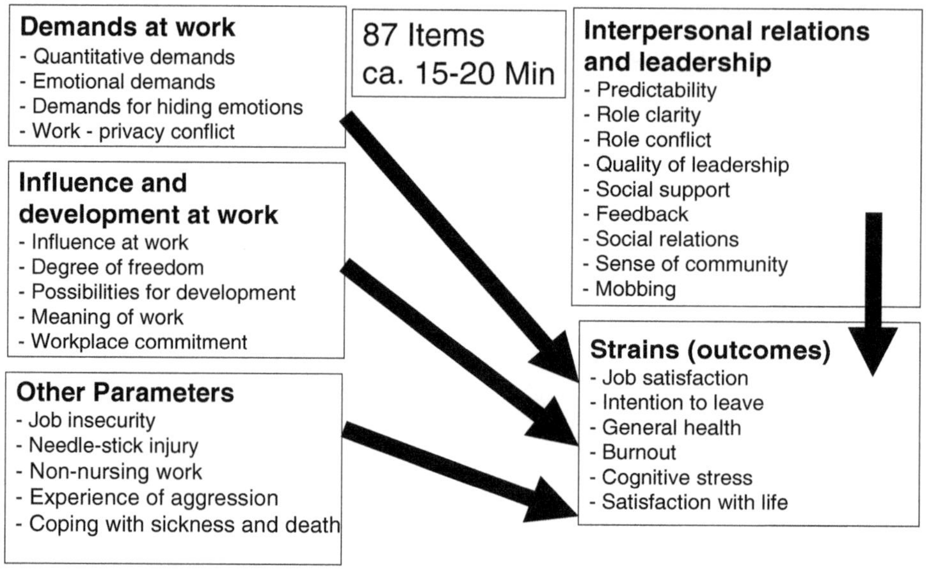

Figure 1 Dimensions of the COPSOQ questionnaire, with some additional dialysis items.

There are no current analyses of the working situation of dialysis staff in Germany. The last German study on the job strain and job satisfaction of dialysis nurses was published more than 20 years ago [4]. This study yielded the following results: the main sources of stress were the principle of maximum therapy, the consumerism of some patients and intra-team tensions. Almost two thirds of the employee confirmed the necessity of psychosocial staff training.

The objective of the present study is to examine the current psychological stress and strain on dialysis employees. The survey results for the dialysis staff were assessed by comparison with those for hospital nurses and for geriatric nurses to facilitate better interpretation and comparability.

Methods

Study sample

The total sample consisted of 20 dialysis facilities. Of these, 14 were from a random sample and six were from an opportunity sample located in North and Central Germany. For the random sample, 30 dialysis facilities insured at the Institution for Statutory Accident Insurance and Prevention in the Healthcare and Welfare Services (BGW) were randomly selected and requested to participate. The survey took place between October 2010 and April 2011. The two samples exhibit a difference in sociodemographics: In the random sample the proportion of women was higher (92.5% vs. 83%, $p = 0.009$) than in the opportunity sample. The two samples differ only in one scale of the COPSOQ scales, namely in the scale social relations (47 vs. 36, $p > 0.001$). The study was approved by Hamburg Ethics Committee. Each of the dialysis facilities was sent a report of the results, on the basis of which appropriate measures could be deduced. In addition, the dialysis facilities were offered counselling and support in the context of this study. All facilities accepted these offers.

Measurement

The survey was performed with the German standard version of the Copenhagen Psychosocial Questionnaire (COPSOQ) - a well validated and internationally recognised survey instrument for the measurement of psychosocial stress at work [22]. The questionnaire includes 87 items, mapped in 25 constructs: 22 scales and three single items. Mostly, a five-point Likert scale is used, where the first category represents the maximal value (for example, "always") and the last the minimal value (for example, "never"). These categories were allocated point scores (maximum = 100, minimum = 0). This transformation of the categories into point values is in accordance with a standardised procedure that was already used in the German validation study [23].

Data from a lot of studies done since 2005 applying this questionnaire is entered into a steadily growing COPSOQ database. In this database the data is weighted und classified by professional groups [24,25]. Surveys with the COPSOQ questionnaire thus allow a comparison of the results with profession specific reference values. The COPSOQ questionnaire consists of four main dimensions: demands at work, influence and development, interpersonal relations and leadership, strain (effects, outcomes) and one additional scale (job insecurity; Figure 1). The professional groups of hospital nurses and geriatric nurses, who were also from Germany, were included for comparison and to facilitate the interpretation of the psychosocial situation at work. At the time of the analysis (01 Oct. 2012), the COPSOQ database included 3,037 hospital nurses and 866 geriatric nurses. Of the group of hospital nurses, 84% were female and 16% male. One third of the employees (33%), were aged 40–49 years. 51% of the hospital employees worked full time. Of the group of geriatric care nurses, 88% of the employees were female and 12% were male. Two fifths of the geriatric care nurses (40%) were aged 40–49 years. 46% of the geriatric care nurses worked full time. In the surveys with the hospital and geriatric care nurses, not all the same information was collected as in the dialysis study.

Table 1 Description of the sample (N = 367)

Variable	Categories	n (%)
Sex	Female	329 (90%)
	Male	38 (10%)
Age (years)	< 30	57 (16%)
	30–39	64 (17%)
	40–49	125 (34%)
	≥ 50	110 (30%)
	No information	11 (3%)
Type of employment	Full time (> 34 h)	189 (51%)
	Part time (15–34 h)	164 (45%)
	Part time (< 15 h)	13 (4%)
On-call duties (per month)	None	267 (73%)
	1–5 times	89 (24%)
	> 5 times	11 (3%)
Night shifts (per month)	Never	219 (60%)
	1–5 times	118 (32%)
	> 5 times	30 (8%)
Split shifts (per month)	Never	348 (95%)
	1–5 times	12 (3%)
	> 5 times	7 (2%)
Variable shifts (per month)	Never	79 (21%)
	1–5 times	91 (25%)
	> 5 times	197 (54%)
Job experience (years)	≤ 5	96 (26%)
	6–10	77 (21%)
	11–15	55 (15%)
	16–20	66 (18%)
	> 20	73 (20%)
Professional group	Certified nurse	260 (71%)
	Trained nurse	22 (6%)
	Other nurse	25 (7%)
	Other professions (e.g. administration)	60 (16%)

Other parameters

To assess dialysis specific working conditions (hazards and demands), this questionnaire was extended by seven questions, which were based on a literature search [16], as well as qualitative interviews with experts. The following three questions had dichotomous response categories (yes/no):

- Within the last 12 months, have you had a needlestick injury?
- During the last 12 months, have you experienced physical aggression from a patient?
- During the last 12 months, have you experienced verbal aggression from a patient?

Four additional questions could be answered on a five-point Likert scale. The answers ranged from 1 ("to a very high degree") to 5 ("to a very low degree"):

- Are you scared of becoming infected with a blood-borne disease during work?
- Do you feel stressed by the verbal or physical aggression of your patients or their families?
- Are you expected to perform many tasks that are remote from the patients (e.g. organisation or documentation)?
- Are you stressed by having to cope with the patients' suffering or death?

Persons are rated as highly stressed if they answer the individual dialysis-specific questions with "to a high degree" or "to a very high degree".

Statistical analysis

To evaluate the observed differences between dialysis staff, hospital nursing and geriatric nursing, a nomenclature was employed that is already regularly used in COPSOQ studies: a difference of at least 5 points in the mean values of groups is evaluated as a clear difference, a deviation of 10 or more points is evaluated as a very clear deviation [12]. This rule of thumb is based on the effect size measure (Cohen's d): COPSOQ scales have usually standard deviations of 15–25 points, thus 5 points represent a small to intermediate effect size of 0.2 – 0.33 and 10 point represent middle to strong effect sizes 0.4 to 0.66.

When interpreting COPSOQ scale values it must be borne in mind that high values stand for "a lot" and low values for "a little". Whether this is favourable or unfavourable depends on the content of the individual scale.

Differences between the professional groups were examined by analysis of variance (ANOVA). Mean value differences were tested with Scheffé's post hoc test. The values were described as statistically significant if $p < 0.05$. Only results being statistically significant and fulfilling the 5

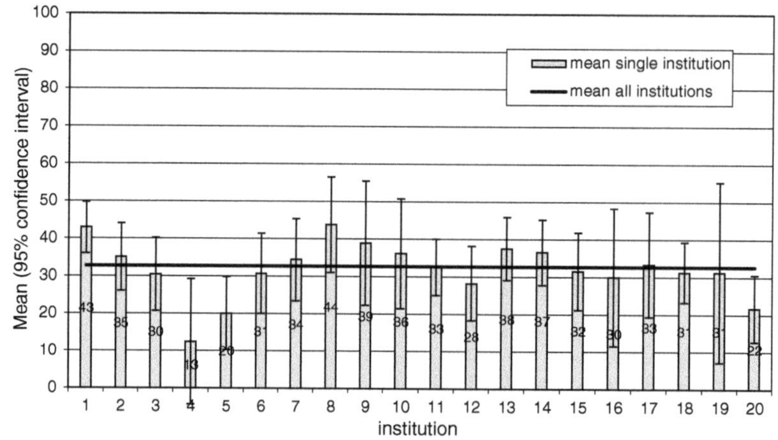

Figure 2 Rating of all dialysis facilities concerning the "fear of blood-borne diseases".

points difference criterion (see above) are interpreted. The data analysis was performed with the IBM SPSS Statistics 21 program. The potential influence of different response rates on the study results was assessed by dichotomising the sample in persons from facilities with a response rate below or above the median response rate and performing non- parametric tests for the comparison of distributions of the 25 outcome scales or variables of the COPSOQ. As we have a random and an opportunity sample, the influence of the two different sampling methods was assessed in a similar way.

Results

A total of 669 questionnaires were issued; 367 employees took part in the study. The response rate was 55%. The interquartile range of the response rate was 45 to 65% and the total range 22 to 96%. With the exception of social relations, no statistically significant difference in the scales and variables of the COPSOQ was observed between the two groups with high or low response rates. The participating dialysis facilities had between 13 and 55 employees. Table 1 describes the study population. Most of the participants were female (90%). The mean age was 43.7 years (±10.4). About one third of the participants was 50 years or older. More than half the interviewees had full time jobs. 27% of the participants performed on-call duties. 40% of the participants stated that they had a night shift at least once a month. Split shifts were rare in the study population (5%). Most participants were registered nurses (71%).

The dialysis-specific questions were answered as follows: 9% reported that they had suffered from needle-stick injuries in the previous 12 months. 11% of employees reported that they were very scared of becoming infected with a blood-borne disease. Though, 26% of employees reported that they were occasionally scared of an infection. 25% of participants reported that they had suffered physical aggression within the previous 12 months. The majority (72%) of employees had suffered verbal aggression. 15% of employees felt under severe stress from physical or verbal aggression from the patients or their families. Almost half the participants (48%) felt that they were under severe stress due to non-nursing tasks. 25% of employees were under stress from coping with the patients' suffering or death.

For the dialysis-specific items, there are no comparative values from other professional groups. Therefore a mean value was calculated for each dialysis facility and compared with the mean for all dialysis facilities. The following illustration shows the variability in the answers among the dialysis facilities, using the question, "Are you scared of becoming infected with a blood-borne disease during work?" as an example. The mean value was 33, with a minimum at 13 points and a maximum at 44 points (Figure 2).

The following table (Table 2) shows the differences in the means for the different COPSOQ scales for dialysis staff, hospital nursing and geriatric nursing.

Employees in dialysis can best be compared to hospital employees, as most of the sample had similar education (Table 1). The greatest significant positive effects (dialysis versus hospital nursing) with at least a small effect size were found in the following aspects: lower quantitative demands (55 vs. 60) and lower emotional demands (60 vs. 65), as well as lower work-privacy conflicts (48 vs. 53).

Overall, it was found that the influence and the degree of freedom at work in dialysis facilities was rated markedly lower in dialysis facilities than in hospital nursing: Influence at work (29 vs. 38), degree of freedom at work (33 vs. 40) and possibilities for development (58 vs. 70). As regards the dimension of social relations and leadership, it was found that the quality of leadership (47 vs. 54), feedback (37 vs. 44) and predictability (50 vs. 55) were also rated as being poorer. Dialysis staff also felt that they were more exposed to mobbing (27 vs. 20).

Table 2 Differences in means for the different COPSOQ scales

Scale	COPSOQ dialysis n = 367 Mean (SD)	COPSOQ nursing n = 3037 Mean (SD)	Difference dialysis-nursing Points	p value (Scheffé)	COPSOQ geriatric nursing n = 866 Mean (SD)	Difference dialysis-geriatric nursing Points	p value (Scheffé)
Demands at work							
Quantitative demands	55 (16)	60 (17)	−5	< 0.001	51 (21)	4	0.003
Emotional demands	60 (19)	65 (18)	−5	< 0.001	54 (20)	6	< 0.001
Demands for hiding emotions	53 (23)	53 (21)	0	n.s.	43 (22)	10	< 0.001
Work-privacy conflict	48 (25)	53 (27)	−5	0.011	43 (29)	5	0.003
Influence and development at work							
Influence at work	29 (19)	38 (20)	−9	< 0.001	42 (21)	−13	< 0.001
Degree of freedom	33 (16)	40 (19)	−7	< 0.001	41 (19)	−8	< 0.001
Possibilities for development	58 (17)	70 (17)	−12	< 0.001	71 (17)	−13	< 0.001
Meaning of work	77 (17)	80 (17)	−3	0.006	86 (15)	−9	< 0.001
Workplace commitment	55 (18)	55 (19)	0	n.s.	63 (20)	−8	< 0.001
Interpersonal relations and leadership							
Predictability	50 (22)	55 (21)	−5	< 0.001	64 (21)	−14	< 0.001
Role clarity	74 (16)	76 (16)	−2	0.018	80 (15)	−6	< 0.001
Role conflict	44 (20)	48 (21)	−4	0.002	39 (21)	5	0.004
Quality of leadership	47 (24)	54 (25)	−7	< 0.001	64 (24)	−17	< 0.001
Social support	65 (20)	69 (20)	−4	0.002	73 (19)	−8	< 0.001
Feedback	37 (21)	44 (22)	−7	< 0.001	53 (23)	−16	< 0.001
Social relations (quantity)	46 (17)	48 (28)	-2	n.s.	34 (30)	12	< 0.001
Sense of community	73 (16)	76 (17)	−3	0.010	78 (18)	−5	< 0.001
Mobbing	27 (26)	20 (23)	7	< 0.001	19 (23)	8	< 0.001
Insecurity at work	28 (22)	30 (22)	−2	n.s.	31 (24)	−3	n.s.
Strain (effects, outcomes)							
Job satisfaction	62 (14)	61 (15)	1	n.s.	67 (15)	−5	< 0.001
Intension to leave	17 (23)	18 (23)	−1	n.s.	12 (19)	5	0.014
General health	70 (19)	72 (19)	−2	n.s.	70 (20)	0	n.s.
Personal burnout	48 (19)	48 (18)	0	n.s.	42 (19)	6	< 0.001
Cognitive stress	32 (19)	29 (19)	3	n.s.	26 (19)	6	< 0.001
Satisfaction with life	66 (19)	66 (19)	0	n.s.	66 (20)	0	n.s.

Note. ≥5 points difference in mean corresponds to a small effect size (0.2-0.33) and ≥10 points to an intermediate or high (0.4-0.66) effect size.

A comparison was also made with geriatric nursing. Staff at dialysis facilities was found to have a more critical view of the stress and strain than the geriatric nurses, with respect to almost all psychosocial aspects. The exception was the quantity of social relations at work, which was viewed much more favourably by the dialysis employees (46 vs. 34).

In all the scales, there was striking variability between the individual dialysis facilities (N = 20). For example, the Figure 3 shows the variability between the facilities with respect to the scale "influence at work" (overall mean = 29 points).

Discussion

This is the first study for more than 20 years to record the psychological stress and strain on dialysis staff in Germany. By means of a survey with the COPSOQ questionnaire, the psychosocial occupational stress and strain were recorded in 367 employees working in 20 different dialysis facilities. To facilitate the classification of the dialysis survey, the results were compared with those for other health care professions. The dialysis results were less favourable than those for institutional geriatric care in almost all aspects. In the comparison with hospital nursing, the dialysis results were more

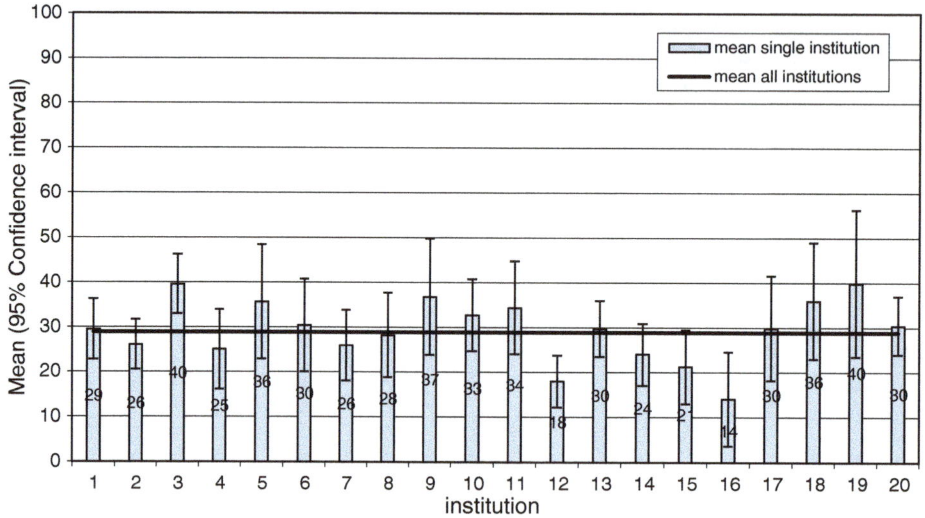

Figure 3 Mean values of 20 dialysis facilities for the scale "influence at work".

favourable in the dimension of demands at work (quantitative demands, emotional demands and work-privacy conflict). More critical values were mainly found in the dimension influence and development at work (influence at work, degree of freedom, possibilities for development), as well as the dimension interpersonal relations and leadership (predictability, quality of leadership, feedback, mobbing).

The dialysis staff rated the quantitative demands considerably lower than did the geriatric nurses. However, the values for the dialysis staff were the same as for the COPSOQ mean (the weighted mean for all employees who answered the questionnaire; database 01. Oct. 12). In spite of the favourable comparison with hospital nursing, this indicates that the quantitative demands are in need of improvement. Many studies show clearly that quantitative demands are a critical issue, particularly in the context of staff reductions [5,17] or limited number of staff [10,26]. As for the emotional demands, the hospital nurses rated this aspect considerably higher than the other two professional groups. In a study among different professionals groups, jobs with client work scored highest on both aspects: emotional demand and demands for hiding emotions [27]. Ashker et al. examined the work-related emotional stressors among dialysis staff and concluded that four factors influence the emotional well-being: intensive and long-term relationships with the patients, development of the disease and near-death experiences, deterioration in the patient's physical and psychological well-being and pressure at work [2].

Although some aspects of demands at work were generally rated better in dialysis than in hospital nursing, there is still need for action. The stress may rise in dialysis setting, as a result of possible staff reductions in the health care system, reductions in budgets, the increase in the number of dialysis-dependent patients with multiple diseases, as well as the complex technical handling of modern instruments.

As discussed in Karasek's demand-control-support model (as extended by: Karasek, R. & Theorell, T. [28]), it is not inevitable that high demands at work are inherently negative, if balanced by high degree of freedom and social support at work. However, the dialysis employees rated their influence and the degree of freedom as being significantly lower than did hospital nurses, thus a compensation of the relatively high demands by high control or support is not given. An obvious conclusion is that the standardized work processes allow little possibility of influencing the work; the employees themselves described their work as routine [17]. Other studies also have shown that dialysis staff would like to be more actively involved in the decision making process [1,17,29]. There are major possibilities for development in this dimension. The view of the 20 dialysis facilities in this survey makes it clear that some facilities exhibit much better values in this respect than do others.

The results indicate that it is easier for dialysis staff to combine work and private life than it is for hospital nurses. Other studies have emphasised night shifts [20] or shift work [18] as stressors. In Germany night shifts are performed by nearly very nurse in hospital and geriatric care. The lower number of dialysis nurses (40%) performing night shifts might explain the positive effect on the compatibility between private and professional lives in our study.

Aspects of the dimension of interpersonal relations and leadership were more critically rated than by hospital nurses (e.g. predictability, quality of leadership, feedback and mobbing). These aspects have hardly been considered or have not been explicitly queried in the literature on the occupational situation in dialysis. Apart from that, these findings provide the first evidence for possible interventions in dialysis facilities. Enhancement of leadership competence and establishment of a constructive feedback culture could lead to improvements in these aspects, supported by better adapted planning and work management, optimised to the requirements of the employees. According to a current research with the COPSOQ dataset, the quality of leadership contributed significantly to job satisfaction [30]. Gregersen et al. found in their review the first empirical evidence on the influence of various leadership style on the health of employees [31]. However, more research is needed on this aspect in the dialysis setting.

As regards the dialysis-specific questions, it was found that 25% of the employees had high or very high fear of blood-borne diseases. In contrast, Brokalaki et al. found that 79% of participants had high fear of blood-borne diseases [1]. Similar results were also found by Nakahara et al. [17]. According to data from the compensation board in Germany (BGW), blood-borne viral diseases have become rarer in health service employees [32]. It is unfortunately unknown how frequently dialysis employees are affected. If safe products are used in dialysis, this may help to alleviate employees' fear of blood-borne viral diseases.

In our study, the majority of participants (72%) reported that they had experienced verbal aggression during the preceding 12 months. 25% of participants reported that they had suffered physical aggression. In a qualitative study, Murphy reported that most employees had suffered verbal and physical aggression during their working lives [18]. The comparison between dialysis staff and hospital nurses led to the following picture: Schablon et al. recorded that 79% of hospital nurses had suffered verbal aggression [33]. This is consistent with the percentage (72%) in the present study. Moreover, 25% of dialysis staff reported physical aggression, which is much lower than the value found for the hospital nurses (56%). On the other hand, 15% of dialysis staff felt that they were under severe stress due to verbal or physical aggression. It is therefore important that dialysis employees should have training in de-escalation and coping strategies, in particular for situations in which employees have been attacked.

Almost every second dialysis employee felt under severe stress from non-nursing tasks. Lewis et al. also reported occupational stress from non-nursing tasks [5]. Other studies do not differentiate between nursing and non-nursing tasks, but just report high occupational stress [1,8,17].

Twenty-five per cent of participants were stressed by having to cope with sickness and death. Other studies have found higher values for stress from near-death experiences or the death of patients [1,2,5,6].

When comparing dialysis staff with geriatric nurses, it should be considered that in the COPSOQ database the professions or occupations are classified according to the system of job classification of the German Federal Statistical Office. Thus, there is no differentiation between out-patient and in-patient geriatric care. The values for both sectors are combined to a single mean value, which can bias our conclusion. In a study by Nübling et al. these two groups were separately examined [12]. They found that out-patient personnel had a much better opinion of their psychosocial situation than did in-patient personnel. However, we were surprised by the relatively poor results for dialysis staff in comparison to geriatric nurses in nearly all aspects. It would be interesting to analyse whether and to what extent these differences can be explained by individual *characteristics* or by differences in the organisations.

To our knowledge, there is no comprehensive data to compare our sample with the total population of German dialyses employees. Therefore, we cannot proof the representativeness of the study sample. In the present cross-sectional study, stress and strain were recorded at the same time, which can lead to a common method bias. Moreover, mean comparisons cannot be used to identify factors that may be linked to possible impairments in well-being, i.e. no relationships are established between psychosocial occupational stress and outcomes. Nevertheless, the results provide some indications of possible approaches to reduce stress on employees in dialysis.

Conclusions

In conclusion, dialysis staff rated their possibilities for influence and development, the social relations and quality of leadership poorer than did hospital and geriatric nursing. Improvement in feedback culture and emphasis by superior on greater employee participation and involvement could decrease the stress suffered by dialysis employees, as the differences from hospital and geriatric nursing are greatest in these areas. The high variance of the results between the facilities indicates that the observed deficits are not inherent to dialysis, but can be favourably influenced by the individual facilities.

Abbreviations

BGW: Institution for Statutory Accident Insurance and Prevention in the Healthcare and Welfare Services in Germany (Berufsgenossenschaft für Gesundheitsdienst und Wohlfahrtspflege); COPSOQ: Copenhagen Psychosocial Questionnaire.

Competing interests

The authors declare that they have no competing interests.

Authors' contributions

AN and MK conceived the study after a systematic review. Data collection and analysis were performed by MN, AK, DW and MK. The first draft of the paper was written by: MK and AK. Important suggestions for the improvement of the first draft were provided by DW, LP, MN and AN. All authors read and approved the manuscript.

Acknowledgements
We want to thank all dialysis nurses who participate in this study.

Author details
[1]Institution for Statutory Accident Insurance and Prevention in the Healthcare and Welfare Services, Pappelallee 33-37, 22089 Hamburg, Germany. [2]University Medical Center Hamburg-Eppendorf Competence Centre for Epidemiology and Health Services Research in Nursing (CVcare), Martinistr. 52, 20246 Hamburg, Germany. [3]University of Applied Science in Hamburg, Lohbrügger Kirchstraße 65, 21033 Hamburg, Germany. [4]Freiburg research centre for occupational and social medicine, Bertoldstr. 27, D 79098 Freiburg, Germany.

References

1. Brokalaki H, Matziou V, Thanou J, Zirogiannis P, Dafni U, Papadatou D: **Job-related stress among nursing personnel in greek dialysis units.** *EDTNA ERCA J* 2001, **27:**181–186.
2. Ashker VE, Penprase B, Salman A: **Work-related emotional stressors and coping strategies that affect the well-being of nurses working in hemodialysis units.** *Nephrol Nurs J* 2012, **39:**231–236.
3. Bilgic A, Akgul A, Sezer S, Arat Z, Ozdemir FN, Haberal M: **Nutritional status and depression, sleep disorder, and quality of life in hemodialysis patients.** *J Ren Nutr* 2007, **17:**381–388.
4. Muthny FA: **Job strains and job satisfaction of dialysis nurses.** *Psychother Psychosom* 1989, **51:**150–155.
5. Lewis SL, Campbell MA, Becktell PJ, Cooper CL, Bonner PN, Hunt WC: **Work stress, burnout, and sense of coherence among dialysis nurses.** *ANNA J* 1992, **19:**545–53. discussion.
6. Lewis SL, Bonner PN, Campbell MA, Cooper CL, Willard A: **Personality, stress, coping, and sense of coherence among nephrology nurses in dialysis settings.** *ANNA J* 1994, **21:**325–335.
7. Anderson JE, Torres JR, Bitter DC, Anderson SC, Briefel GR: **Role of physician assistants in dialysis units and nephrology.** *Am J Kidney Dis* 1999, **33:**647–651.
8. O'Brien JL: **Relationships among structural empowerment, psychological empowerment, and burnout in registered staff nurses working in outpatient dialysis centers.** *Nephrol Nurs J* 2011, **38:**475–481.
9. Kotzabassaki S, Parissopoulos S: **Burnout in renal care professionals.** *EDTNA ERCA J* 2003, **29:**209–213.
10. Dermody K, Bennett PN: **Nurse stress in hospital and satellite haemodialysis units.** *J Ren Care* 2008, **34:**28–32.
11. Glaser J, Lampert B, Weigl M: *Arbeit in der Stationären Altenpflege - Analyse und Förderung von Arbeitsbedingungen, Interaktion, Gesundheit und Qualität. Abschlussbericht zum Forschungsvorhaben F1977 zur Vorlage an die Bundesanstalt für Arbeitsschutz und Arbeitsmedizin - Projekt BELUGA (Belastungsanalyse und Gesundheitsförderliche Arbeit in der Altenpflege).* München, Bericht Nr. 86: Lehrstuhl für Psychologie, Technische Universität München; 2007.
12. Nübling M, Vomstein M, Schmidt SG, Gregersen S, Dulon M, Nienhaus A: **Psychosocial work load and stress in the geriatric care.** *BMC Public Health* 2010, **10:**428.
13. Hasselhorn HM, Conway PM, Widerszal-Bazyl M, Simon M, Tackenberg P, Schmidt S, Camerino D, Müller BH: **Contribution of job strain to nurses' consideration of leaving the profession - results from the longitudinal European nurses' early exit study.** *Scand J Work Environ Health Suppl* 2008, **6:**75–82.
14. Bakker AB, Killmer CH, Siegrist J, Schaufeli WB: **Effort-reward imbalance and burnout among nurses.** *J Adv Nurs* 2000, **31:**884–891.
15. Ross J, Jones J, Callaghan P, Eales S, Ashman N: **A survey of stress, job satisfaction and burnout among haemodialysis staff.** *J Ren Care* 2009, **35:**127–133.
16. Böhmert M, Kuhnert S, Nienhaus A: **Psychological stress and strain in dialysis staff - a systematic review.** *J Ren Care* 2011, **37:**178–189.
17. Nakahara N, Morita N, Uchida M, Kishimoto T, Miura K: **Nursing care for dialysis patients in Japan.** *EDTNA ERCA J* 2004, **30:**217–221.
18. Murphy F: **Stress among nephrology nurses in Northern Ireland.** *Nephrol Nurs J* 2004, **31:**423–431.
19. Klersy C, Callegari A, Martinelli V, Vizzardi V, Navino C, Malberti F, Tarchini R, Montagna G, Guastoni C, Bellazzi R, Rampino T, David S, Barbieri C, Dal Canton A, Politi P: **Burnout in health care providers of dialysis service in Northern Italy-a multicentre study.** *Nephrol Dial Transpl* 2007, **22:**2283–2290.
20. Arikan F, Köksal CD, Gökce C: **Work-related stress, burnout, and job satisfaction of dialysis nurses in association with perceived relations with professional contacts.** *Dialysis & Transplantation* 2007, **36:**182–191.
21. Schulz KH, Thaiss F: **Long-term outcome with end-stage renal disease - survival is not enough: does dialysis or kidney transplantation matter?** *Bundesgesungheitsbl Gesundheitsforsch Gesundheitsschutz* 2012, **55:**543–551.
22. Nübling M, Stößel U, Hasselhorn HM, Michaelis M, Hofmann F: *Methoden zur Erfassung Psychischer Belastungen - Erprobung Eines Messinstrumentes (COPSOQ).* Dortmund/Berlin/Dresden: Wirtschaftsverlag NW, Verlag für neue Wissenschaften; 2005.
23. Nübling M, Stössel U, Hasselhorn HM, Michaelis M, Hofmann F: **Measuring psychological stress and strain at work - evaluation of the COPSOQ questionnaire in Germany.** *Psychol Med* 2006, **3:**Doc05.
24. Nübling M, Hasselhorn HM: **The Copenhagen psychosocial questionnaire in Germany: from the validation of the instrument to the formation of a job-specific database of psychosocial factors at work.** *Scand J Public Health* 2010, **38:**120–124.
25. Nübling M, Vomstein M, Nübling T, Stößel U, Hasselhorn HM, Hofmann F: *Referenzdaten zu psychischen Belastungen – die COPSOQ online-Datenbank*, 4. Umweltmed: Arbeitsmed.Sozialmed; 2012:3–S. 180.
26. Flynn L, Thomas-Hawkins C, Clarke SP: **Organizational traits, care processes, and burnout among chronic hemodialysis nurses.** *West J Nurs Res* 2009, **31:**569–582.
27. Kristensen TS, Borritz M, Villadsen E, Christensen KB: **The copenhagen burnout inventory: a new tool for the assessment of burnout.** *Work Stress* 2005, **19:**192–207.
28. Karasek RA, Theorell T: *Healthy work, stress, productivity, and the reconstruction of working life.* New York: Basic Books; 1990.
29. Di Iorio B, Cillo N, Cucciniello E, Bellizzi V: **Burn-out in the dialysis unit.** *J Nephrol* 2008, **21**(Suppl 13):S158–S162.
30. Nübling M, Stössel U, Michaelis M: **Messung von Führungsqualität und Belastungen am Arbeitsplatz: Die Deutsche Standardversion des COPSOQ (Copenhagen Psychosocial Questionnaire) Fehlzeiten-Report 2009.** In Edited by Badura B, Schröder H, Klose J, Macco K. Berlin Heidelberg: Springer; 2010:pp.253–261.
31. Gregersen S, Kuhnert S, Zimber A, Nienhaus A: **Leadership behaviour and health - current research state.** *Gesundheitswesen* 2011, **73:**3–12.
32. Nienhaus A, Kesavachandran C, Wendeler D, Haamann F, Dulon M: **Infectious diseases in healthcare workers - an analysis of the standardised data set of a German compensation board.** *J Occup Med Toxicol* 2012, **7:**8.
33. Schablon A, Zeh A, Wendeler D, Peters C, Wohlert C, Harling M, Nienhaus A: **Frequency and consequences of violence and aggression towards employees in the German healthcare and welfare system: a cross-sectional study.** *BMJ Open* 2012, **2:**e001420.

21

Brachial plexopathy: a case–control study of the relation to physical exposures at work

Jørgen Riis Jepsen[1,2]

Abstract

Background: Work-related upper limb disorders constitute a diagnostic challenge. However, patterns of neurological abnormalities that reflect brachial plexus dysfunction are frequent in limbs with pain, weakness and/or numbness/ tingling. There is limited evidence about the association between occupational physical exposures and brachial plexopathy.

Methods: 80 patients with brachial plexopathy according to defined criteria and 65 controls of similar age and sex without upper limb complaints were recruited by general practitioners. Patients and controls completed a questionnaire on physical and psychosocial work-exposures and provided psychophysical ratings of their perceived exposures. The exposures of cases and controls were compared by a Wilcoxon rank sum test. Odds ratios and dose–response relationships were studied by logistic regression.

Results: Whether assessed as the extent during the workday or days/week, most physical exposures, in particular upper limb posture and repetition, were significant risk indicators with clear dose–response relationships. These findings were supported by psychophysical responses that also identified perceived work pace and the use of force as risk indicators. The identified psychosocial relations were limited to measures reflecting physical exposures.

Conclusions: While the identified risk indicators have previously been associated to upper limb *symptoms* as well as to diagnosed *disorders* other than brachial plexopathy, this study indicates an association between physical and work-exposures and brachial plexopathy. Longitudinal studies should be conducted in order to exclude bias from information and selection, both of which may occur with the applied case–control design.

Background

In addition to pain, which is often of a neuropathic character, people with upper limb complaints frequently report weakness and/or numbness/tingling. The character of pain may be nagging, stabbing, burning, "like tooth ache" and/or shooting [1]. This combination of symptoms suggests neural involvement and may represent a disorder of the brachial plexus.

Few studies, however, have established a relation between physical exposures and brachial plexopathy [2], although many have suggested hypothetical relations [3-7]. The limited evidence for the existence and frequency of relation to work of brachial plexopathy argues for further research in this field.

Studies of occupational risk indicators for upper limb disorders should rely on both signs and symptoms [8]. Still, epidemiological studies have mainly been restricted to studies of the relation to regional symptoms [9] or to the so-called "specific" disorders such as, e.g. carpal tunnel syndrome [10,11], wrist tendinitis [11,12], epicondylitis [11] and shoulder tendinitis [13,14]. The challenge is that a major group of so-called "non-specific" disorders (that do not meet the criteria for "specific" conditions) are only characterised by symptoms [1]. In a study of upper extremity musculoskeletal complaints, a specific diagnosis was made in only 25% and 16% of patients were not given any diagnosis. The remaining 59% patients (n = 389) were labelled as "non-specific", i.e. "repetitive strain syndrome", by the clinician. The pain in this group of patients was equally distributed among

Correspondence: joergen.riis.jepsen@svs.regionsyddanmark.dk
[1]Department of Occupational Medicine, Hospital of South-western Jutland, Østergade 81-83, DK-6700 Esbjerg, Denmark
[2]Center of Maritime Health and Society, Institute of Public Health, University of Southern Denmark, DK-6700 Esbjerg, Denmark

neck, shoulder, upper arm, elbow, forearm, and wrist/hand and shared the characteristics of neuropathic pain described above. "Repetitive strain syndrome" was significantly associated with activities with elevated arms, repetitive and extreme movements [1]. In a French population, more than 50% of workers participating in an epidemiologic surveillance system presented non-specific symptoms during the preceding 12 months, and only 13% had a defined upper limb musculoskeletal condition, in particular rotator cuff syndrome, carpal tunnel syndrome and epicondylitis [15].

The application in people with upper limb pain in the primary health sector [16] and in clinical occupational medicine [17-19] of a physical examination consisting of semi-quantitative ratings of selective muscle weakness, sensory deviations from normal in homonymous innervation territories and disturbed mechano-sensitivity of nerve trunks has revealed high frequencies of neurological patterns in accordance with neuropathies with various locations. The clinical applicability and feasibility of this approach, which is based on the classical neurological examination, is indicated by good inter-examiner reliability [17,20-22], construct validity in terms of correlation of physical findings to symptoms [19], and significant interrelations of locations of defined focal neuropathy [23]. The majority of the patients that were subjected to this examination displayed neurological physical patterns in accordance with brachial plexopathy with a prevailing infraclavicular location [16,20]. This observation suggests the importance of identifying, managing and preventing this condition.

Brachial plexopathy remains a controversial diagnosis. Some researchers and clinicians argue that the clinical assessment has a limited validity [24] and that the diagnosis mostly cannot be confirmed by electrophysiological studies [25,26]. They therefore reject the frequency of brachial plexopathy [27] Other researchers and clinicians recognize brachial plexopathy as a common condition [28,29] – also in the context of occupational health [30]. Sheth and Belzberg regard brachial plexopathy as the most underrated, overlooked, misdiagnosed, and difficult to manage peripheral nerve compression in the upper extremity [31].

Clinicians tend to emphasize brachial plexopathy as a condition related to an affliction of the brachial plexus on its passage through the scalene triangle and pay less attention to a compromise more distally, e.g. at the passage of the brachial plexus behind the pectoralis minor muscle (pectoralis minor syndrome) [32,33]. In the clinical setting as well as in epidemiological research distorted diagnostics due to this focus would be unfortunate, in particular in case of the latter location being more common.

Brachial plexopathy can be defined as a combination of symptoms (pain or subjective weakness or sensory abnormalities) and physical findings (weakness in defined muscles, mechanical allodynia at the brachial plexus, and sensory deviations from normal with specific locations). This physical approach permits the examiner to diagnose brachial plexopathy and to define its location precisely [17,20] and accurately [19,23] in a significant number of symptomatic patients, including patients that are diagnostically unclassifiable according to standard diagnostic criteria [17,20,34]. With the application of this diagnostic approach, brachial plexopathy with an infraclavicular location was found to be the most frequent diagnosis in a sample of people with upper limb pain in the primary health sector [16] as well as among patients referred to a department of occupational medicine [19,20].

Such physical diagnostic approach based on symptoms and neurological findings permits the identification of proximally located upper limb neuropathic conditions and makes better sense than alternative diagnostic classification systems in common use [16], e.g. those suggested by Sluiter et al. [35]. It would therefore be essential to include physical neurologic signs that can identify brachial plexopathies in diagnostic classification systems for upper limb disorders.

This study aims to assess the association of brachial plexopathy to physical and psychophysical exposures at work.

Material and methods

Study design

This case–control study was based on a case group of people with non-traumatic upper limb pain fulfilling defined criteria for brachial plexopathy and a control group without upper limb complaints. The cases and the controls answered the same questionnaire on work exposures. The distribution of exposures was compared for cases and controls.

Study subjects

Cases: Out of 277 patients with upper limb pain, of 16–65 years of age and in active occupation that were identified by 21 general practitioners, 169 agreed to participate in the study. Eight patients were excluded due to a history of previous acute trauma, or information on medical conditions that may predispose to upper limb disorders (pregnancy, alcoholism, rheumatoid arthritis, cardiac disease, hypothyroidism, diabetes, amyloidosis, polyneuropathy, vitamin B12 deficiency). The remaining 161 patients were physically examined by a single examiner and classified diagnostically according to previously defined criteria [16].

The neurological part of the physical examination has been previously described in details [17,20]. This examination consisted of manual testing of 17 upper limb muscles, assessment of sensation (light touch, pinprick, vibration 256 Hz) in five homonymously innervated territories of the skin corresponding to the peripheral nerves, and assessment of mechanical allodynia at ten defined nerve-locations [16]. Abnormal sensation was recorded with hypo- as well as hyperexitability and/or abnormal perception of vibration. Brachial plexopathy was defined in the presence of the following characteristics [16]:

Symptoms

Pain, subjective weakness or sensory disturbances in either/or the neck, shoulder, arm, or hand.

Brachial plexopathy at the infraclavicular level (pectoralis minor syndrome)

The definition of this condition required all three of the following findings:

- Weakness of the posterior deltoid, biceps brachii, and radial flexor of wrist muscles and one or more of the following muscles: Triceps, short radial extensor of wrist, long extensor of thumb, long flexor of thumb, short abductor of thumb, pectorals, deep flexor to the 5th digit, small adductor of the 5th digit.
- Mechanical allodynia with mild pressure at the infraclavicular brachial plexus on the passage behind the pectoralis minor muscle.
- Sensory abnormalities in the deltoid region.

Brachial plexopathy at the supraclavicular level (scalene triangle syndrome)

The definition of this condition required all three of the following findings:

- Weakness of the infraspinatus, posterior deltoid, and biceps brachii muscles. Normal strength in the radial flexor of wrist (unless concomitant more distal neuropathy).
- Mechanical allodynia with mild pressure at the brachial plexus at the passage through the scalene triangle
- Sensory abnormalities in the deltoid region.

139 patients were diagnosed with brachial plexopathy, and the affliction within the plexus was localized. Based on the same protocol [16] additional upper limb disorders were diagnosed (Figure 1).

Out of patients defined with brachial plexopathy, 80 patients who answered the exposure questionnaire [36] constituted the case group (Figure 1) giving a response rate for cases of 58%. The mean age (SD) of the cases was 43.9 (10.1) years for 61 females and 46.3 (9.1) years for 19 males, respectively.

Controls: 86 control subjects were recruited from the same general practitioners. For each case, the selected control subject was the first subsequent patient after each enrolled case who belonged to the same sex and age-group and who agreed to participate. The controls fulfilled identical inclusion and exclusion criteria as the cases. They could have any occupation and call for any complaint, work-related or not except for the requirement of the absence of any neck or upper limb complaints.

Out of these, 65 control subjects who answered the exposure questionnaire [36] constituted the final group of controls (Figure 2) giving a response rate for controls of 81%. The mean age (SD) of the 65 controls was 41.9 (10.4) years for 49 females and 47.3 (9.9) years for 16 males, respectively.

Assessment of work exposures

A questionnaire was developed for the assessment of physical and psychosocial work exposures and rating of psychophysical perceptions [36]. This questionnaire combined previously published questionnaires, out of which two addressed physical exposures [37,38], one psychophysical items [39] and one psychosocial issues [40]. The final questionnaire included questions to which answers were to be ranked in terms of duration or intensity. Some psychophysical ratings assessed the respondents' perceptions for each side while others did not (e.g. work pace and back position). All scores were ordinal as reflected by the legends for Tables 1, 2, 3, 4 and 5.

Various ways to validate these questionnaires have been previously applied. The ability to predict symptoms and the usefulness of psychophysical perceptions for preventive purposes was demonstrated for the questionnaire based on psychophysical items. One of the questionnaires on mechanical exposure was shown to be reliable in use [38]. The advantages of combining questions relating to the exposure and psychophysical perceptions has been documented [41].

Questions regarding psychosocial issues were included in order to assess their potential role as confounders rather than individual risk indicators for brachial plexopathy.

Statistics

The presence of brachial plexopathy on any or both sides was compared to the reported exposures. The relation between case status and individual ordinal scores for exposures according to Wiktorin et al. [37] was analysed by a Wilcoxon Mann–Whitney rank sum test (Table 1).

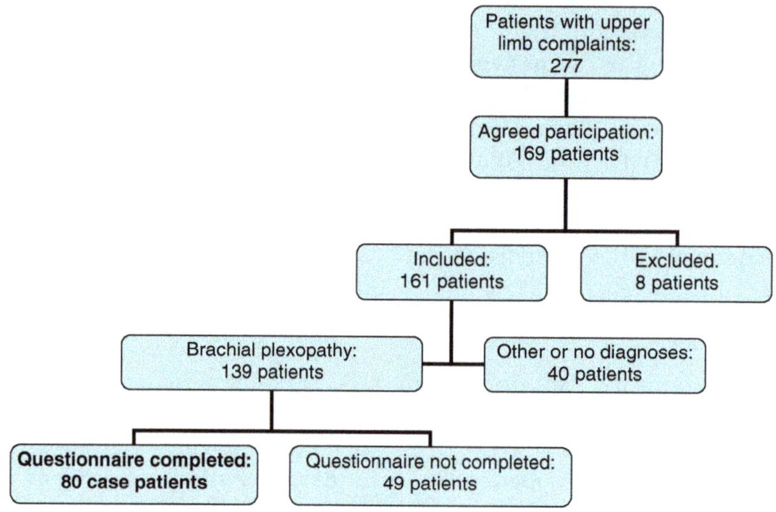

Figure 1 Study sample.

In addition, the magnitude of risk expressed by the odds ratios for selected mechanical exposures according to Torgén et al. [38] was calculated with logistic regression and the dose–response relationships estimated. For this calculation, the influence of the proportion of the workday with exposure to each risk factor was assessed with three exposure levels, except for work with vibrating hand tools, which was assessed dichotomously (Table 2). The effect of the number of exposure days per week was assessed with five exposure categories (Table 3). All exposure categories were compared to "Almost never/not at all".

A Wilcoxon Mann–Whitney rank sum test was also applied for the comparison of the psychophysical ratings [39] in between cases and controls. When applicable, separate analyses were made for the right and left side.

Data were processed by Stata ver. 12.1.

Ethics

The study complied with the Helsinki declaration. The clinical examination protocol was approved by the local ethics committee (De Videnskabsetiske Komittéer for Region Syddanmark) and signed informed consent was obtained from all participants.

Results

According to the defined criteria, 9 and12 limbs were diagnosed as right and left supraclavicular brachial plexopathy, respectively, with bilateral affliction in five. 52 and 37 limbs were diagnosed as right and left infraclavicular brachial plexopathy, respectively, with bilateral involvement in 12. Nine and eight patients had a combination of supraclavicular and infraclavicular plexopathy on the right and left side, respectively.

According to the applied diagnostic criteria [16], a high proportion of cases had additional non-neuropathic diagnoses with the major concomitant diagnoses on the right/left side being rotator cuff disorder (12/8), and epicondylitis (19/12), respectively [16]. Simultaneous presence of epicondylitis and rotator cuff disorder was identified in one right limb. All except one limb with brachial plexopathy had additional peripheral neuropathy, which was mainly involving the median and the radial/interosseous nerves at elbow level.

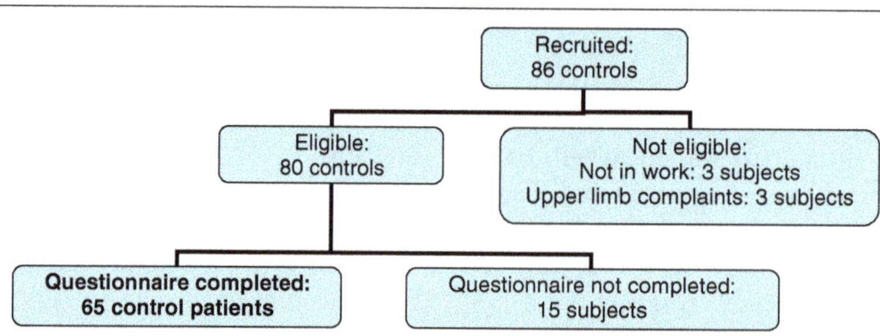

Figure 2 Sample of controls.

Table 1 Extent of time for various job tasks and exposures according to Wiktorin [37]

Exposure	U	Controls		Cases		p
		N	Median	N	Median	
A. Sitting (a)	−4.2	65	3	77	1	0.0000
B. Standing (a)	5.3	64	2	80	5	0.0000
C. Walking (a)	3.1	63	2	78	3	0.0023
D. Operating a computer (a)	−3.7	64	2	80	1	0.0003
E. Work with vibrating hand tools (a)	2.1	64	1	79	1	0.0385
F. Work with arms in or over shoulder level (a)	3.4	65	1	80	1	0.0006
G. Work with stretched arms ≥ 45 degrees forward or laterally (a)	3.6	63	1	80	2	0.0004
H. Work with almost maximally flexed neck (a)	3.0	63	1	79	2	0.0025
I. Work with identical arm movements many times per minute (a)	4.4	64	1	79	3	0.0000
J. Work with identical hand/finger movements many times/minute (a)	2.7	64	2	79	3	0.0074
K. Precision work > 2 hours/day (b)	1.2	65	1	80	1	0.2441
L. Work with arms in or over shoulder height > ½ hour/day (b)	3.5	65	1	80	1	0.0004
M. Work with arm extension ≥ 45 degrees forward or laterally > ½ hour/day (b)	3.3	63	1	78	4	0.0010
N. Work with identical arm movements many times/minute > 2 hours/day (b)	4.8	63	1	80	5	0.0000
O. Work with identical hand or finger movements many times/minute > 2 hours/day (b)	2.6	65	1	79	5	0.0088
P. Fingers exposed to cold (b)	2.9	65	1	76	1	0.0041

The questions read: (a) How big a proportion of a normal work-day did you …..? Answers on a five step scale: Almost never/not at all (1), approx. 1/4 of the time (2), approx. 1/2 of the time (3), approx. 3/4 of the time (4), almost all the time (5). (b) Did you have………? Answers on a five step scale: Almost never/not at all (1), 1–3 days/months (2), 1 day/week (3), 2–4 days/week (4), every day (5).
U = test magnitude. p = significance level.
Wilcoxon Mann–Whitney rank sum test.

Relation between cases and controls in terms of ordinally grouped individual exposures, exposures grouped into indices and psychophysical ratings

Assessment of the daily amount of exposure by the application of the mechanical exposure questions by Wiktorin [37] showed that sitting and computer work appeared to be protective in terms of brachial plexopathy. Working with arms at or over shoulder height, stretched arms 45° or more forward or laterally, neck flexion and repetitive arm and hand/finger work all constituted highly significant physical risk exposures while vibrating hand tools had a relatively minor influence on the prevalence of brachial plexopathy (Table 1).

The extension of work tasks with the limb extended more than 45° forward or laterally more than a half hour/day and of repetitive arm, hand or finger work more than 2 hours/day was also strongly associated to case status. Cold exposure was also a risk factor. Precision work exceeding 2 hours/day was not significantly related to brachial plexopathy (Table 1).

The distribution in controls and cases of the extent of the various job tasks is illustrated in the box plot in Figure 3.

The risk estimates for the various job tasks and exposures according to Torgén et al. [38] as illustrated in Table 2 (Proportion of workday exposed) and Table 3 (Number of days/week exposed) showed similar results. There was a dose–response relationship with increasing exposure during the workday for standing, arms in or over shoulder height, arms extended more than 45° forward or laterally, almost maximal neck flexion, identical arm movements many times/minute, and identical finger movements many times/minute. At the maximal exposure levels, the risk estimates for all these variables were significant. There was an increasing risk with increasing amount of walking and work with vibrating hand tools, but the risk estimates did not reach significance. Again, sitting and computer work appeared to be protective in this sample (Table 2).

Except for precision work exceeding 2 hours/day, the analyses of the influence of the amount of days/week exposed showed a similar picture with significantly elevated risk estimates for work over shoulder level more than a half hour/day, arms extended more than 45^0 forward or laterally more than a half hour/day, identical arm movements many times/minute exceeding 2 hours/day, and identical finger movements many times/minute during more than 2 hours/day. Exposure to cold was also a significant risk factor. There was a dose–response relationship to the number of days exposed per week for all exposures except precision work (Table 3).

All psychophysical measures [39] that relate to work pace, postures, the use of force, the usual weight of manually handled items, and local pressure were significantly related to case status. Local vibration was

Table 2 Odds ratios depending of the temporal extent of exposure during the workday according to Torgén et al. [38]

Risk factor (Proportion of workday)	Controls(N)	Cases (N)	OR (95% CI)
Sitting			
Almost never/not at all	11	42	1.00
Approx. ¼ - ½ of workday	27	18	0.54 (0.24 1.21)
More than ½ of workday	27	17	0.18 (0.05-0.71)
Standing			
Almost never/not at all	20	11	1.00
Approx. ¼ - ½ of workday	31	18	1.11 (0.44-2.82)
More than ½ of workday	13	51	7.49 (2.90-19.37)
Walking			
Almost never/not at all	18	16	1.00
Approx. ¼ - ½ of workday	35	32	1.02 (0.46-2.25)
More than ½ of workday	10	30	3.33 (0.69-7.15)
Operating a computer			
Almost never/not at all	23	54	1.00
Approx. ¼ - ½ of workday	24	15	0.28 (0.12-0.62)
More than ½ of workday	17	11	0.29 (0.123-0.71)
Extent of work with vibrating hand tools			
Almost never/not at all	63	71	1.00
Approx. ¼ of workday or more	1	8	7.11 (0.87-58.42)
Extent of work with arms in or over shoulders			
Almost never/not at all	51	43	1.00
Approx. ¼ - ½ of workday	13	25	2.28 (1.04-4.99)
More than ½ workday or more	1	12	14.23 (1.77-113.91)
Extent of work with arms extended more than 45^{0} forward or to the side			
Almost never/not at all	37	27	1.00
Approx. ¼ - ½ of workday	21	26	1.79 (0.84-3.80)
More than ½ of workday	2	18	7.80 (2.67-22.80)
Extent of work with almost maximal neck flexion			
Almost never/not at all	44	39	1.00
Approx. ¼ - ½ of workday	17	22	1.49 (0.69-3.19)
More than ½ of workday	1	10	10.35 (2.26-47.37)
Extent of work with identical arm movements many times per minute			
Almost never/not at all	41	24	1.00
Approx. ¼ - ½ of workday	13	22	2.84 (1.22-6.62)
More than ½ of workday	10	33	5.54 (2.34-13.15)
Extent of work with identical hand/finger movements many times per minute			
Almost never/not at all	25	19	1.00
Approx. ¼ - ½ of workday	21	22	1.36 (0.59-3.14)
More than ½ of workday	18	38	2.74 (1.22-6.16)

Logistic regression.

borderline not significantly related to brachial plexopathy. Whole body vibrations, the weight and balance of the usual tool and the weight of the heaviest handled items were unrelated to case status (Table 4).

Psychosocial exposures [40], for which the distribution differed significantly between cases and controls are illustrated in Table 5. The distribution was the same in the two samples for all other variables (emotional

Table 3 Odds ratios relating to the amounts of workdays for various job tasks and exposures according to Torgén et al. [38]

Risk factor (Amount of days with job tasks and exposures)	Controls (N)	Cases(N)	OR (95% CI)
Precision work > 2 hours/day			
Almost never/not at all	54	61	1.00
1-3 days/month	3	2	0.43 (0.15-1.30)
1 day/week	2	1	0.26 (0.03-2.02)
2-4 days/week	1	3	0.19 (0.01-2.62)
Every day	5	13	1.15 (0.10-13.88)
Working over shoulder level > ½ hour/day			
Almost never/not at all	51	42	1.00
1-3 days/month	1	3	3.64 (0.37-36.32)
1 day/week	4	3	0.91 (0.19-4.30)
2-4 days/week	4	6	1.82 (0.48-6.88)
Every day	5	26	6.31 (2.23-17.87)
Working with extended arms > 45^0 or more forward or laterally > ½ hour/day			
Almost never/not at all	39	26	1.00
1-3 days/month	2	4	2.92 (0.50-17.09)
1 day/week	3	1	0.49 (0.05-4.94)
2-4 days/week	2	9	6.59 (1.32-32.82)
Every day	17	38	3.27 (1.55-6.91)
Working with identical arm movements many times/minute > 2 hours/day			
Almost never/not at all	45	27	1.00
1-3 days/month	4	1	0.42 (0.04-3.92)
1 day/week	2	3	2.50 (0.39-15.93)
2-4 days/week	4	6	2.50 (0.65-9.66)
Every day	10	43	7.17 (3.10-16.56)
Working with identical hand/finger movements many times/minute > 2 hours/day			
Almost never/not at all	34	25	1.00
1-3 days/month	2	3	1.96 (0.31-12.60)
1 day/week	1	2	2.62 (0.22-30.43)
2-4 days/week	6	6	1.31 (0.38-4.53)
Every day	22	43	2.56 (1.24-5.27)
Fingers exposed to cold			
Almost never/not at all	55	50	1.00
1-3 days/month	5	5	1.02 (0.28-3.72)
1 day/week	3	1	0.33 (0.03-3.37)
2-4 days/week	0	4	-
Every day	2	16	8.15 (1.78-37.15)

Logistic regression.

demands, meaning and commitment, collaboration and leadership, interaction between the individual and work, stress and depression).

Discussion

The high frequency of brachial plexopathies in the original sample of patients from which the cases for this study was drawn [16] is in accordance with previous studies [16,19,20]. With the applied diagnostic definition [16], this study has clearly indicated a number of risk indicators for brachial plexopathy. Whether based on assessments of physical exposures or of psychophysical perceptions, highly significant relations were demonstrated for adverse upper limb

Table 4 Psychophysical measures according to Punnett et al. [39]

Exposure	U		Controls				Cases				p	
			N		Median		N		Median			
	Right	Left	Right	Left	Right	Left	Right	Left	Right	Left	Right	Left
Work pace (a)	2.925		65		6		80		8		0.0034	
Back positions (b)	4.319		65		3		80		5		0.0000	
Neck positions (b)	4.505		64		3		79		5		0.0000	
Shoulder positions (b)	5.235	4.958	65	65	3	2	80	80	6	5	0.0000	0.0000
Arm positions (b)	4.651	5.304	65	65	3	2	80	80	6	5	0.0000	0.0000
Hand positions (b)	3.625	4.211	65	65	4	2	80	80	5.5	5	0.0000	0.0003
Whole body vibration (c)	1.093		64		0		80		0		0.2743	
Local vibration (c)	1.942	1.848	65	65	0	0	80	79	0	0	0.0521	0.0646
Applied hand force (d)	4.746	4.993	65	65	2	2	80	80	6	5	0.0000	0.0000
Applied hand force in uncomfortable positions	4,211	4.281	65	65	1	1	76	76	2	1	0.0000	0.0000
Pressure on hand or arm (d)	3.976		65		0		78		0		0.0001	
Usual weight with manual handling (e)	2.094		33		4		63		5		0.0362	
Heaviest weight with manual handling (e)	1.228		32		6.5		62		7.5		0.2194	
Weight of usual tool (e)	1.503		24		2		36		3		0.1329	
Balance of usual tool (f)	1.824		24		1		36		2.5		0.0681	
Force required for holding and using tool (g)	2.901		24		1.5		35		5		0.0037	

Wilcoxon Mann–Whitney rank sum test. All ordinal measures on a VAS-scale 0–10.
(a) Very slow - too fast, (b) (Very comfortable - very uncomfortable, (c) None - a lot, (d) None/very small - very large, (e) Very light – very heavy, (f) Perfect – major imbalance, (g) Very small – very large. NB Calculations for perceptions related to the limbs made for each side.
U = test magnitude. p = significance level.

Table 5 Psychosocial exposure measures according to Søndergaard [40]

Psychosocial exposure	U	Controls		Cases		p
		N	Median	N	Median	
A. Required to work at high pace (a)	2.9	61	3	77	2	0.003
B. Influence on decisions about the work (b)	−2.8	63	2	77	3	0.005
C. Possibilities for learning (b)	−2.8	63	2	79	3	0.005
D. Influence on the content of work (b)	−2.1	63	3	78	3	0.038
E. Support from immediate superior (a)	−2.6	63	2	75	3	0.009
F. Frequency of consultation with superior of quality of job performance (a)	−2.4	63	3	75	4	0.015
G. Conflict solving skills with superior (b)	−2.0	63	3	75	3	0.047
H. Satisfied with physical work environment (c)	−4.5	53	2	77	2	0.000
I. Satisfied with the way your skills are used (c)	−3.4	63	2	76	2	0.001
J. Self-rating of health (d)	−4.6	65	2	79	3	0.000
K. Happy and satisfied during the last four weeks	−2.3	64	2	79	3	0.024
L. Enthusiastic and full of life during the last four weeks	−3.6	64	3	78	4	0.000
M. Full of energy during the last four weeks	−3.8	64	3	77	4	0.000
N. Warn during the last four weeks	3.5	64	5	78	4	0.000
O. Tired during the last four weeks	2.4	64	5	79	4	0.01

Wilcoxon Mann–Whitney rank sum test.
(a) Always, frequently, at times, rarely, never/almost never, (b) to very high degree, to high degree, partly, to small degree, to very small degree, (c) very satisfied, satisfied, unsatisfied, very unsatisfied, (d) excellent, very good, good, not so good, bad, (e) All the time, most of the time, a lot of the time, some times, little of the time, never.
U = test magnitude. p = significance level.

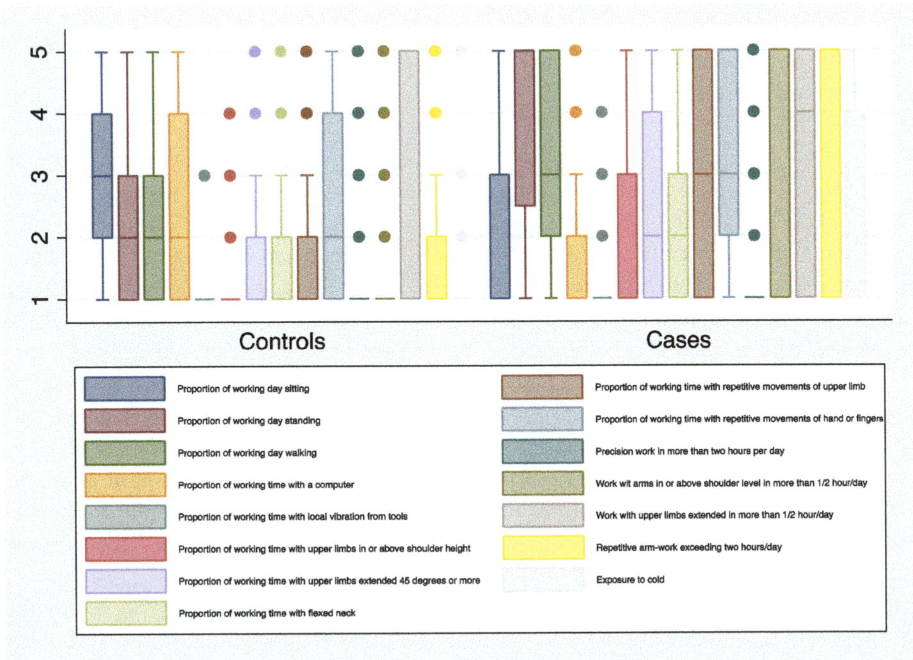

Figure 3 Boxplot illustrating the distribution of the extent of job tasks and exposures in Table 1. The boxes illustrate the interquartile range. The horizontal line represents the median. The vertical lines illustrate the maximal and minimal values excluding outliers, and the dots represent outliers.

postures, repetitive work, work pace and the use of strength.

Two of the identified risk factors, walking and exposure of the fingers to cold (Table 1), can hardly be explained in terms of pathophysiological mechanisms, but may rather be related to the character of work, which may combine walking and cold exposure with other identified risk indicators.

Surprisingly, two exposures were more prevalent among controls than cases: sitting and computer work. The effect of sitting may be explained by the fact that most sitting work does not involve adverse positions and repetitive work, although undertaking sitting tasks that do involve these exposures may in fact contribute to further adverse upper limb postures, e.g. by requiring further arm elevation than working in the standing position. Brachial plexopathy has been demonstrated in a series of patients with intensive computer work [42], and neurological patterns in accordance with brachial plexopathy were common in symptomatic computer operators in active occupation [43]. A meta-analysis found moderate evidence for the relation between computer use and upper limb pain but limited relation to specific musculoskeletal disorders out of which brachial plexopathy was not addressed [44]. The current findings might be explained by an exposure to computer work of a low intensity, which does not constitute a risk for brachial plexopathy.

The relation between local vibration and upper limb nerve afflictions is well documented [45], but the effect on brachial plexopathy in the current study was limited. The minor impact of vibration may relate to the distance between the hand and the brachial plexus. A more likely explanation, however, is the limited number of subjects in the sample that were exposed to local vibration (Table 2).

The analyses assessed the association between the exposures and brachial plexopathy with a supraclavicular as well as an infraclavicular location. Due to the dominance of infraclavicular locations in this sample, the conclusions concern infraclavicular rather than supraclavicular brachial plexopathy. This observation demonstrates the importance of studying the brachial plexus at several locations – not only at the scalene triangle.

The assessment of exposure by a questionnaire based on questions developed and validated by others included physical, psychophysical, and psychosocial issues. Although a questionnaire approach to exposure assessment is generally regarded as inferior to direct observations, the former has major advantages in terms of costs and practical execution. A French study found that the questionnaire was superior to direct observations in identifying workers at high risk of upper limb work-related musculoskeletal disorders [46]. The inclusion of the psychophysical questions was regarded advantageous due to the ability of these to qualify questions addressing physical exposures [41]. The ability of the physical and psychophysical ratings to identify comparable risk indicators supports the consistency of the presented findings.

Validity

Non-experimental research has a number of innate methodological constraints. One point of importance is the potential confounding that may occur when the frequency of risk indicators other than those studied differs in between cases and controls. This potential for bias is an acknowledged weakness of the case–control design.

Bias of information

The collection on a cross-sectional basis of questionnaire information on exposure may result in information bias. Such bias would be differential and lead to spuriously increased risk estimates if, compared to controls, cases would overrate their exposures. The absence of differential misclassification has been demonstrated for some of the posed questions [37] while the risk for differential misclassification cannot be excluded in the remaining questions on mechanical exposure [37,47]. It has, however, been shown that questions addressing physical risk exposures for upper limb disorders seem to cause less misclassification than is the case for low back disorders [48]. In this context, the absence of a relation between symptoms and exposures, which the responders would be likely to regard as related to upper limb symptoms (e.g. precision work or computer work) is noteworthy. Information bias cannot therefore be excluded but is regarded as less likely to seriously distort the results.

Bias of selection

The selection of the studied samples of patients and controls is another potential source of bias. In spite of instructions, the general practitioners may not have selected all eligible patients. For example, although the practitioners were asked to enrol as cases all patients with non-traumatic upper limb symptoms, there could be a reluctance to enrol those with milder or easily interpreted symptoms rather than patients for which they may have been more inclined to request a second opinion from the research team [16]. Bias from the selection of controls can also not be excluded. While the general practitioner was asked to select as control subject the first eligible patient who was willing to complete the questionnaire, one cannot be sure if this really happened. Whether the occupations differed in between cases and controls is not known. A higher share of manual workers in the case group could induce a bias of selection. Consequently, although the response rate and the distribution on age and sex were comparable in cases and controls, a potential differential selection may have influenced the composition of the final sample of controls.

Psychosocial issues

It is noticeable that answers to questions about psychosocial issues [40] that differed between cases and controls (Table 5) reflect either the physical exposure or conditions that can either be linked to circumstances that characterize the physical work-environment such as repetitive work (Tables 1, 2 and 3), or the psychophysical perceptions, e.g. the requirement of working at high pace (Table 4-A). Most responses to psychosocial issues, however, were not linked to these factors. This applies for, e.g. the perceived emotional demands from work, the meaning and commitment of work, the collaboration and leadership, the interaction between the individual and the work, as well as for perceptions that reflect stress and depression.

This study supports previous longitudinal studies that have shown evidence for a link between upper limb symptoms and the influence of high work demands [49], little control at work [49], and low job satisfaction [50]. The adverse influence of little job control and additionally of supervisor support has also been demonstrated in a cross-sectional study that, however, estimated the magnitude of the population attributable fraction of upper limb disorders for exposure to psychological factors to 12% [51]. While several physical risk indicators for arm pain were identified, no psychosocial stressors were identified in a case–control study of patients presenting to primary care, in which, however, a number of mental health variables were linked to case status [52].

High work demands, little control, low job satisfaction, and supervisor support are common terms in trades with repetitive and paced work with adverse upper limb positions. Consequently, the demonstration in the present study of the role of these psychosocial exposures is not surprising. On the other hand, the absence of an influence of psychosocial exposures that are not linked to physical risk indicators suggests psychosocial factors in themselves to be less likely risk indicators for brachial plexopathy. This observation supports the validity of the identified relations to mechanical exposures.

Physical examination and case-definition

With a high inter-observer reproducibility, a detailed neurological examination of patients with and without upper limb symptoms has indicated frequent neurological patterns in accordance with brachial plexopathies [19,20]. In a sample of people with upper limb pain and people with other disorders, this examination predicted with a high accuracy the presence or absence of symptoms [19]. The neurological items studied in this validity study were comparable to those included in the current definitions of brachial plexopathy. This definition permitted the diagnosis of brachial plexopathy in a high number of people with upper limb pain in clinical occupational medicine [19] and general practice [16].

Still, the endpoints in terms of defined disease outcome may be challenged. Brachial plexopathy is a controversial diagnostic construct, and there is neither consensus about its diagnosis, frequency nor potential work-relatedness. The main challenge is the absence in most brachial plexopathies of electrophysiological abnormalities [25], which tends to be interpreted as its nonexistence. This is unfortunate because brachial plexopathy should be diagnosed based on clinical findings rather than electrophysiological studies [53]. Although the latter are regarded by many as the "gold standard" for peripheral neuropathy, a mixed and partial nerve affliction with few myelinated fibers intact and reinnervation taking place may result in entirely normal findings [54].

Characteristic symptoms in these patients include pain, which is often of a neuropathic character, weakness and/or numbness/tingling. The content of the applied neurological examination was derived from anatomical facts and pathophysiology that has led to an established paradigm on which the traditional neurologic bedside examination is based: Focal neuropathy with a certain location is likely to result in rather specific neurological deviations from normal. These abnormalities may well be minor and include weakness and sensory deviations from normal distal to the nerve affliction, and a maximal mechanical allodynia of nerve trunks where, according to the neurological patterns, the affliction is located.

The case definition for infraclavicular brachial plexopathy (pectoralis minor syndrome) that was applied in this study is based on anatomical facts. A compromise at this location is likely to involve the lateral-most portion of the brachial plexus because the available space for passage behind the pectoralis minor muscle is more limited laterally than medially. This portion of the brachial plexus contains neurons from the axillary, musculocutaneous and radial nerves that supply motor innervation to the deltoid, biceps, and radial flexor of wrist muscles as well as the cutaneous axillary nerve innervation of the deltoid region. With a supraclavicular location of brachial plexopathy (scalene triangle syndrome), the neurons supplying the suprascapular nerve that innervates the infraspinatus muscle are at risk because of the location in the top of the scalene triangle.

The applied diagnostic criteria for brachial plexopathy cannot be satisfied with any other upper limb condition. On the other hand, when these criteria are met, concomitant disorders of a neuropathic or a non-neuropathic character may also be present. Concomitant disorders, in particular rotator cuff disorders, epicondylitis, and peripheral upper limb neuropathies were frequent in the studied sample [16]. Their relative influence as dependant variables cannot be determined in this study. It can, however, be argued that rotator cuff disorders and epicondylitis may share similar risk indicators and that these conditions may complicate or predispose to brachial plexopathy. This study cannot determine the potential relation and succession of such events.

It is noticeable that the criteria for diagnosing a concomitant peripheral neuropathic condition were fulfilled for all except one limb with brachial plexopathy. This observation is in accordance with clinical experiences as well as with the "double crush" theory [55], which can explain neurological patterns and symptoms that may appear confusing to the clinician. According to the diagnostic criteria applied in this study [16], the identification of a peripheral neuropathic condition required a defined combination of motor and sensory outcomes as well as allodynia with gentle palpation of the nerve trunk at the location of entrapment. The latter suggests a peripheral nerve involvement at this specific location.

The correlation of regional pain to physical findings in the same region characterises much analytical research targeting upper limb disorders. However, epidemiological studies that aim to correlate the location of symptoms with physical findings at the same location may be distorted because upper limb pathology may be situated at a distance to the dominant location(s) of symptoms such as pain. This is particularly true with involvement of the peripheral nerves (referred pain [56]). Upper limb symptoms are often of a fluctuant character and intensity, and their locations are likely to change and spread. Consequently, the physical examination should include the whole limb as well as the neck and include a careful examination of the peripheral nervous system [57]. Such comprehensive physical approach can identify proximally located neuropathic conditions such as at the brachial plexus, and explain the fluctuating symptoms by a dynamic compression. In the absence of such examination, the correlation between exposures and symptoms with certain locations is likely to be diluted.

Causality

Viewing the findings of this study in the context of the considerations of causality by Bradford Hill [58], it can be positively concluded that the documented associations are strong, dose–response related, and that the time-relation is clear through the design. The relation between brachial plexopathy and the identified physical exposures and psychophysical perceptions is biologically plausible and there is evidence for the relation of physical findings in the examination of the peripheral nerves to minor or major impacts on nerve tissue. In a literature review, Rempel et al. highlighted the cascade of effects resulting from low level nerve pressure, consisting of inhibition of intraneurial microvascular blood flow, axonal transport and nerve function as well as endoneurial oedema and displacement of myelin. Higher pressure have more profound effects including demyelination, inflammation, fibrosis, growth of new axons and remyelination [59]. Schmid et al. have reviewed the pathophysiological mechanisms [60] and shown that even mild nerve compression in animals is sufficient to induce intraneural inflammation, which is associated with neuropathic pain behaviour [61].

Still, some weak points should be mentioned. Consistency in terms of similar results from other studies is lacking as no other studies have yet demonstrated the relation of brachial plexopathy to mechanical exposures at work. The specificity in terms of causation may also be questioned. A variety of exposures were attributed to brachial plexopathy. In addition, other upper limb conditions may share the risk indicators as here reported for brachial plexopathy. Consequently, this study has demonstrated associations to work exposures but cannot conclude about causality, which needs to be examined in prospective studies of patients with brachial plexopathy without other concomitant disease. In addition, the aggregated effects of the various mechanical exposures, and the interaction in between them should be studied. Most importantly, the demonstration of a reduced occurrence of disease following elimination or reduction of the identified risk exposures would represent an important step for improved prevention of brachial plexopathy.

Conclusions

This study has demonstrated several adverse physical exposures at work, in particular upper limb posture and repetitive movements of the arm, hand and fingers to be risk indicators for brachial plexopathy with significant dose–response relationships. These findings were supported by psychophysical responses that additionally indicated work pace and the use of force as risk indicators. The identified relations to psychosocial measures were limited to those reflecting physical exposures.

This study has two major clinical implications. With acceptance of the applied diagnostic criteria, brachial plexopathy is a frequent condition, which should not be overlooked. A simple screening of the upper limb nerves can exclude this condition [62]. The diagnosis of brachial plexopathy can provide directions for management and, taking into account the demonstrated risk indicators, for preventive interventions at workplaces.

It can therefore be concluded that this study provides evidence of a relation of mechanical work-exposures to brachial plexopathy. The identified risk indicators for upper limb disorders have previously been associated to *symptoms* as well as to diagnosed "specific" upper limb *disorders* other than brachial plexopathy. Longitudinal studies should be conducted in order to provide evidence of causality and for excluding bias from information and selection, both of which may occur with the applied case–control design.

Competing interests
The author declares that he has no competing interests.

References

1. Sluiter JK, Rest KM, Frings-Dresen MHW. Criteria document for evaluation of the work-relatedness of upper extremity musculoskeletal disorders. Amsterdam: Coronel Institute for occupational and environmental health, academic medical center, University of Amsterdam. 2000. p. 1–194.
2. Ohlsson K, Attewell RG, Pålsson B, Karlsson B, Balogh I, Johnsson B, et al. Repetitive industrial work and neck and upper limb disorders in females. Am J Ind Med. 1995;27:731–47.
3. Feldman RG, Goldman R, Keyserling WM. Classical syndromes in occupational medicine. Peripheral nerve entrapment syndromes and ergonomic factors. Am J Ind Med. 1983;4:661–81.
4. Hagberg M, Wegman DH. Prevalence rates and odds ratios of shoulder-neck diseases in different occupational groups. Br J Ind Med. 1987;44:602–10.
5. Mackinnon SE, Patterson GA, Novak CB. Thoracic outlet syndrome: a current overview. Semin Thor Cardiovasv Surg. 1996;8:176–82.
6. Mandel S. Neurologic syndromes from repetitive trauma at work. Postgrad Med. 1987;82:87–92.
7. Wright IS. The neurovascular syndrome produced by hyperabduction of the arms. Am Heart J. 1945;29:1–19.
8. Gold JE, Piligian G, Glutting JJ, Hanlon A, Frings-Dresen MH, Sluiter JK. Cluster analysis of symptoms among patients with upper extremity musculoskeletal disorders. J Occup Rehabil. 2010;20:526–36.
9. Musculoskeletal disorders and workplace factors - A critical review of epidemiological evidence for work-related musculoskeletal disorders of the neck, upper extremity and low back. Cincinnati (OH): National Institue for Occupational Safety and Health. 1997.
10. Thomsen JF, Hansson GA, Mikkelsen S, Lauritzen M. Carpal tunnel syndrome in repetitive work: a follow-up study. Am J Ind Med. 2002;42:344–53.
11. Leclerc A, Landre MF, Chastang JF, Niedhammer I, Roquelaure Y. Upper-limb disorders in repetitive work. Scand J Work Environ Health. 2001;27:268–78.
12. Thomsen JF, Mikkelsen S, Andersen JH, Fallentin N, Loft IP, Frost P, et al. Risk factors for hand-wrist disorders in repetitive work. Occup Environ Med. 2007;64:527–33.
13. Frost P, Bonde JP, Mikkelsen S, Andersen JH, Fallentin N, Kaergaard A, et al. Risk of shoulder tendinitis in relation to shoulder loads in monotonous repetitive work. Am J Ind Med. 2002;41:11–8.
14. Miranda H, Punnett L, Viikari-Juntura E, Heliovaara M, Knekt P. Physical work and chronic shoulder disorder. Results of a prospective population-based study. Ann Rheum Dis. 2008;67:218–23.
15. Cruccu G, Truini A. Assessment of neuropathic pain. Neurol Sci. 2006;27 Suppl 4:s288–90.
16. Laursen LH, Sjogaard G, Hagert CG, Jepsen JR. Diagnostic distribution of non-traumatic upper limb disorders: vibrotactile sense in the evaluation of structured examination for optimal diagnostic criteria. Med Lav. 2007;98:127–44.
17. Jepsen J, Laursen L, Larsen A, Hagert CG. Manual strength testing in 14 upper limb muscles. A study of the inter-rater reliability. Acta Orthop Scand. 2004;75:442–8.
18. Greening J, Smart S, Leary R, Hall-Craggs M, O'Higgins P, Lynn B. Reduced movement of median nerve in carpal tunnel during wrist flexion in patients with non-specific arm pain: a magnetic resonance imaging study. Lancet. 1999;354:217–8.
19. Jepsen JR, Laursen LH, Hagert C-G, Kreiner S, Larsen AI. Diagnostic accuracy of the neurological upper limb examination II. The relation to symptoms of patterns of findings. BMC Neurol. 2006;6:10.
20. Jepsen JR, Laursen LH, Hagert C-G, Kreiner S, Larsen AI. Diagnostic accuracy of the neurological upper limb examination I. Inter-rater reproducibility of findings and patterns. BMC Neurol. 2006;6:8.

21. Schmid AB, Brunner F, Luomajoki H, Held U, Bachmann LM, Künzer S, et al. Reliability of clinical tests to evaluate nerve function and mechanosensitivity of the upper limb peripheral nervous system. BMC Musculoskelet Disord. 2009;10:11.
22. Thaller M, Hughes T. Inter-rater agreement of observable and elicitable neurological signs. Clin Med. 2014;14:264–7.
23. Jepsen JR, Laursen LH, Kreiner S, Larsen AI. Neurological examination of the upper limb: A study of construct validity. Open Neurol J. 2009;3:54–63.
24. Warrens AN, Heaton JM. Thoracic outlet syndrome: the lack of reliability of its clinical assessment. Ann R Coll Surg Engl. 1987;69:203–4.
25. Aminoff MJ, Olney RK, Parry GF, Raskin NH. Relative utility of different electrophysiologic techniques in the evaluation of brachial plexopathies. Neurology. 1988;38:546–50.
26. Daube JR. Nerve conduction studies in thoracic outlet syndrome. Neurology. 1975;25:347.
27. Wilbourn AJ. The thoracic outlet syndrome is overdiagnosed. Arch Neurol. 1990;47:328–30.
28. Poole GV, Thomae KR. Thoracic outlet syndrome reconsidered. Am Surg. 1996;62:287–91.
29. Roos DB. The thoracic outlet syndrome is underrated. Arch Neurol. 1990;47:327–8.
30. Pascarelli EF, Hsu YP. Understanding work-related upper extremity disorders: clinical findings in 485 computer users, musicians, and others. J Occup Rehabil. 2001;11:1–21.
31. Sheth RN, Belzberg AJ. Diagnosis and treatment of thoracic outlet syndrome. Neurosurg Clin North Am. 2001;12:295–310.
32. Sanders RJ. Recurrent neurogenic thoracic outlet syndrome stressing the importance of pectoralis minor syndrome. Vasc Endovascular Surg. 2011;45:33–8.
33. Sanders RJ, Rao NM. The forgotten pectoralis minor syndrome: 100 operations for pectoralis minor syndrome alone or accompanied by neurogenic thoracic outlet syndrome. Ann Vasc Surg. 2010;24:701–8.
34. Palmer K, Cooper C. Repeated movement and repeated trauma affecting the musculoskeletal disorders of the upper limbs. In: Baxter P, Adams P, Aw T, Cockcroft A, Harrington J, editors. Hunter's diseases of occupations. London: Arnold; 2000. p. 453–75.
35. Sluiter JK, Rest KM, Frings-Dresen MH. Criteria document for evaluating the work-relatedness of upper-extremity musculoskeletal disorders. Scand J Work Environ Health. 2001;27:1–102.
36. Jepsen JR. Udvikling af et spørgeskema til belysning af arbejdsmæssige risikofaktorer for belastningslidelser i overekstremiteten. Esbjerg: Arbejdsmedicinsk afdeling; 2002. p. 1–139.
37. Wiktorin C, Vingård E, Mortimer M, Pernold G, Wigaeus-Hjelm E, Kilbom A, et al. Interview versus questionnaire for assessing physical loads in the population-based MUSIC-Norrtälje Study. Am J Ind Med. 1999;35:441–55.
38. Torgén M, Alfredsson L, Köster M, Wiktorin C, Smith KF, Kilbom Å. Reproduceability of a questionnaire for assessment of present and past physical activities. Int Arch Occup Environ Health. 1997;70:107–18.
39. Punnett L. Ergonomic stressors and upper extremity disorders in vehicle manufacturing: cross sectional exposure-response trends. Occup Environ Med. 1998;55:414–20.
40. Søndergaard T. AMI's spørgeskema om psykisk arbejdsmiljø. København: Arbejdsmiljøinstituttet; 2002.
41. Moore JS, Garg A. The strain index: A proposed method to analyze jobs for risk of distal upper extremity disorders. Am Ind Hyg Assoc J. 1995;56:443–58.
42. Jepsen JR. Upper limb neuropathy in computer operators? A clinical case study of 21 patients. BMC Musculoskelet Disord. 2004;5:26.
43. Jepsen JR, Thomsen G. A cross-sectional study of the relation between symptoms and physical findings in computer operators. BMC Neurol. 2006;6:40.
44. Andersen JH, Fallentin N, Thomsen JF, Mikkelsen S. Risk factors for neck and upper extremity disorders among computers users and the effect of interventions: an overview of systematic reviews. PLoS One. 2011;6:e19691.
45. Bovenzi M, Giannini F, Rossi S. Vibration-induced multifocal neuropathy in forestry workers: electrophysiological findings in relation to vibration exposure and finger circulation. Int Arch Occup Environ Health. 2000;73:519–27.
46. Descatha A, Roquelaure Y, Caroly S, Evanoff B, Cyr D, Mariel J, et al. Self-administered questionnaire and direct observation by checklist: Comparing two methods for physical exposure surveillance in a highly repetitive tasks plant. Appl Ergon. 2009;40:194–8.
47. Wiktorin C, Selin K, Ekenvall L, Alfredsson L, The MUSIC - Norrtälje Study Group. An interview technique for recording work postures in epidemiological studies. Int J Epidemiol. 1996;25:171–80.
48. Viikari-Juntura E, Rauas S, Martikainen R, Kuosma E, Riihimäki H, Takala EP, et al. Validity of self-reported physical work load in epidemiologic studies on musculoskeletal disorders. Scand J Work Environ Health. 1996;22:251–9.
49. Bongers PM, Ijmker S, Vanden HS, Blatter BM. Epidemiology of work related neck and upper limb problems: Psychosocial and personal risk factors (Part I) and effective interventions from a bio behavioural perspective (Part II). J Occup Rehabil. 2006;16:279–302.
50. Andersen JH, Haahr JP, Frost P. Risk factors for more severe regional musculoskeletal symptoms: a two-year prospective study of a general working population. Arthritis Rheum. 2007;56:1355–64.
51. Sim J, Lacey RJ, Lewis M. The impact of workplace risk factors on the occurrence of neck and upper limb pain: a general population study. BMC Public Health. 2006;6:234.
52. Ryall C, Coggon D, Peveler R, Reading I, Palmer KT. A case–control study of risk factors for arm pain presenting to primary care services. Occup Med (Lond). 2006;56:137–43.
53. Parziale JR, Akelman E, Weiss AP, Green A. Thoracic outlet syndrome. Am J Orthop. 2000;29:353–60.
54. Krarup C. Pitfalls in electrodiagnosis. J Neurol. 1999;246:1115–26.
55. Novak CB, Mackinnon SE. Multilevel nerve compression and muscle imbalance in work-related neuromuscular disorders. Am J Ind Med. 2002;41:343–52.
56. Quintner JL, Cohen ML. Referred pain of peripheral nerve origin: an alternative to the "myofascial pain" construct. Clin J Pain. 1994;10:243–51.
57. Jepsen JR. Work-related upper limb pain and its diagnosis: Contribution from the neurological examination. In: Pain in perspective. Gosh Sth ed. Rijeka: InTech; 2012. p. 11–34.
58. Hill AB. The environment and disease: association or causation? Proc R Soc Med. 1965;58:295–300.
59. Rempel D, Dahlin L, Lundborg G. Pathophysiology of nerve compression syndromes: response of peripheral nerves to loading. J Bone Joint Surg (Am). 1999;81:1600–10.
60. Schmid AB, Nee RJ, Coppieters MW. Reappraising entrapment neuropathies - Mechanisms, diagnosis and management. Man Ther. 2013;18:449–57.
61. Schmid AB, Coppieters MW, Ruitenberg MJ, McLachlan EM. Local and remote immune-mediated inflammation after mild peripheral nerve compression in rats. J Neuropathol Exp Neurol. 2013;72:662–80.
62. Jepsen JR. Can testing of six individual muscles represent a screening approach to upper limb neuropathic conditions? BMC Neurol. 2014;14:90.

22

A study of the association between urinary aluminum concentration and pre-clinical findings among aluminum-handling and non-handling workers

Masanori Ogawa[1*] and Fujio Kayama[2]

Abstract

Background: Aluminum is considered to be a relatively safe metal for humans. However, there are some reports that aluminum can be toxic to humans and animals. In order to estimate the toxicity of aluminum with respect to humans, we measured the aluminum concentration in urine of aluminum-handling and non-handling workers and investigated the relationships between their urinary aluminum concentrations and pre-clinical findings.

Methods: Twenty-three healthy aluminum-handling workers and 10 healthy non-aluminum-handling workers participated in this study. Their medical examinations, which were otherwise unremarkable, included the collection of urine and blood. Urinary aluminum levels were analyzed using ICP analysis. As pre-clinical tests, we measured KL-6, SP-D, TRCP-5b, IL-6, and IL-8 in blood and δ-ALA and β2-microglobulin in urine. These were considered to be lung, bone, kidney and inflammation markers. Moreover, we measured 8-OHdG in urine as an oxidative DNA damage marker.

Results: The aluminum concentration in urine ranged from 6.9 to 55.1 μg/g cre (median: 20.1 μg/g cre) in the aluminum-handling workers and from 5.6 to 15.6 μg/g cre (median: 8.8 μg/g cre) in the non-aluminum-handling workers, with a significant difference between them. In the pre-clinical findings, there were no significant differences between these two groups except in the case of δ-ALA. However, there were no significant relationships between aluminum concentration and the pre-clinical findings, work years, age or 8-OHdG in the aluminum-handling workers.

Conclusions: While the excretion of aluminum in urine was elevated in aluminum-handling workers, our findings suggest that low-dose aluminum is not directly harmful to humans, at least when workers' urinary aluminum concentration is below 55 μg/g cre.

Keywords: Aluminum, Biological monitoring, Pre-clinical marker

Background

Aluminum is widely used in everyday life and is considered to be a relatively safe metal for humans compared with other metals such as cadmium, mercury and arsenic, based on the toxicological guideline values of the Joint FAO/WHO Expert Committee on Food Additives (JECFA) [1,2]. Moreover, it is not classifiable as a human carcinogen [3].

However, there have been reports that aluminum is toxic to the lungs and nerves of humans, to the bones in humans who undergo hemodialysis, and to myelopoietic organs in animals. Pulmonary fibrosis has been reported in relation to aluminum exposure [4,5]. Significant changes in neuropsychological tests and dose-dependent central nervous dysfunction have been observed in aluminum-handling workers [6,7]. In patients treated with hemodialysis, aluminum accumulates in the bone with

* Correspondence: masa-oga@jichi.ac.jp
[1]Health Service Center, Jichi Medical University, 3311-1, Yakushiji, Shimotsuke, Tochigi 329-0498, Japan
Full list of author information is available at the end of the article

high turnover, and the effects of aluminum on bone, such as osteomalacia, have been found to be dose-dependent and time-dependent [8,9]. Aluminum has been shown to affect δ-aminolevulinic acid dehydratase levels in the blood of mice and the bone marrow of rats [10,11]. Moreover, there are some reports that aluminum nanoparticles affect inflammatory cytokines such as IL-6 and IL-8 and elevate oxygen-reactive species *in vitro* [12,13].

It is important to prevent occupational poisoning before clinical findings appear. Biological monitoring is thought to be a useful tool to detect the effects of exposure on organs before distinct organ damage occurs. However, there are few reports in which the associations between aluminum concentrations in blood or urine and clinical findings have been studied, except for associations with neurological findings.

Various pre-clinical markers show abnormalities before organ damage becomes obvious. Therefore, in order to examine the effect of aluminum on organs, we measured the urinary aluminum concentrations among aluminum-handling and non-handling workers and investigated the relationships between these concentrations and these pre-clinical markers. We focused on the effect of aluminum on lungs, bones, and kidneys and on inflammation and oxidative DNA damage.

Pulmonary fibrosis and neurological findings have been evident under high-dose aluminum exposure [4,14]. Therefore, it is appropriate for pre-clinical markers to be studied in the field under lower aluminum exposure levels.

This study was carried out in a workplace where dust concentration is appropriately controlled under Japanese regulations.

Methods

Participants

Twenty-three healthy aluminum-handling workers who were not taking any medications and 10 age-adjusted, healthy non-aluminum-handling workers participated in this study. No significant findings had been made for any of the subjects in the medical examinations, which were carried out annually. Moreover, they had not had any illnesses of the lungs, kidneys, blood or bones. The aluminum-handling workers were engaged in aluminum casting, and the non-handling workers were desk workers at the same facility.

This study was approved by the Ethics Committee of Jichi Medical University. All subjects gave their informed consent.

Samples

We collected urine and blood samples in examining rooms at a medical facility, not at the aluminum casting factory. The aluminum-handling workers' blood and urine were collected in the latter half of a work-day in the latter part of the work-week. The non-handling workers' blood and urine were collected at their convenience.

Aluminum in urine was analyzed using inductively coupled plasma mass spectrometry (ICP-MS). We assigned this analysis to a commissioned company (La Belle Vie, Inc., Tokyo, Japan). This measurement method has a limit of quantification for aluminum in urine of 1.4 ppb.

In order to check the pre-clinical findings, we measured KL-6, SP-D, TRCP-5b, IL-6, and IL-8 in blood and δ-ALA and β2-microglobulin in urine. These markers were intended to indicate lung fibrosis, bone metabolites, inflammation, hematopoietic injury and glomerular damage to the kidney, respectively. These markers were measured by a commercial company (LSI Medience Co., Tokyo, Japan) using their routine method. Moreover, 8-hydroxy-2'-deoxyguanosine (8-OHdG) in urine was measured as an oxidative DNA damage marker using an ELISA kit, the New 8-OHdG Check (Japan Institute for The Control of Aging). Urease treatment was carried out to cancel the effect of urea on the data.

The marker measurements are listed in Table 1.

Work environmental measurement in the aluminum-handling location

The geometric means of the measurement of aluminum dust in various aluminum-handling locations in the work environment ranged from 0.09–0.31 mg/m^3. These values fall under Control Class 1 in Japan, which indicates that the workplace is appropriately controlled [15]. Moreover, these values are under the occupational exposure limit of aluminum dust (0.5 mg/m^3) [16] set by the Japan Society for Occupational Health.

Statistical analysis

Statistical analyses were performed using Stat View 5.0 (SAS Institute, Inc., Cary, NC, USA). A comparison of each pre-clinical marker and of age between the aluminum-handling workers and non-handling workers was analyzed by the Mann–Whitney *U* test. In the aluminum-handling workers, the relationships between urinary aluminum concentration and each pre-clinical marker, age and work-years were analyzed by Spearman's rank correlation. The results were considered statistically significant if the p values were <0.05.

Results

The aluminum concentration in urine in the aluminum-handling and non-handling workers are summarized in Table 2, and the distribution of these data are shown in Figure 1. It ranged from 6.9 to 55.1 μg/g cre (median concentration: 20.1 μg/g cre) in the aluminum-handling workers and from 5.6 to 15.6 μg/g cre (median concentration: 8.8 μg/g cre) in the non-handling workers. The

Table 1 The markers measured in this study

Markers	Blood	Urine	Remarks
Aluminum		o	Measured by inductively coupled plasma analysis
KL-6	o (serum)		Marker of lung fibrosis
SP-D	o (serum)		Marker of lung fibrosis
TRACP-5b	o (serum)		Marker of influence on bone
IL-6	o (plasma)		Marker of inflammation
IL-8	o (plasma)		Marker of inflammation
δ-ALA		o	Marker of influence on myelopoietic organ
β2-MG		o	Marker of influence on kidney
8-OHdG		o	Marker of oxidative DNA damage

difference between aluminum-handling and non-handling workers was statistically significant.

In the pre-clinical findings, although there was a significant difference in δ-ALA, there were no significant differences in KL-6, SP-D, TRCP-5b, IL-6, IL-8, β2-microglobulin or 8-OHdG between the two groups (Figure 2). The data under the detection limit were assumed to be half of the detection limit.

In the aluminum-handling workers, no significant relationship was found between aluminum concentration and each pre-clinical marker, work-years or age.

Discussion

The excretion of aluminum in urine was elevated in aluminum-handling workers. However, there was no significant relationship between aluminum concentration and work-years, age, or any pre-clinical finding or 8-OHdG in this study. From these findings, no health effects of aluminum at urinary concentrations below 55 μg/g cre could be observed.

Threshold levels have been reported for the association between urinary aluminum and neurological effects. Pre-clinical neurotoxic effects are observed when serum aluminum levels exceed 10 μg/l [6]. Serum aluminum levels of 0.25–0.35 μmol/l (6.8–9.5 μg/l), and urinary aluminum

Table 2 Urinary aluminum concentrations in the aluminum-handling and non-handling workers

	Aluminum-handling workers					Non-handling workers		
	Age	Al	Al	Work-year		Age	Al	Al
	y.o.	μg/g cre	μmol/l	Year		y.o.	μg/g cre	μmol/l
	27	6.9	0.62	6		36	5.6	0.33
	38	8.1	1.02	7		54	7.6	0.57
	30	10.9	0.54	2		52	7.8	0.42
	46	11.5	0.48	20		58	8.3	0.41
	48	11.6	0.68	22		34	8.4	0.43
	24	12.3	0.66	5		30	9.1	0.18
	52	12.3	0.81	31		44	10.2	0.39
	55	15.1	0.82	36		40	11.0	0.37
	34	16.1	0.95	15		23	12.3	0.22
	37	17.4	1.49	1		47	15.6	0.56
	19	18.4	1.48	1	Median		8.8	0.40
	43	20.1	1.69	8				
	40	20.7	1.31	21				
	52	24.0	2.10	31				
	29	24.2	2.10	4				
	36	26.8	2.18	17				
	47	27.9	1.70	19				
	33	30.2	1.59	3				
	54	33.4	3.99	35				
	53	36.8	1.12	25				
	54	37.3	0.56	36				
	60	54.4	1.95	31				
	41	55.1	1.68	7				
Median		20.1	1.31					

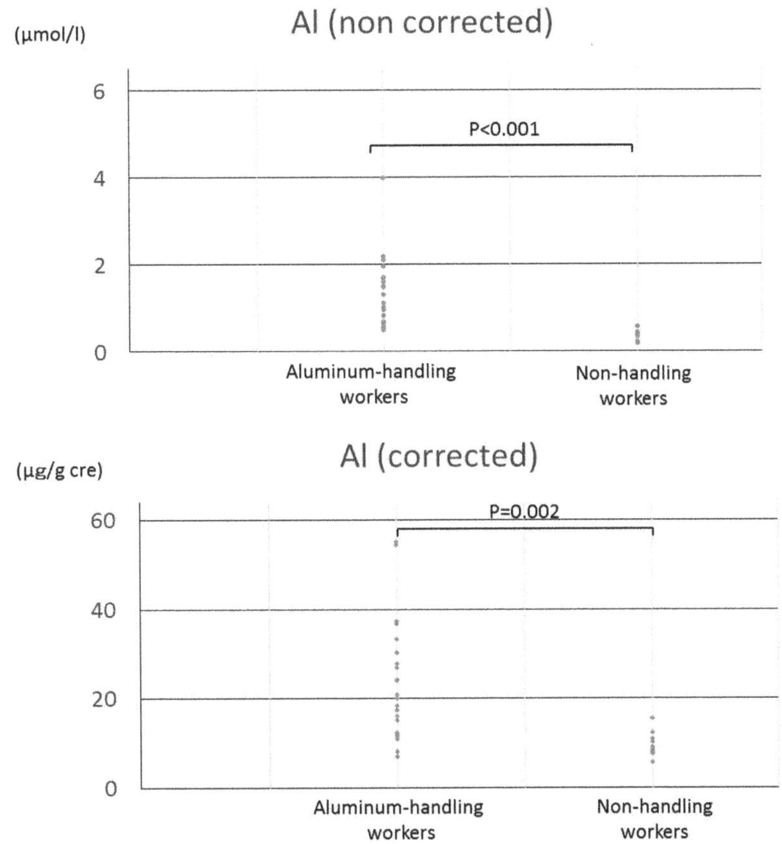

Figure 1 The distribution of aluminum concentrations in aluminum-handling and non-handling workers. The upper graph is raw data and the lower is data corrected by urinary creatinine.

levels of 4–6 μmol/l (108–162 μg/l) appear to represent a threshold for observed adverse neurological effects [7]. Iregren et al. [17] indicated that a urinary level of 100 μg/l was a critical concentration for the development of neurological effects. However, there are few reports in which the associations between the aluminum concentration in blood or urine and clinical findings have been studied, except for associations with neurological findings. The urinary aluminum concentration in aluminum-handling workers observed in this study was much lower than the threshold for neurological effects. This is due to the low dust concentration in the air at the workplace studied.

Sjögern et al. [18] reported a difference in urinary aluminum concentrations between welders with 0.08 to 2 years' exposure and those with 18 to 20 years' exposure. On the other hand, our study found no relationship between urinary aluminum and work-years. The aluminum concentration in the air in the study by Sjögren et al. was relatively high, at 2.4 mg/m^3 (8 h-TWA). In our study, the total dust concentration in the air was much lower, at 0.09–0.31 mg/m^3. All workers in this study have at least 16 hours between shifts. There are reports suggesting that about 1% of aluminum in welding fumes is rapidly absorbed from the lungs [19], and about 45% of that is cleared from the lungs after one day [20]. We suppose that no relationship between urinary aluminum concentration and work-years could be detected because the concentration of inhaled aluminum was not very high and the time interval to the next work shift was relatively long.

Many studies have been done on pulmonary fibrosis in aluminum-handling workers [4,5]. Aluminum induces the impairment of bone formation [21], and this occurs mostly in patients with chronic renal disease who are undergoing renal dialysis [3]. In an *in vitro* study, aluminum nanoparticles were shown to inhibit the inflammation reaction (e.g. IL-6, IL-8) to methicillin-resistant *Staphylococcus aureus* [12]. Dey et al. [13] reported that aluminum nanoparticles shifted into the cells and elevated the level of reactive oxygen species. An animal experiment showed that aluminum has a distinct effect on blood δ-aminolevulinic acid dehydratase (ALA-D) activity according to the aluminum concentration in the blood [10]. No significant differences in KL-6, SP-D, TRCP-5b, IL-6, IL-8, or 8-OHdG were detected between aluminum-handling and non-handling workers; therefore, although the excretion of aluminum in urine was elevated in aluminum-handling workers, this study suggests that aluminum is not harmful to humans.

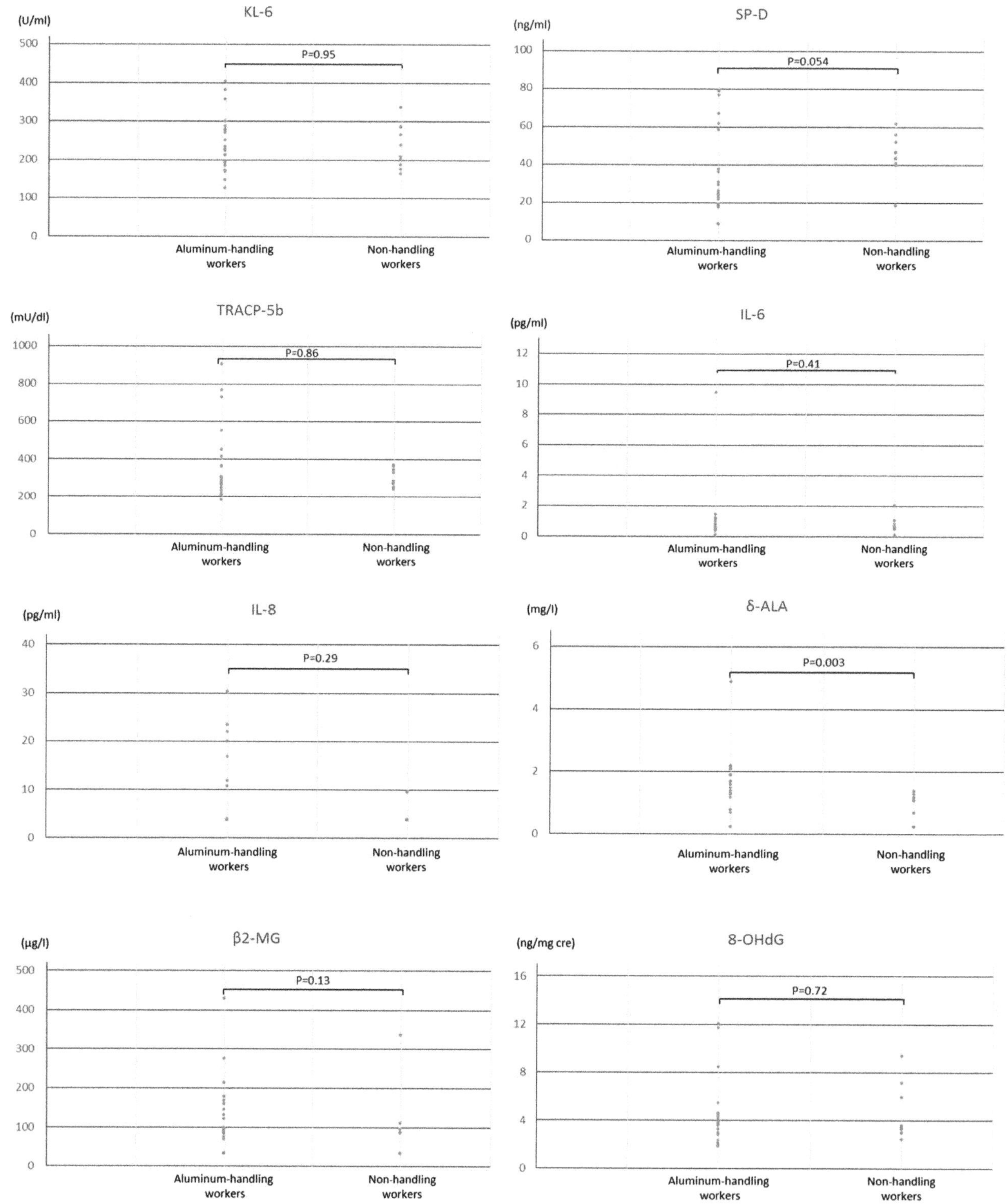

Figure 2 Distributions of pre-clinical markers in aluminum-handling and non-handling workers. There were no significant differences in KL-6, SP-D, TRCP-5b, IL-6, IL-8, β2-microglobulin and 8-OHdG between these two groups. A significant difference was found in δ-ALA levels.

Some metals do cause kidney damage and an elevation of urinary β2 microglobulin [22,23] but no reports have yet shown that aluminum causes renal dysfunction in healthy people. Urinary β2 microglobulin was measured in the present study; however, it was not elevated in aluminum-handling workers compared with non-handling workers.

Some stomach medicines and foods contain aluminum, and the ingestion of these may affect the urinary aluminum concentration. Generally, the aluminum concentration in food is lower than that in aluminum-containing medicine, and the absorption of aluminum from the gastrointestinal tract has been reported to be very low [24,25]. Therefore, we had the participants restrain their intake of aluminum-containing drugs, but we did not limit their food intake. Because of this restriction, we suspected that the elevation of urinary aluminum in the aluminum-handling workers resulted mainly from inhalation.

In this study, there were some smokers among both the aluminum-handling and non-handling workers. Iarmarcovai et al. mentioned that although cadmium was significantly more prevalent in smokers [26], the concentrations of other metals including aluminum did not differ between smokers and non-smokers. Therefore, we did not distinguish between smokers and non-smokers in our analysis.

As for the sampling time, one report found that although urinary aluminum concentrations were not significantly different between the beginning and end of the work-week, the concentration at the end of the week was higher [26]. Therefore, the samples used in this study were collected in the latter half of the work-day in the latter part of the work-week.

The primary objectives of biological monitoring of aluminum are to detect excessive aluminum entering the lungs and to prevent the harmful accumulation of aluminum in target organs. Biological monitoring of aluminum can be effectively used for these purposes [26]. When performing biological monitoring, the determination of aluminum in urine is recommended due to the higher sensitivity and robustness of this measure compared to the measurement of aluminum in plasma [27,28]. This is why urinary aluminum was used to assess the aluminum concentration in our study.

Among the pre-clinical markers, only δ-ALA showed a significant difference between the aluminum-handling and non-handling workers. Lead is well known for inhibiting ALA-D activity and increasing the excretion of δ-ALA into urine [23]. In order to rule out the effect of lead on δ-ALA in aluminum-handling workers, lead in urine was also measured by ICP-MS. There was no significant difference in urinary lead levels between the two groups. Consequently, the elevation of δ-ALA in aluminum-handling workers' urine may have been due to aluminum. However, the elevation of δ-ALA in urine did not exceed the occupational exposure limits based on biological monitoring issued by the Japan Society for Occupational Health [16], and the level of elevation observed in this study has not shown any health effects.

There are some limitations to this study. First, the aluminum concentration in the air in this particular workplace is low. Thus, the urinary aluminum concentration is lower than that seen in cases with obvious adverse effects. However, it is appropriate for pre-clinical markers to be studied in the field under lower aluminum levels. Second, the sample size may be small. However, the urinary aluminum concentration in aluminum-handling workers was found to be significantly higher than that in non-handling workers. Thus, the effect of aluminum on the pre-clinical markers could be assessed. Since no previous studies have focused on the effect of pre-clinical markers under the aluminum exposure, this study is useful from the viewpoint of occupational health.

From these findings, no health effects of aluminum at urinary concentrations below 55 μg/g cre (4 μmol/l) could be observed. Aluminum has low toxicity to humans; however, it is still important to try to reduce aluminum exposure as much as possible. It has been reported that workers in workplaces without collective protection devices showed significantly higher urinary aluminum concentrations than those in workplaces equipped with smoke-extraction systems [26]. Therefore, equipping workers and workplaces with appropriate collective protective devices, such as local exhaust ventilation, is an effective measure for reducing workers' exposure to aluminum; wearing personal protective equipment, such as a dust mask, is also recommended.

Conclusions

The excretion of aluminum in urine was elevated in aluminum-handling workers. Although our sample study was small and the workplace relatively free of aluminium dust, our findings suggest that the aluminum in such a workplace is not directly harmful to the lungs, bones, and kidneys and it does not cause inflammation and oxidative DNA damage in humans, at least when urinary aluminum is below 55 μg/g cre.

Competing interests

The authors declare that they have no competing interests.

Authors' contributions

MO participated in the design of the study and the collection of samples, performed the statistical analysis and drafted the manuscript. FK gave professional advice for data processing. Both authors read and approved the final manuscript.

Author details

[1]Health Service Center, Jichi Medical University, 3311-1, Yakushiji, Shimotsuke, Tochigi 329-0498, Japan. [2]Department of Environmental and Preventive Medicine, Jichi Medical University, 3311-1, Yakushiji, Shimotsuke, Tochigi 329-0498, Japan.

References

1. Food and Agriculture Organization of the United Nations: Summary report of the seventy-fourth meeting of JECFA [ftp://ftp.fao.org/ag/agn/jecfa/JECFA_74_Summary_Report_4July2011.pdf]
2. Food and Agriculture Organization of the United Nations: Joint FAO/WHO food standards programme codex committee on contaminants in foods fifth session [ftp://ftp.fao.org/codex/meetings/CCCF/cccf5/cf05_INF.pdf]
3. American Conference of Governmental Industrial Hygienists (ACGIH). Aluminum metal and insoluble compounds. In: Documentation of the TLVs and BEIs with other worldwide occupational exposure values [CD-ROM]. Cincinnati: ACGIH; 2014.
4. Jederlinic PJ, Abraham JL, Churg A, Himmelstein JS, Epler GR, Gaensler EA. Pulmonary fibrosis in aluminum oxide workers. Investigation of nine workers, with pathologic examination and microanalysis in three of them. Am Rev Respir Dis. 1990;142:1179–84.
5. Al-Masalkhi A, Walton SP. Pulmonary fibrosis and occupational exposure to aluminum. J Ky Med Assoc. 1994;92:59–61.
6. Polizzi S, Pira E, Ferrara M, Bugiani M, Papaleo A, Albera R, et al. Neurotoxic effects of aluminium among foundry workers and Alzheimer's disease. Neurotoxicology. 2002;23:761–74.
7. Riihimäki V, Hänninen H, Akila R, Kovala T, Kuosma E, Paakkulainen H, et al. Body burden of aluminum in relation to central nervous system function among metal inert-gas welders. Scand J Work Environ Health. 2000;26:118–30.
8. Ellis HA, McCarthy JH, Herrington J. Bone aluminium in haemodialysed patients and in rats injected with aluminium chloride: relationship to impaired bone mineralisation. J Clin Pathol. 1979;32:832–44.
9. Dahl E, Nordal KP, Halse J, Flatmark A. The early effects of aluminium deposition and dialysis on bone in chronic renal failure: a cross-sectional bone-histomorphometric study. Nephrol Dial Transplant. 1990;5:449–56.
10. Pimentel Vieira VL, Rocha JB, Schetinger MR, Morsch VM, Rodrigues SR, Tuerlinckz SM, et al. Effect of aluminum on delta-aminolevulinic acid dehydratase from mouse blood. Toxicol Lett. 2000;117:45–52.
11. Farina M, Rotta LN, Soares FA, Jardim F, Jacques R, Souza DO, et al. Hematological changes in rats chronically exposed to oral aluminum. Toxicology. 2005;209:29–37.
12. Braydich-Stolle LK, Speshock JL, Castle A, Smith M, Murdock RC, Hussain SM. Nanosized aluminum altered immune function. ACS Nano. 2010;4:3661–70.
13. Dey S, Bakthavatchalu V, Tseng MT, Wu P, Florence RL, Grulke EA, et al. Interactions between SIRT1 and AP-1 reveal a mechanistic insight into the growth promoting properties of alumina (Al_2O_3) nanoparticles in mouse skin epithelial cells. Carcinogenesis. 2008;29:1920–9.
14. Rifat SL, Eastwood MR, McLachlan DR, Corey PN. Effect of exposure of miners to aluminium powder. Lancet. 1990;336:1162–5.
15. Hori H. Work environment control and occupational hygienist in Japan. Ind Health. 2013;51:143–4.
16. The Japanese Society of Occupational Health. Recommendation of occupational exposure limits (2014–2015). J Occup Health. 2014;56:401–20.
17. Iregren A, Sjögren B, Gustafsson K, Hagman M, Nylén L, Frech W, et al. Effects on the nervous system in different groups of workers exposed to aluminium. Occup Environ Med. 2001;58:453–60.
18. Sjögren B, Lidums V, Håkansson M, Hedström L. Exposure and urinary excretion of aluminum during welding. Scand J Work Environ Health. 1985;11:39–43.
19. Riihimäki V, Valkonen S, Engström B, Tossavainen A, Mutanen P, Aitio A. Behavior of aluminum in aluminum welders and manufacturers of aluminum sulfate–impact on biological monitoring. Scand J Work Environ Health. 2008;34:451–62.
20. Priest ND. The biological behaviour and bioavailability of aluminium in man, with special reference to studies employing aluminium-26 as a tracer: review and study update. J Environ Monit. 2004;6:375–403.
21. Aaseth J, Boivin G, Andersen O. Osteoporosis and trace elements–an overview. J Trace Elem Med Biol. 2012;26:149–52.
22. Bernard A. Renal dysfunction induced by cadmium: biomarkers of critical effects. Biometals. 2004;17:519–23.
23. International Programme on Chemical Safety (ICPS). Inorganic lead. In: environmental health criteria 165. Geneva: WHO; 1995.
24. Greger JL, Powers CF. Assessment of exposure to parenteral and oral aluminum with and without citrate using a desferrioxamine test in rats. Toxicology. 1992;76:119–32.
25. International Programme on Chemical Safety (IPCS). Aluminum. Environmental health criteria 194. Geneva: WHO; 1997.
26. Iarmarcovai G, Sari-Minodier I, Chaspoul F, Botta C, De Méo M, Orsière T, et al. Risk assessment of welders using analysis of eight metals by ICP-MS in blood and urine and DNA damage evaluation by the comet and micronucleus assays; influence of XRCC1 and XRCC3 polymorphisms. Mutagenesis. 2005;20:425–32.
27. Riihimäki V, Aitio A. Occupational exposure to aluminum and its biomonitoring in perspective. Crit Rev Toxicol. 2012;42:827–53.
28. Rossbach B, Buchta M, Csanády GA, Filser JG, Hilla W, Windorfer K, et al. Biological monitoring of welders exposed to aluminium. Toxicol Lett. 2006;162:239–45.

23

The impact of multi-site musculoskeletal pain on work ability among health care providers

Chanwit Phongamwong* and Hemwarun Deema

Abstract

Background: Epidemiologic studies have reported that multi-site musculoskeletal pain threatens work ability. However, no study has been conducted on this topic among health care providers. The aim of the present study was to determine the association between multi-site pain and poor work ability among health care providers.

Methods: A cross-sectional study was conducted. Participants completed a self-administered questionnaire including basic characteristics, job satisfaction, stress screening, musculoskeletal pain at neck, upper extremities, low back, and lower extremities within the last month, and work ability index. Pain intensity was dichotomized according to a numerical pain rating scale score: less than five (no) and at least five (yes). Musculoskeletal pain was divided in three groups: 1) no pain, 2) few pain sites (one to two sites), and 3) many pain sites (three to four sites). The association of the number of pain sites with poor work ability was explored through multivariable logistic regression analysis.

Results: A total of 254 health care providers participated in the present study. The majority of participants were female (73.2 %) with mean age of 33.9 (SD 9.5) years. Few pain sites and many pain sites were reported by 79 (31.1 %) and 39 participants (15.4 %), respectively. The adjusted odds ratio for poor work ability of participants who had few pain sites and many pain sites were 1.85 (95 % CI: 0.91 – 3.76) and 2.41 (95 % CI: 1.04 – 5.58), respectively.

Conclusion: The present study showed that multi-site musculoskeletal pain had an association with poor work ability. The magnitude of association was likely to increase by a higher number of pain sites.

Keywords: Multi-site pain, Number of pain sites, Musculoskeletal pain, Work ability, Health care providers

Introduction

Currently, musculoskeletal pain has become a major health problem around the world [1]. The most recent report of the global burden caused by the 25 leading diseases and injuries in 2010 showed that low back pain ranked as the seventh with 80,667,000 of disability-adjusted life-years (DALYs), followed by neck pain as the twenty-first with 32,651,000 of DALYs. Other musculoskeletal disorders was ranked the twenty-third with 30,877,000 of DALYs, whereas ischemic heart disease ranked as the first with 129,795,000 of DALYs [2].

In the recent decade, many epidemiologic studies focused on multi-site musculoskeletal pain, and their findings revealed that the prevalence of multi-site pain is high in both general and working populations including hospital workers [3–11]. The prevalence among health care providers is about 40 – 50 % depending on definition of pain site and study population [4, 6].

Epidemiologic studies found the multi-site pain associates with poor work ability in working populations [12–14]. A prospective study among food-industrial workers demonstrated that the number of pain sites predicted poor work ability after 4 years of follow-up with a dose–response manner [13]. However, no epidemiologic evidence is available among the hospital working population. Hence, the aim of the present study was to confirm whether the number of pain sites has an association with poor work ability among health care providers.

* Correspondence: sengsmart@hotmail.com
Department of Rehabilitation Medicine, Phramongkutklao Hospital and Phramongkutklao College of Medicine, Bangkok, Thailand

Methods

Study design and participants

The present study was cross-sectional study conducted among health care providers of a tertiary hospital in Thailand between April 2014 and June 2014. The self-administered paper questionnaires were distributed in the hospital with convenient sampling. There was no reminder to complete the questionnaires. Eligibility criteria included being a health care provider including physicians, nurses, pharmacists, dentists, medical technicians, and physical/occupational therapists who worked in the hospital at least six months, were able to communicate in Thai, and consented to participate in the present study. Retired workers, outsourced personnel, and those suffering from tumors, fracture, chronic infection or systemic and neurologic diseases were excluded. The present study protocol was approved by the Institutional Review Board, Royal Thai Army Medical Department.

Outcome

The outcome in the present study was work ability assessed by the work ability index (WAI). This questionnaire was developed by the Finnish Institute of Occupational Health in the 1980s comprising seven items including current work ability compared with the lifetime best, work ability in relation to the demands of the job, number of current diseases diagnosed by a physician, estimated work impairment due to diseases, sick leave during the past year (12 months), own prognosis of work ability 2 years from now, and mental resources [15]. All items were weighted and summed up to a total score of seven (the poorest) to 49 (the best). The present study used a short version with 14 groups of diseases in the third item (51 diseases in the original version) [16]. In the present study, the work ability index was dichotomized as good (37 – 49) and poor (7 – 36) [17].

Exposure

The exposure in the present study was the number of pain sites assessed by self-administered paper questionnaire with a question on pain symptom in four-different anatomical regions including neck, upper extremities, low back, and lower extremities within the last month. Pain at the upper and lower extremities was recorded including the right, left, or both sides [12]. Pain intensity of each region was measured by zero (no pain) to ten (the worst pain) on a numerical pain rating scale. Each answer was dichotomized according to a numerical pain rating scale: less than five (no) and at least five (yes). Binary outcome of four-different anatomical regions was computed as the number of pain sites and categorized in three groups including no pain (0), few pain sites (1 – 2 sites), and many pain sites (3 – 4 sites).

Confounders

Age, stress problem, and satisfaction in workload, payment, rest time, teamwork, and working environment were included in multivariable logistic regression analysis as confounders of the association between the number of pain sites and poor work ability [9, 18–21]. Age was categorized in two groups: less than 40 years and at least 40 years old. Stress problem was evaluated by a stress test (ST5) questionnarie which was developed by Department of Mental Health, Ministry of Public Health of Thailand comprising five items: sleep problem, decreased concentration, irritability, boredom, and social isolation. Each item was scored between zero and three, so its total score of ST5 questionnaire ranged from 0 to 15. Scores were dichotomized into categorical data of stress problem (No = not more than four, and Yes = more than four) [22]. Each topic of job satisfaction was measured by a 5-level Likert scale: highly satisfied, satisfied, partially satisfied, not satisfied, or not at all satisfied. However, in statistical analysis, these data were divided into two categories of satisfaction (Satisfied = highly satisfied or satisfied, and Not satisfied = partially satisfied, not satisfied, or not at all satisfied).

Statistical analysis

The sample size was calculated based on the results of the study conducted by Neupane *et al.* [13]. Power of 80 % was selected for the Chi-square test. To detect computed effect size of 0.054 with an alpha level of 0.05, a total required sample of 222 participants was expected. Assuming a 70 % rate of response, a total of 318 participants would be required.

Logistic regression was conducted to determine the number of pain sites associated with poor work ability. The association was presented by odds ratio and its 95 % confident interval. Dummy variables were used to put number of pain sites (no pain = reference group) in the model. As potential confounders, sex (0 = male, 1 = female), age (0 = <40 years, 1 = ≥40), stress problem (No = 0, Yes = 1), satisfaction in workload (Satisfied = 0, Not satisfied = 1), satisfaction in payment (Satisfied = 0, Not satisfied = 1), satisfaction in rest time (Satisfied = 0, Not satisfied = 1), satisfaction in teamwork (Satisfied = 0, Not satisfied = 1), and satisfaction in working environment (Satisfied = 0, Not satisfied = 1) were included in the logistic regression analysis. In addition, before conducting the regression model, all potential confounders were tested by a formal-detection tolerance for multicollinearity diagnostics. A tolerance of less than 0.2 indicates a multicollinearity problem. All statistical analyses were performed using STATA version 10.

Results

Participant characteristics

A total of 254 health care providers participated in the study and completed all questionnaires (response rate of 79.9 %). According to the demographic characteristics (Table 1), the majority of participants were female (73.2 %) with a mean age of 33.9 (9.5) years ranging from 18 to 58 years. Of these, 28.7 %, 23.2 %, 20.5 %, 11.8 %, 10.6 %, and 5.1 % were nurses, physicians, pharmacists, medical technician, dentist, and physical/occupational therapist, respectively.

Musculoskeletal pain and work ability

Among 254 participants, poor work ability was reported by 65 participants (25.6 %). The prevalence of any musculoskeletal pain during the past month was 46.5 %. Pain in the lower extremities was most frequently reported (28.3 %), followed by low back pain (26.6 %), neck pain (24.8 %) and upper extremities pain (17.8 %). In all, 31.1 % of participants had few pain sites (1 – 2 sites), whereas 15.4 % had many pain sites (3 – 4 sites).

Impact of the number of pain sites on work ability

As shown in Table 2, the prevalence of poor work ability in participants who had no pain, few pain sites, and many pain sites were 18.4 %, 30.4 %, and 41.0 %, respectively. In crude analysis, a statistically significant association was found between the number of pain sites and work ability. Odds ratio of poor work ability in participants who had few pain sites was 1.9 (95 % CI 1.01 – 3.69), while in those who had many pain sites was 3.0 (95 % CI 1.42 – 6.68).

To eliminate the effect of confounders, logistic regression analysis was conducted. All of the potential confounders were tested for multicollinearity diagnostics. A formal-detection tolerance of all of these ranged from 0.6 to 0.9, so there was no multicollinearity problem. After adjustment for many confounders, odds ratio in those who had few pain sites showed no statistical significance (1.89 (95 % CI 0.93 – 3.80)), whereas those who had many pain sites still showed statistical significance although its odds ratio showed a small decrease (2.44 (95 % CI 1.06 – 5.66)).

Table 1 Demographic characteristics of the participants

Variable	N	%
Age (year) – mean (SD)		33.9 (9.5)
Female	186	73.2
BMI		
<18.5 kg/m^2	20	7.9
18.5 – 24.99 kg/m^2	165	65.2
≥25 kg/m^2	68	26.9
Occupation		
Physician	59	23.2
Pharmacist	52	20.5
Nurse	73	28.7
Dentist	27	10.6
Medical technician	30	11.8
Physical and occupational therapist	13	5.1
No stress problem	122	48.0
Satisfied in workload	148	58.3
Satisfied in payment	76	29.9
Satisfied in rest time	109	42.9
Satisfied in teamwork	165	65.0
Satisfied in working environment	141	55.5
Neck pain	63	24.8
Upper extremities pain	45	17.8
Low back pain	67	26.6
Lower extremities pain	72	28.3
Number of pain sites		
No pain	136	53.5
Few pain sites	79	31.1
Many pain sites	39	15.4

Discussion

The present study is the first to reveal the negative impact of the number of pain sites on work ability among health care providers. The hypothesis in this study was the association between musculoskeletal pain and poor work ability would be stronger when the number of pain sites increased. The main findings supported this hypothesis.

The main results showed that participants who had few pain sites were 1.9 time more likely to develop poor

Table 2 Odds ratio of poor work ability from multivariable logistic regression analysis

	All subjects	No. of subjects with poor work ability (%)	Crude OR (95 % CI)	Adjusted OR[a] (95 % CI)
No pain	136	25 (18.4)	1	1
Few pain sites	79	24 (30.4)	1.9 (1.01 – 3.69)**	1.85 (0.91 – 3.76)
Many pain sites	39	16 (41.0)	3.0 (1.42 – 6.68)**	2.41 (1.04 – 5.58)**

[a]Adjusted for sex, age group, stress, satisfaction in workload, satisfaction in payment, satisfaction in rest time, satisfaction in teamwork, satisfaction in working environment

**P *value* <0.05

work ability than those who had none, while this probability increased to 3.0 times in participants who had many pain sites by crude analysis. After adjustment for age, stress problem, and job sattisfaction in the regression model, the tendency for this result still remained. Hence, the number of pain sites could predict the probabity of poor work ability among health care providers. However, the results in those who had few pain sites were not significant by multivariable analysis. This was likely caused by the small sample size resulting in a wide 95 % confident interval. To compare with previous studies, these findings were similar to the health survey among Finnish general workers, and the prospective study conducted among Finnish industrial workers [12, 13].

The present study had several stengths. Firstly, this study focused on musculoskeletal pain within the last month to reduce the recall bias. Next, the WAI, one of the the validated international questionnaires of work ability assessment, was used to determine poor work ability [15]. Importantly, this study was concerned with the effect of some potential confounders and included them in the logistic regression model.

On the other hand, some weaknesses were observed in this study. The major limitation was the lack of a temporal relationship between the number of pain sites (exposure) and work ability (outcome) because this study employed a cross-sectional design. In addition, This study was carried out only in a tertiary care center involving a great workload and number of responsibilities, so the results from this study could not be applied to other hospital care settings such as a primary care unit. Moreover, all data were collected by the self-administered questionnaire without objective assessment, for example, a physical examination to determine musculoskeletal pain. Hence, information bias or invalidation of data might occur, but a questionnaire survey seem to be the practical way to assess musculoskeletal pain in epidemiological studies [13]. Finally, Participants who had many pain sites tended to have chronic pain which might have affected work ability [3]. Therefore, a subgroup analysis divided by pain duration could be conducted in further studies.

Conclusions

The probability of poor work ability would be higher when the number of pain sites increased. Multi-site musculoskeletal pain should be concerned not only in industrial working populations but also in hospital working populations, and should be specially attended in occupational health services, for example, annual health examination, ergonomic concerns, and walk-through survey. In addition, among health care providers, the self-administered questionnaire for simply counting the number of pain sites could be a screening instrument to detect workers who have the risk of poor work ability.

Abbreviations

DALYs: Disability-adjusted life-years; WAI: Work ability index.

Competing interests

The authors declare that they have no competing interests.

Authors' contributions

CP: correspondent author, participated in the design of the study, performed the statistical analysis, drafted the manuscript and finished the manuscript. HD: participated in the design of the study, performed the data collection. Both authors read and approved the final manuscript.

Acknowledgements

We would like to thank Assoc. Prof. Jariya Boonhong, M.D. for her contribution in the design of the study. This study was finacially supported by Phramongkutklao Hospital.

References

1. Brooks PM. The burden of musculoskeletal disease–a global perspective. Clin Rheumatol. 2006;25(6):778–81.
2. Murray CJ, Lopez AD. Measuring the global burden of disease. N Engl J Med. 2013;369(5):448–57.
3. Carnes D, Parson S, Ashby D, Breen A, Foster NE, Pincus T, et al. Chronic musculoskeletal pain rarely presents in a single body site: results from a UK population study. Rheumatology (Oxford). 2007;46(7):1168–70.
4. Freimann T, Coggon D, Merisalu E, Animagi L, Paasuke M. Risk factors for musculoskeletal pain amongst nurses in Estonia: a cross-sectional study. BMC Musculoskelet Disord. 2013;14:334.
5. Hoftun GB, Romundstad PR, Zwart JA, Rygg M. Chronic idiopathic pain in adolescence–high prevalence and disability: the young HUNT Study 2008. Pain. 2011;152(10):2259–66.
6. Phongamwong C, Mungkumpa A, Pawapootanon W, Saiyotha D, Duangtapha C. The impact of musculoskeletal pain on health-related quality of life in Fort Prajaksilapakom Hospital. J Med Assoc Thai. 2014;97 Suppl 2:S181–7.
7. Solidaki E, Chatzi L, Bitsios P, Coggon D, Palmer KT, Kogevinas M. Risk factors for new onset and persistence of multi-site musculoskeletal pain in a longitudinal study of workers in Crete. Occup Environ Med. 2013;70(1):29–34.
8. Solidaki E, Chatzi L, Bitsios P, Markatzi I, Plana E, Castro F, et al. Work-related and psychological determinants of multisite musculoskeletal pain. Scand J Work Environ Health. 2010;36(1):54–61.
9. Sembajwe G, Tveito TH, Hopcia K, Kenwood C, O'Day ET, Stoddard AM, et al. Psychosocial stress and multi-site musculoskeletal pain: a cross-sectional survey of patient care workers. Workplace Health Saf. 2013;61(3):117–25.
10. Kamaleri Y, Natvig B, Ihlebaek CM, Benth JS, Bruusgaard D, et al. Change in the number of musculoskeletal pain sites: a 14-year prospective study. Pain. 2009;141(1–2):25–30.
11. Picavet HS, Hoeymans N. Health related quality of life in multiple musculoskeletal diseases: SF-36 and EQ-5D in the DMC3 study. Ann Rheum Dis. 2004;63(6):723–9.
12. Miranda H, Kaila-Kangas L, Heliovaara M, Leino-Arjas P, Haukka E, Liira J, et al. Musculoskeletal pain at multiple sites and its effects on work ability in a general working population. Occup Environ Med. 2010;67(7):449–55.
13. Neupane S, Miranda H, Virtanen P, Siukola A, Nygard CH. Multi-site pain and work ability among an industrial population. Occup Med (Lond). 2011;61(8):563–9.
14. Neupane S, Virtanen P, Leino-Arjas P, Miranda H, Siukola A, Nygard CH. Multi-site pain and working conditions as predictors of work ability in a 4-year follow-up among food industry employees. Eur J Pain. 2013;17(3):444–51.
15. Ilmarinen J. The work ability index (WAI). Occup Med. 2007;57(2):160.
16. Roelen CA, van Rhenen W, Groothoff JW, van der Klink JJ, Twisk JW, Heymans MW. Work ability as prognostic risk marker of disability pension: single-item work ability score versus multi-item work ability index. Scand J Work Environ Health. 2014;40(4):428–31.
17. El Fassi M, Bocquet V, Majery N, Lair ML, Couffignal S, Mairiaux P. Work ability assessment in a worker population: comparison and determinants of Work Ability Index and Work Ability score. BMC Public Health. 2013;13:305.

18. van den Berg TI, Elders LA, de Zwart BC, Burdorf A. The effects of work-related and individual factors on the Work Ability Index: a systematic review. Occup Environ Med. 2009;66(4):211–20.
19. Kamaleri Y, Natvig B, Ihlebaek CM, Benth JS, Bruusgaard D. Number of pain sites is associated with demographic, lifestyle, and health-related factors in the general population. Eur J Pain. 2008;12(6):742–8.
20. Lindegard A, Larsman P, Hadzibajramovic E, Ahlborg Jr G. The influence of perceived stress and musculoskeletal pain on work performance and work ability in Swedish health care workers. Int Arch Occup Environ Health. 2014;87(4):373–9.
21. Magnusson K, Osteras N, Mowinckel P, Natvig B, Hagen KB. No strong temporal relationship between obesity and multisite pain - results from a population-based 20-year follow-up study. Eur J Pain. 2014;18(1):120–7.
22. Silpakit O. Srithanya stress scale. J Mental Health Thai. 2012;16(3):177–85.

Permissions

All chapters in this book were first published in JOMT, by BioMed Central; hereby published with permission under the Creative Commons Attribution License or equivalent. Every chapter published in this book has been scrutinized by our experts. Their significance has been extensively debated. The topics covered herein carry significant findings which will fuel the growth of the discipline. They may even be implemented as practical applications or may be referred to as a beginning point for another development.

The contributors of this book come from diverse backgrounds, making this book a truly international effort. This book will bring forth new frontiers with its revolutionizing research information and detailed analysis of the nascent developments around the world.

We would like to thank all the contributing authors for lending their expertise to make the book truly unique. They have played a crucial role in the development of this book. Without their invaluable contributions this book wouldn't have been possible. They have made vital efforts to compile up to date information on the varied aspects of this subject to make this book a valuable addition to the collection of many professionals and students.

This book was conceptualized with the vision of imparting up-to-date information and advanced data in this field. To ensure the same, a matchless editorial board was set up. Every individual on the board went through rigorous rounds of assessment to prove their worth. After which they invested a large part of their time researching and compiling the most relevant data for our readers.

The editorial board has been involved in producing this book since its inception. They have spent rigorous hours researching and exploring the diverse topics which have resulted in the successful publishing of this book. They have passed on their knowledge of decades through this book. To expedite this challenging task, the publisher supported the team at every step. A small team of assistant editors was also appointed to further simplify the editing procedure and attain best results for the readers.

Apart from the editorial board, the designing team has also invested a significant amount of their time in understanding the subject and creating the most relevant covers. They scrutinized every image to scout for the most suitable representation of the subject and create an appropriate cover for the book.

The publishing team has been an ardent support to the editorial, designing and production team. Their endless efforts to recruit the best for this project, has resulted in the accomplishment of this book. They are a veteran in the field of academics and their pool of knowledge is as vast as their experience in printing. Their expertise and guidance has proved useful at every step. Their uncompromising quality standards have made this book an exceptional effort. Their encouragement from time to time has been an inspiration for everyone.

The publisher and the editorial board hope that this book will prove to be a valuable piece of knowledge for researchers, students, practitioners and scholars across the globe.

List of Contributors

Muhammad Khisroon, Aisha Gul, Ajmal Khan, Naheed Ali, Farah Zaidi, Syed Basit Rasheed and Ahmadullah
Department of Zoology, University of Peshawar, Peshawar, Pakistan

Huma Akbar
Institute of Chemical Sciences, University of Peshawar, Peshawar, Pakistan

Agnessa Kozak
University Medical Center Hamburg-Eppendorf Competence Centre for Epidemiology and Health Services Research in Nursing (CVcare), Martinistr. 52, 20246 Hamburg, Germany

Lara Paderow
University of Applied Science in Hamburg, Lohbrügger Kirchstraße 65, 21033 Hamburg, Germany

Matthias Nübling
Freiburg research centre for occupational and social medicine, Bertoldstr. 27, D 79098 Freiburg, Germany

Jørgen Riis Jepsen
Department of Occupational Medicine, Hospital of South-western Jutland, Østergade 81-83, DK-6700 Esbjerg, Denmark
Center of Maritime Health and Society, Institute of Public Health, University of Southern Denmark, DK-6700 Esbjerg, Denmark

Masanori Ogawa
Health Service Center, Jichi Medical University, 3311-1, Yakushiji, Shimotsuke, Tochigi 329-0498, Japan

Fujio Kayama
Department of Environmental and Preventive Medicine, Jichi Medical University, 3311-1, Yakushiji, Shimotsuke, Tochigi 329-0498, Japan

Alexandra M Preisser
Institute for Occupational and Maritime Medicine, University Medical Center Hamburg-Eppendorf (UKE), Hamburg, Germany

Maren Kersten and Dana Wendeler
Institution for Statutory Accident Insurance and Prevention in the Healthcare and Welfare Services, Pappelallee 33-37, 22089 Hamburg, Germany

Albert Nienhaus
Institution for Statutory Accident Insurance and Prevention in the Healthcare and Welfare Services, Pappelallee 33-37, 22089 Hamburg, Germany
University Medical Center Hamburg-Eppendorf Competence Centre for Epidemiology and Health Services Research in Nursing (CVcare), Martinistr. 52, 20246 Hamburg, Germany

Hiroya Terui, Satoshi Konno and Masaharu Nishimura
First Department of Medicine, Hokkaido University School of Medicine, Kita-15 Nishi-7 Kita-Ku, Sapporo, Hokkaido 060-8638, Japan

Kichizo Kaga
Cardiovascular and Thoracic Surgery, Hokkaido University School of Medicine, Sapporo, Hokkaido 060-8638, Japan

Yoshihiro Matsuno, Kanako C. Hatanaka and Hiromi Kanno
Department of Surgical Pathology, Hokkaido University Hospital, Sapporo, Hokkaido 060-8638, Japan

Hiroshi Moriyama
Niigata University Medical & Dental Hospital Bioscience Medical Research Center, Niigata, Niigata 951-8520, Japan

Motohiro Uo
Advanced Biomaterials, Department of Restorative Sciences, Division of Oral Health Sciences, Graduate School of Medical and Dental Sciences, Tokyo Medical and Dental University, Bunkyo-ku, Tokyo 113-8549, Japan

Felix C Ringshausen
Department of Respiratory Medicine, Hanover Medical School, Hanover, Germany

Peter Morfeld
Institute and Policlinic for Occupational Medicine, Environmental Medicine and Prevention Research of Cologne University, Kerpener Str. 62, 50937 Köln, Germany
Institute for Occupational Epidemiology and Risk Assessment (IERA) of Evonik Industries AG, Rellinghauser Str. 1-11, D-45128 Essen, Germany

Michael Spallek
Institute for Occupational, Social and Environmental Medicine of the Goethe University Frankfurt/Main, Theodor-Stern-Kai 7, 60590 Frankfurt am Main, Germany
European Research Group on Environment and Health in the Transport Sector (EUGT e.V.), Fritschestr. 35, 10627 Berlin, Germany

Sebsibe Tadesse and Zemichael Gizaw
Institute of Public Health, The University of Gondar, Gondar, Ethiopia

Kamil Ebrahim
Labour and social affairs, Oromia Regional State, Addis Ababa, Ethiopia

David A. Groneberg, Matthias Bundschuh, Mario Schwarzer and Alexander Gerber
Department of Health Economics, The Institute of Occupational Medicine, Social Medicine and Environmental Medicine, Goethe University Frankfurt, Theodor-Stern-Kai 7, 60590 Frankfurt, Germany

Shaghayegh Rahimian
Institute of Occupational Medicine, Charité School of Medicine, Thielallee 73, 14195 Berlin, Germany

Beatrix Kloft
Health Economics, Department of Gynecology and Obstetrics, Goethe University Frankfurt, Theodor-Stern-Kai 7, 60590 Frankfurt, Germany

C. Roedlich, M. Fouquet and C. Geraut
External Consultation on Occupational and Environmental Health, Department of Occupational and Environmental Health, Nantes University Hospital, 5 rue du Doyen Boquien, Nantes F 44 093, France

D. Tripodi and B. Cougot
External Consultation on Occupational and Environmental Health, Department of Occupational and Environmental Health, Nantes University Hospital, 5 rue du Doyen Boquien, Nantes F 44 093, France
Laboratory of Psychology of Pays de la Loire (LPPL - UPRES EA 4638), Nantes University - Faculty of Psychology, Nantes F 44 312, France

G. Fleury-Bahi
Laboratory of Psychology of Pays de la Loire (LPPL - UPRES EA 4638), Nantes University - Faculty of Psychology, Nantes F 44 312, France

A. Petit, C. Paget and Y. Roquelaure
Laboratory of Ergonomics & Epidemiology in Occupational Health, LEEST, UA-InVS - IFR 132, UPRES EA 4336 Faculty of Medicine, University of Angers, Angers F 49 000, France

P. Menu and C. Dubois
Physical Medicine Rehabilitation Department, Nantes University Hospital, 85 rue Saint Jacques, Nantes F 44 093, France

Christian Geraut
Department of Occupational Medicine and Environment Health, HCWs Research Laboratory, 5 rue du doyen Boquien, Nantes University Hospital, Nantes 44 093, France

Doina Ileana Giurgiu
Department of Occupational Medicine and Environment Health, HCWs Research Laboratory, 5 rue du doyen Boquien, Nantes University Hospital, Nantes 44 093, France
"Lucian Blaga" University of Sibiu, 10 Victoriei Boulevard, Sibiu 550024, Romania

Benjamin Grasset and Dominique Tripodi
Department of Occupational Medicine and Environment Health, HCWs Research Laboratory, 5 rue du doyen Boquien, Nantes University Hospital, Nantes 44 093, France
Psychology Laboratory of Pays de la Loire (LPPL - UPRES EA 4638), Department of Psychology, University of Nantes, BP 81 227 44312 Nantes cedex 3, France

Christine Jeoffrion
Psychology Laboratory of Pays de la Loire (LPPL - UPRES EA 4638), Department of Psychology, University of Nantes, BP 81 227 44312 Nantes cedex 3, France

Christine Roland-Lévy
Cognition, Health, Socialization, EA6291 University of Reims Champagne-Ardenne, 57, rue Pierre-Taittinger, Reims 51 096, France

Brigitte Keriven Dessomme and Leila Moret
Department of Public Health, Nantes University Hospital, 35 rue Saint Jacques, Nantes 44 000, France

Yves Roquelaure
Laboratory of Ergonomics Epidemiology Health and Work, LEEST-UA InVS - IFR 132- UPRES EA 4336, University of Angers, Faculty of Medicine, University Hospital, 4 rue Larrey, 49933 Angers Cedex, France

Alain Caubet and Christian Verger
Occupational Medicine Department, 6 rue Henri Le Guilloux, University Hospital of Rennes, Rennes 35 000, France

Chakib El Houssine Laraqui
Graduate School of Health Engineering and Project Management, 24 rue Lafontaine, Quartier Racine, Casablanca 20 100, Morocco

Pierre Lombrail
Public Health Department, SMBH, Paris 13 University, 74 avenue Marcel Cachin, Bobigny93017, France

Tanja Wirth and Grita Schedlbauer
Institution for Statutory Accident Insurance and Prevention in the Health and Welfare Services, Department for the Principle of Prevention and Rehabilitation, Pappelallee 33/35/37, 22089 Hamburg, Germany

Albert Nienhaus
Institution for Statutory Accident Insurance and Prevention in the Health and Welfare Services, Department for the Principle of Prevention and Rehabilitation, Pappelallee 33/35/37, 22089 Hamburg, Germany
University Medical Centre Hamburg-Eppendorf, Institute for Health Services Research in Dermatology and Nursing, Martinistraße 52, 20246 Hamburg, Germany

Agnessa Kozak
University Medical Centre Hamburg-Eppendorf, Institute for Health Services Research in Dermatology and Nursing, Martinistraße 52, 20246 Hamburg, Germany

Dorte Jessing Agerby Hanskov and Charlotte Brauer
Department of Occupational and Environmental Medicine, Bispebjerg Hospital, Copenhagen, Denmark

Lilli Kirkeskov
Department of Occupational and Environmental Medicine, Bispebjerg Hospital, Copenhagen, Denmark
Department of Occupational and Environmental Medicine, Unit of Social Medicine, Frederiksberg Hospital, Nordre Fasanvej 57, 2000 Copenhagen F, Denmark

Maria Girbig, Alice Freiberg, Stefanie Deckert, Diana Druschke, Christian Kopkow and Andreas Seidler
Institute and Policlinic of Occupational and Social Medicine, Faculty of Medicine Carl Gustav Carus, TU Dresden, Fetscherstr 74, 01307 Dresden, Germany

Albert Nienhaus
Institute for Health Services Research in Dermatology and Nursing, Hamburg Center for Health Economics, University Hamburg, Hamburg, Germany

Jessica Bengtsson and Pernille Søgaard Thygesen
Department of Occupational and Environmental Medicine, Frederiksberg and Bispebjerg Hospitals, Bispebjerg Bakke 23, Copenhagen, NV DK-2400, Denmark

Jens Peter Bonde
Department of Occupational and Environmental Medicine, Frederiksberg and Bispebjerg Hospitals, Bispebjerg Bakke 23, Copenhagen, NV DK-2400, Denmark
Department of Public Health, Section of Environmental Health, University of Copenhagen, Copenhagen, Denmark

Linda Kaerlev
Research Unit of Clinical Epidemiology, Institute of Clinical Research, University of Southern Denmark, Odense, Denmark
Center for Clinical Epidemiology, Odense University Hospital, Odense, Denmark

Lisbeth E. Knudsen
Department of Public Health, Section of Environmental Health, University of Copenhagen, Copenhagen, Denmark

Patricia Appel, Michael Schuler, Heiner Vogel and Hermann Faller
Department of Medical Psychology and Psychotherapy, Medical Sociology and Rehabilitation Sciences, University of Würzburg, Klinikstrasse 3, 97070 Würzburg, Germany

Amina Oezelsel
Center for Occupational Health and Psychology, hanza resources, Hammerbrookstr. 93, 20097 Hamburg, Germany

Xiali Zhong, Ming Zeng, Caigao Zhong and Fang Xiao
Department of Health Toxicology, Xiangya School of Public Health, Central South University, NO. 238 Shangmayuanling Road, Kaifu District, Changsha 410078, Hunan, People's Republic of China

Huanfeng Bian
Shajing Institution of Health Supervision of Baoan District, Shenzhen 518104, People's Republic of China

Åse Dalseth Austigard
Municipality of Trondheim, Working Environment Office, Trondheim, Norway

Kristin Svendsen
Institute of Industrial Economics and Technology Management, Norwegian University of Science and Technology, Alfred Getz vei 3, 7491 Trondheim, Norway

Kari K. Heldal
The National Institute of Occupational Health, Oslo, Norway

Shiming Cheng, Guangxue He, Hui Guo, Lixia Wang, Dongmei Hu, Haiying Fan, Fei Zhao and Yu Wang
China Center for Disease Control and Prevention, 155 Changbai Road Changping District, Beijing 102206, People's Republic of China

Deanna Tollefson and Emily Bloss
U.S. Centers for Disease Control and Prevention (CDC), 1600 Clifton Road NE, MS-93, Atlanta, GA 30329, USA

Shua Chai, Jay K. Varma and Carol Y. Rao
U.S. Centers for Disease Control and Prevention (CDC), 1600 Clifton Road NE, MS-93, Atlanta, GA 30329, USA
U.S. Centers for Disease Control and Prevention (CDC), Beijing, China

Yuan Li
U.S. Centers for Disease Control and Prevention (CDC), Beijing, China

Fangfang Gao, Fei Gao, Guoxin Han, Liping Ren and Yulin Ren
Inner Mongolia Center for Tuberculosis Control and Prevention, Middle Hugao Rd, New District, Hohhot, Inner Mongolia 010080, People's Republic of China

Jianbo Li
Ulanqab General Hospital, No.157, Jiefang Road, Jining District, Ulanqab, Inner Mongolia 012000, People's Republic of China

Amare W Nigatu, Magne Bråtveit and Bente E Moen
Department of Global Public Health and Primary Care, University of Bergen, Bergen, Norway

Wakgari Deressa
School of Public Health, Addis Ababa University, Addis Ababa, Ethiopia

Naomi J Anderson, David K Bonauto and Darrin Adams
Washington State Department of Labor & Industries, Safety & Health Assessment & Research for Prevention (SHARP) Program, Olympia, WA 98504-4330, USA

Marcus Oldenburg, Ralf Wegner and Bernd Poschadel
Institute for Occupational and Maritime Medicine, Hamburg State Department for Health and Consumer Protection, ZfAM, University Medical Center Hamburg-Eppendorf, Seewartenstrasse10, D-20459 Hamburg, Germany

Dennis Wilken
Department of Pulmonary Medicine, Asklepios Hospital Harburg, Hamburg, Germany

Xaver Baur
Institute for Occupational Medicine, Charité University Medicine Berlin and EOM Society, Berlin, Germany

Anja Schablon
Institute for Health Service Research in Dermatology and Nursing (IVDP), Center of Excellence for Epidemiology and Health Service Research forHealthcare Professionals (CVcare), University Medical Center Hamburg-Eppendorf, Martinistraße 52, Hamburg 20246, Germany

Albert Nienhaus
Institute for Health Service Research in Dermatology and Nursing (IVDP), Center of Excellence for Epidemiology and Health Service Research forHealthcare Professionals (CVcare), University Medical Center Hamburg-Eppendorf, Martinistraße 52, Hamburg 20246, Germany
Principles of Prevention and Rehabilitation Department (GPR), Institute for Statutory Accident Insurance and Prevention in the Health and Welfare Services (BGW), Hamburg, Germany

Roland Diel
Institute of Epidemiology, University Medical Center Schleswig-Holstein (UKSH), Kiel Campus, Kiel, Germany
Lung Clinic Grosshansdorf, Member of the German Center for Lung Research (DZL), Grosshansdorf, Germany

Chanwit Phongamwong and Hemwarun Deema
Department of Rehabilitation Medicine, Phramongkutklao Hospital and Phramongkutklao College of Medicine, Bangkok, Thailand

Index

CPSIA information can be obtained
at www.ICGtesting.com
Printed in the USA
LVHW062015100122
708212LV00002B/247

9 781639 274505